Extension of Healthy Life Span of Dialysis Patients in the Era of a 100-Year Life

Extension of Healthy Life Span of Dialysis Patients in the Era of a 100-Year Life

Editors

Katsuhiko Mori
Masaaki Inaba

MDPI • Basel • Beijing • Wuhan • Barcelona • Belgrade • Manchester • Tokyo • Cluj • Tianjin

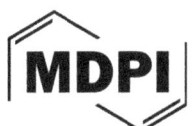

Editors
Katsuhiko Mori
Nephrology
Osaka City University Graduate
School of Medicine
Osaka
Japan

Masaaki Inaba
Nephrology
Osaka City University Graduate
School of Medicine
Osaka
Japan

Editorial Office
MDPI
St. Alban-Anlage 66
4052 Basel, Switzerland

This is a reprint of articles from the Special Issue published online in the open access journal *Nutrients* (ISSN 2072-6643) (available at: www.mdpi.com/journal/nutrients/special_issues/selected_papers_on_nutrition_from_2020_annual_meeting_of_the_japanese_society_of_dialysis_therapy).

For citation purposes, cite each article independently as indicated on the article page online and as indicated below:

LastName, A.A.; LastName, B.B.; LastName, C.C. Article Title. *Journal Name* **Year**, *Volume Number*, Page Range.

ISBN 978-3-0365-2346-0 (Hbk)
ISBN 978-3-0365-2345-3 (PDF)

© 2021 by the authors. Articles in this book are Open Access and distributed under the Creative Commons Attribution (CC BY) license, which allows users to download, copy and build upon published articles, as long as the author and publisher are properly credited, which ensures maximum dissemination and a wider impact of our publications.

The book as a whole is distributed by MDPI under the terms and conditions of the Creative Commons license CC BY-NC-ND.

Contents

Masaaki Inaba and Katsuhito Mori
Extension of Healthy Life Span of Dialysis Patients in the Era of a 100-Year Life
Reprinted from: *Nutrients* **2021**, *13*, 2693, doi:10.3390/nu13082693 1

Masaaki Inaba, Senji Okuno and Yoshiteru Ohno
Importance of Considering Malnutrition and Sarcopenia in Order to Improve the QOL of Elderly Hemodialysis Patients in Japan in the Era of 100-Year Life
Reprinted from: *Nutrients* **2021**, *13*, 2377, doi:10.3390/nu13072377 3

Yoshitaka Isaka
Optimal Protein Intake in Pre-Dialysis Chronic Kidney Disease Patients with Sarcopenia: An Overview
Reprinted from: *Nutrients* **2021**, *13*, 1205, doi:10.3390/nu13041205 15

Katsuhito Mori
Maintenance of Skeletal Muscle to Counteract Sarcopenia in Patients with Advanced Chronic Kidney Disease and Especially Those Undergoing Hemodialysis
Reprinted from: *Nutrients* **2021**, *13*, 1538, doi:10.3390/nu13051538 25

Junichi Hoshino
Renal Rehabilitation: Exercise Intervention and Nutritional Support in Dialysis Patients
Reprinted from: *Nutrients* **2021**, *13*, 1444, doi:10.3390/nu13051444 47

Senji Okuno
Significance of Adipose Tissue Maintenance in Patients Undergoing Hemodialysis
Reprinted from: *Nutrients* **2021**, *13*, 1895, doi:10.3390/nu13061895 63

Yoshihiko Kanno, Eiichiro Kanda and Akihiko Kato
Methods and Nutritional Interventions to Improve the Nutritional Status of Dialysis Patients in JAPAN—A Narrative Review
Reprinted from: *Nutrients* **2021**, *13*, 1390, doi:10.3390/nu13051390 81

Ken Tsuchiya and Taro Akihisa
The Importance of Phosphate Control in Chronic Kidney Disease
Reprinted from: *Nutrients* **2021**, *13*, 1670, doi:10.3390/nu13051670 89

Shinsuke Yamada and Masaaki Inaba
Potassium Metabolism and Management in Patients with CKD
Reprinted from: *Nutrients* **2021**, *13*, 1751, doi:10.3390/nu13061751 111

Hiroyuki Takashima, Takashi Maruyama and Masanori Abe
Significance of Levocarnitine Treatment in Dialysis Patients
Reprinted from: *Nutrients* **2021**, *13*, 1219, doi:10.3390/nu13041219 131

Shinya Nakatani, Katsuhito Mori, Tetsuo Shoji and Masanori Emoto
Association of Zinc Deficiency with Development of CVD Events in Patients with CKD
Reprinted from: *Nutrients* **2021**, *13*, 1680, doi:10.3390/nu13051680 155

Yasuyuki Nagasawa
Positive and Negative Aspects of Sodium Intake in Dialysis and Non-Dialysis CKD Patients
Reprinted from: *Nutrients* **2021**, *13*, 951, doi:10.3390/nu13030951 177

Tsutomu Inoue, Eito Kozawa, Masahiro Ishikawa and Hirokazu Okada
Application of Magnetic Resonance Imaging in the Evaluation of Nutritional Status: A Literature Review with Focus on Dialysis Patients
Reprinted from: *Nutrients* **2021**, *13*, 2037, doi:10.3390/nu13062037 . . . . **195**

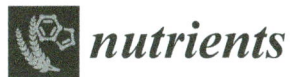

Editorial

Extension of Healthy Life Span of Dialysis Patients in the Era of a 100-Year Life

Masaaki Inaba [1,2,*] and Katsuhito Mori [1]

1. Department of Nephrology, Osaka City University Graduate School of Medicine, Osaka 545-8585, Japan; ktmori@med.osaka-cu.ac.jp
2. Kidney Center, Ohno Memorial Hospital, 1-26-20, Minami-Horie, Osaka 550-0015, Japan
* Correspondence: inaba-m@med.osaka-cu.ac.jp

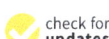

Citation: Inaba, M.; Mori, K. Extension of Healthy Life Span of Dialysis Patients in the Era of a 100-Year Life. *Nutrients* **2021**, *13*, 2693. https://doi.org/10.3390/nu13082693

Received: 23 July 2021
Accepted: 30 July 2021
Published: 4 August 2021

Publisher's Note: MDPI stays neutral with regard to jurisdictional claims in published maps and institutional affiliations.

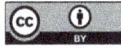

Copyright: © 2021 by the authors. Licensee MDPI, Basel, Switzerland. This article is an open access article distributed under the terms and conditions of the Creative Commons Attribution (CC BY) license (https://creativecommons.org/licenses/by/4.0/).

With both the elongation of hemodialysis (HD) duration resulting from the sophistication of HD technology and the increasing age at the time of HD initiation due to the aging society of Japan, the mean age of prevalent HD patients is increasing at an accelerating rate [1]. Along with the aging of HD patients, presymptomatic conditions such as malnutrition, frailty, sarcopenia, and inflammation have been focused on as important states to help to improve the condition of patients, both those living independently and those requiring physical support or nursing care [1,2], as in the general elderly population. In addition, it should be emphasized that such presymptomatic conditions can often act as a trigger, causing critical events, such as cardiovascular disease (CVD), falls, and fragile fractures, which significantly impair quality of life (QOL) [1].

Since these disorders increase with advancing age, even in a healthy population, it is reasonable to think that a comprehensive approach is required to maintain the QOL of elderly HD patients from the initial stages of these presymptomatic conditions. This Special Issue for the 65th annual meeting of the Japanese Society for Dialysis Therapy (JSDT) focuses on how to overcome these factors in elderly HD patients and how to maintain QOL, with patients potentially enjoying a 100-year long life.

It is increasingly recognized that sarcopenia is one of main factors leading to impaired QOL in the elderly population, such as in HD patients [3]. To counteract age-related development of sarcopenia in HD patients, multifaceted intervention including both nutritional and physical therapy is needed [3,4]. In addition to the maintenance of muscle mass, the importance of maintaining fat mass should be emphasized in elderly undernourished HD patients. Subcutaneous fat in particular, rather than visceral fat, seems to reflect nutritional status [5]. Based on these findings, sufficient calorie/protein intake is essential in undernourished elderly HD patients [6]. Traditionally, protein restriction diet therapy has been recommended to protect against the decline in renal function in pre-dialysis chronic kidney disease (CKD) patients [2]. However, inadequate protein intake may exacerbate malnutrition to induce sarcopenia and emaciation in such patients. Thus, flexible responses are considered regarding whether protein restriction should be continued or loosened in pre-dialysis CKD patients [2]. With an increase in protein intake, hyperphosphatemia is another key factor to be avoided in CKD/HD patients since phosphate overload leads to secondary hyperparathyroidism and vascular calcification, causing fractures and CVD events, respectively [7]. Increased protein intake is usually associated with hyperkalemia, which is an emergent condition leading to lethal arrythmia [8]. The application of new drugs including phosphate binders and potassium chelators may achieve both a high enough intake and balanced levels of phosphate and potassium in elderly undernourished HD patients [7,8].

In CKD and HD patients, the deficiency of certain micronutrients such as carnitine [9] and zinc [10] is often observed and involved in pathological conditions. Therefore, levocarnitine administration and zinc supplementation may be reasonable therapeutic approaches [9,10]. Although the cause of appetite loss is largely unknown in HD patients, a fundamental solution may be an increased food intake in HD patients. In this respect, sodium, which is generally correlated to mortality through hypertension, is an interesting factor. Since sodium stimulates appetite, appropriate salt intake may improve a patient's nutritional condition and subsequent prognosis [11]. The advancement of functional magnetic resonance imaging (MRI), such as blood oxygenation level-dependent MRI, has made it possible to evaluate the activation of the brain and to identify the functional areas associated with appetite, intake, and eating behavior [12]. In the future, new MRI technology may provide clues regarding appetite loss in HD patients. In addition to sufficient energy intake, exercise is also required to prevent muscle protein catabolism [3,4]. Renal rehabilitation has received much attention in clinical practice [4]. Comprehensive care by a wide variety of medical staff is essential for the wellbeing of elderly HD patients.

The theme of the 65th annual meeting of JSDT was the "Extension of Healthy Life Span of Dialysis Patients in the Era of a 100-year Life". The Guest Editors appreciate all of authors' contributions to this Special Issue.

Author Contributions: Conceptualization and writing, M.I. and K.M. Both authors have read and agreed to the published version of the manuscript.

Institutional Review Board Statement: Not applicable.

Informed Consent Statement: Not applicable.

Data Availability Statement: Not applicable.

Conflicts of Interest: The authors declare no conflict of interest.

References

1. Inaba, M.; Okuno, S.; Ohno, Y. Importance of Considering Malnutrition and Sarcopenia in Order to Improve the QOL of Elderly Hemodialysis Patients in Japan in the Era of 100-Year Life. *Nutrients* **2021**, *13*, 2377. [CrossRef]
2. Isaka, Y. Optimal Protein Intake in Pre-Dialysis Chronic Kidney Disease Patients with Sarcopenia: An Overview. *Nutrients* **2021**, *13*, 1205. [CrossRef]
3. Mori, K. Maintenance of Skeletal Muscle to Counteract Sarcopenia in Patients with Advanced Chronic Kidney Disease and Especially Those Undergoing Hemodialysis. *Nutrients* **2021**, *13*, 1538. [CrossRef]
4. Hoshino, J. Renal Rehabilitation: Exercise Intervention and Nutritional Support in Dialysis Patients. *Nutrients* **2021**, *13*, 1444. [CrossRef]
5. Okuno, S. Significance of Adipose Tissue Maintenance in Patients Undergoing Hemodialysis. *Nutrients* **2021**, *13*, 1895. [CrossRef] [PubMed]
6. Kanno, Y.; Kanda, E.; Kato, A. Methods and Nutritional Interventions to Improve the Nutritional Status of Dialysis Patients in JAPAN-A Narrative Review. *Nutrients* **2021**, *13*, 1390. [CrossRef]
7. Tsuchiya, K.; Akihisa, T. The Importance of Phosphate Control in Chronic Kidney Disease. *Nutrients* **2021**, *13*, 1670. [CrossRef]
8. Yamada, S.; Inaba, M. Potassium Metabolism and Management in Patients with CKD. *Nutrients* **2021**, *13*, 1751. [CrossRef] [PubMed]
9. Takashima, H.; Maruyama, T.; Abe, M. Significance of Levocarnitine Treatment in Dialysis Patients. *Nutrients* **2021**, *13*, 1219. [CrossRef]
10. Nakatani, S.; Mori, K.; Shoji, T.; Emoto, M. Association of Zinc Deficiency with Development of CVD Events in Patients with CKD. *Nutrients* **2021**, *13*, 1680. [CrossRef]
11. Nagasawa, Y. Positive and Negative Aspects of Sodium Intake in Dialysis and Non-Dialysis CKD Patients. *Nutrients* **2021**, *13*, 951. [CrossRef] [PubMed]
12. Inoue, T.; Kozawa, E.; Ishikawa, M.; Okada, H. Application of Magnetic Resonance Imaging in the Evaluation of Nutritional Status: A Literature Review with Focus on Dialysis Patients. *Nutrients* **2021**, *13*, 2037. [CrossRef] [PubMed]

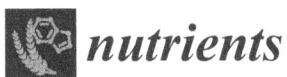

Review

Importance of Considering Malnutrition and Sarcopenia in Order to Improve the QOL of Elderly Hemodialysis Patients in Japan in the Era of 100-Year Life

Masaaki Inaba [1,2,*], Senji Okuno [3] and Yoshiteru Ohno [2]

1. Department of Nephrology, Osaka City University Medical School, 1-4-3 Asahi-machi, Abeno-ku, Osaka 543-8585, Japan
2. Kidney Center, Ohno Memorial Hospital, 1-26-10, Minami-Horie, Nishi-ku, Osaka 550-0015, Japan; teru11090116@yahoo.co.jp
3. Kidney Center, Shirasagi Hospital, 7-11-23, Higashisumiyoshi-ku, Osaka 546-0002, Japan; okuno@shirasagi-hp.or.jp
* Correspondence: inaba-m@med.osaka-cu.ac.jp

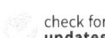

Citation: Inaba, M.; Okuno, S.; Ohno, Y. Importance of Considering Malnutrition and Sarcopenia in Order to Improve the QOL of Elderly Hemodialysis Patients in Japan in the Era of 100-Year Life. *Nutrients* 2021, 13, 2377. https://doi.org/10.3390/nu13072377

Academic Editor: Riccardo Caccialanza

Received: 22 June 2021
Accepted: 8 July 2021
Published: 12 July 2021

Publisher's Note: MDPI stays neutral with regard to jurisdictional claims in published maps and institutional affiliations.

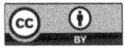

Copyright: © 2021 by the authors. Licensee MDPI, Basel, Switzerland. This article is an open access article distributed under the terms and conditions of the Creative Commons Attribution (CC BY) license (https://creativecommons.org/licenses/by/4.0/).

Abstract: In the current aging society of Japan, malnutrition and resultant sarcopenia have been widely identified as important symptomatic indicators of ill health and can cause impairments of longevity and quality of life in older individuals. Elderly individuals are recommended to have sufficient calorie and protein intake so as to enjoy a satisfactory quality of life, including maintaining activities of daily living in order to avoid emaciation and sarcopenia. The prevalence of emaciation and sarcopenia in elderly hemodialysis (HD) patients in Japan is higher than in non-HD elderly subjects due to the presence of malnutrition and sarcopenia associated with chronic kidney disease (CKD). Furthermore, comorbidities, such as diabetes and osteoporosis, induce malnutrition and sarcopenia in HD patients. This review presents findings regarding the mechanisms of the development of these early symptomatic conditions and their significance for impaired QOL and increased mortality in elderly HD patients.

Keywords: clinical malnutrition; older individuals; hemodialysis; sarcopenia; chronic kidney disease; quality of life; mortality

1. Introduction

The society of Japan is aging, and the percentage of predialysis-chronic kidney disease (CKD) patients is greater in older populations; thus, it is not surprising that the number of elderly CKD patients who require renal replacement therapy (RRT) has been increasing. Since as few as 3% of dialysis patients can be maintained on peritoneal dialysis [1] and kidney transplantation is uncommon [2], nearly all end-stage CKD patients undergo hemodialysis (HD) as RRT. Moreover, over the last three-decade period, the average age of HD patients in Japan remarkably increased from 47 years in 1983 to 69 years in 2017, according to the registry of the Japanese Society of Dialysis Therapy (JSDT) [3]. In fact, the proportion of HD patients in Japan ≥65 years old has increased to 71%, and that of those ≥75 years old has increased to 43% (Figure 1) [4]. An analysis of the annual dialysis data report for the 2018 JSDT renal data registry [4] shows that the increasing age of HD patients in Japan can be accounted for by both elongation of HD duration due to the sophistication of dialysis techniques, and increasing age at the time of HD initiation. The DOPPS study demonstrated that the mortality rate in Japan is the lowest among the DOPPS-participating countries, and has continued to decline given the increasing age of Japanese HD patients. Along with the aging of the HD patient population, the number of co-morbidities that may impair a satisfactory quality of life (QOL), and thus cause emaciation and sarcopenia, is increasing. Impaired QOL in elderly HD patients changes patients' condition from independent living to the requirement of physical support or nursing care [5], thus impairing the quality of a potential 100-year life. This review tries to elucidate the mechanism of the development of these presymptomatic conditions of emaciation/sarcopenia/frailty and their significance for impaired longevity, QOL, and mortality in elderly HD patients. Furthermore, the importance of diabetes and osteoporosis in the development of malnutrition and sarcopenia is emphasized.

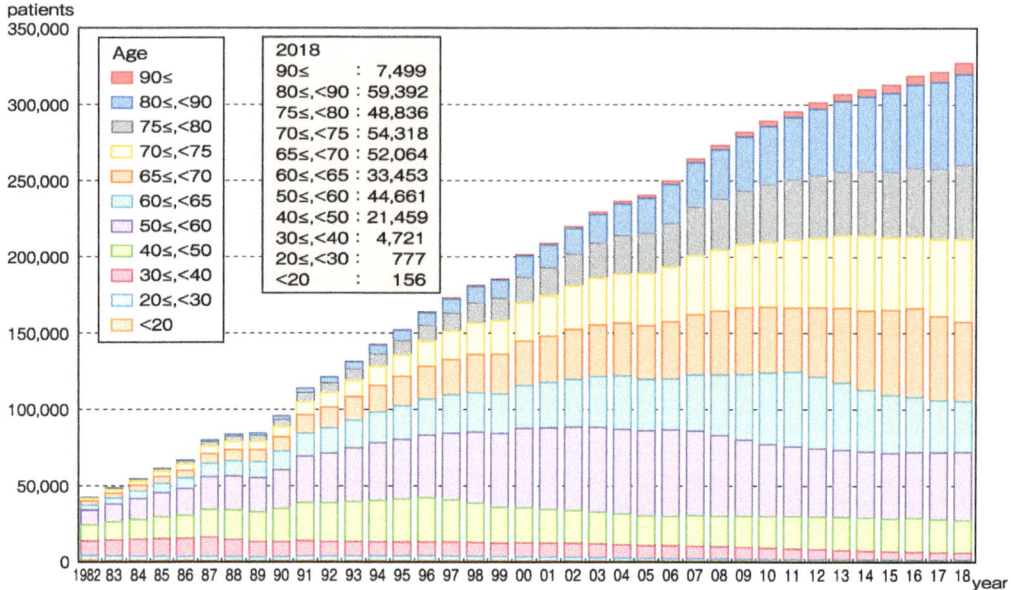

Figure 1. Trends in counts of Japanese hemodialysis patients stratified by age for the period 1982–2018. The proportion of patients aged ≥65 years and ≥75 years has increased up to 71% and 43%, respectively, in Japan. The average age of HD patients in Japan has remarkably increased during the last three decades, from 47 years old in 1983 to 69 years old in 2017 (registry of Japanese Society of Dialysis Therapy).

2. Preferential Occurrence of Malnutrition and Its Mechanism in Pre-Dialysis CKD Patients

Old age is known to be associated with poor nutritional status, while CKD itself is closely associated with malnutrition because of several different mechanisms [6]. First, CKD may be associated with dietary inadequacy in relation to suboptimal energy and protein intake due to poor appetite status, taste perception [7], low diet quality, and/or psychosocial or financial barriers. Furthermore, a reduction in metabolic rate resulting from reduced physical activity and muscle mass can contribute to poor appetite in HD patients [8]. Second, a protein-restricted diet has been recommended for pre-dialysis CKD patients to prevent exacerbation of renal dysfunction, though that might be a risk factor for malnutrition and sarcopenia [9], which is supported by the findings showing the beneficial effects of a high-protein diet or amino acid supplementation on nutritional state, as assessed by improved serum albumin and various nutritional markers [10]. Third, CKD is complicated by a metabolic syndrome termed malnutrition–inflammation complex syndrome (MICS) [11], or protein energy wasting (PEW) syndrome [12], which consist of catabolic inflammatory reactions and cachexia leading to malnutrition. Fourth, it is possible that multiple comorbidities associated with malnutrition and frailty/sarcopenia, such as diabetes mellitus (DM), cardiovascular disease (CVD), cerebrovascular disease, immobility, and insomnia, contribute to malnutrition. Interestingly, a study of common malnutrition in pre-dialysis CKD patients found that more than 50% of nephrologists initiate dialysis for end-stage CKD patients after their nutritional status is impaired [13].

3. Significance of Malnutrition for Various Clinical Outcomes in HD Patients

Along with the common occurrence of malnutrition in end-stage CKD cases, a malnutritional state can continue even when the patient reaches a stable condition on maintenance HD. Although HD initiation allows for a more liberal intake of protein and food so as to improve nutritional state [14,15], dialysis-specific factors still exist that cause malnutrition. These relate to the low adequacy induced by 4-h HD sessions performed three times a week, which causes a persistent uremic state [16], metabolic acidosis [17], and the accumulation of various uremic substances in serum that disturb metabolism. A related study showed that patients in Japan who underwent extended-time HD sessions, based on a treatment policy of extending dialysis time and removing dietary restrictions, exhibited better survival, along with the maintenance of or an increase in body mass index [18]. Furthermore, a massive loss of nutrients and amino acid from circulation to dialysate via the high-performance dialysis membrane, as well as hemodiafiltration, are dialysis-specific mechanisms of malnutrition [19].

At the time of HD initiation, a patient presenting with malnutrition has a high mortality risk on the basis of low nutrition markers, such as geriatric nutritional risk index (GNRI) [20], subjective global assessment [21], low body mass index (BMI) [22], low serum levels of albumin [20] and cholesterol [21], and low food intake [23]. Among these parameters, we reported the clinical utility of GNRI as a relevant predictor for mortality in HD patients [20]. A GNRI value <90 was associated with a significantly lower survival rate in HD patients as compared to those with GNRI $\geq$90 [24]. Furthermore, we previously reported that HD patients who gained fat mass after HD initiation exhibited a better survival rate than those with loss of fat mass after HD initiation [25], and that fat mass gain after HD initiation was significantly associated with reductions in serum CRP, a reliable marker for inflammation and CVD risk. This suggests that the improvement of nutritional status might lead to the suppression of inflammation and atherosclerosis [26], and thus finally a better survival rate.

4. Significance of Sarcopenia in Relation to Harmful Effects of Malnutrition in HD Patients

Sarcopenia was defined in 1988 as an age-related reduction in skeletal muscle mass and function [27], after which the Asia Working Group for Sarcopenia provided a definition for the evaluation of sarcopenia in Asian individuals [28]. Serum albumin, which is reported to be elevated by an increased intake of food, protein, and branched-chain amino acids, also rises with an increase in muscle content. Furthermore, GNRI, a relevant marker for nutrition and mortality, is defined via serum albumin in addition to body weight, which is mainly determined by muscle content. We examined the importance of the creatinine index, another nutritional marker in HD patients without residual renal function, as a predictor of mortality risk [29]. The creatinine index is calculated using the following formula: Cr index = 16.21 ($+1.12$ if male) $- 0.06 \times$ [age (years)] $- 0.08 \times$ (single pool Kt/V) $+ 0.009 \times$ [serum creatinine (μmol/L]. Thus, the creatinine index is a nutritional marker that is mainly determined in HD patients by muscle content, given the lack of apparent residual renal function. We found that lower GNRI and Cr index values were both independently and equally associated with an increased risk of all-cause mortality in a multivariable-adjusted model [29]. Taken together, these findings demonstrate that the mechanism by which malnutrition increases mortality risk in Japanese HD patients can be mostly explained by reduced muscle mass. Therefore, we next focused on the significance of the development of sarcopenia in HD patients.

5. Preferential Occurrence of Sarcopenia, and the Significance of Muscle Strength Rather Than Muscle Mass in HD Patients

Based on our report [30], with the increasing age of Japanese HD patients, the prevalence of sarcopenia among them was found to have increased to as much as 40% (37% in males and 45% in females). Although the definition of sarcopenia is based on muscle mass measurements by the Asian Working Group for Sarcopenia [28], it remains to be determined whether muscle mass or muscle strength is more important in determining the clinical outcome of sarcopenia in humans. Our study found that serum creatinine has a significantly positive correlation with not only muscle mass, determined via dual-energy X-ray absorptiometry (DXA), but also muscle strength measured by handgrip strength [31]. Therefore, we examined whether muscle mass or muscle strength might be a more important determinant of serum creatinine level in HD patients. Multivariate analysis demonstrated that poor arm muscle quality, calculated using the handgrip strength/DXA-determined arm lean mass ratio, rather than reduced DXA-determined arm lean mass, is responsible for the reduction in serum creatinine in HD patients [32]. This indicates that muscle strength is a more important factor than muscle mass as a determinant for serum creatinine level in HD patients. To confirm the harmful effects of reduced muscle strength on mortality in HD patients in Japan, we also examined the effects of impaired muscle quality, assessed by the reduced muscle strength/muscle mass ratio [31]. A total of 272 HD patients were divided into two equal-sized groups (higher and lower) based on muscle quality, and the Kaplan–Meier analysis results demonstrated that the higher group exhibited a significantly lower mortality rate than the lower group. Furthermore, Cox regression hazards analysis identified higher muscle quality as a significant independent predictor for survival in HD patients, independently of the presence of DM, age, and serum albumin level. In another study, higher age, female gender, longer HD duration, presence of DM, lower BMI, and higher CRP were shown to be independent factors associated with lower handgrip strength in HD patients [33]. Our recent findings also suggest that the efficient utility of ketone bodies, which are mainly utilized as an efficient energy source in the muscle tissues of HD patients, is an independent determinant of higher levels of albumin and uric acid in serum [34]. Serum albumin [35] and uric acid [36] are both established as nutritional markers intimately associated with mortality in HD patients. Furthermore, it was reported that a higher level of serum β-hydroxybutyrate, probably due to its impaired metabolism in muscle tissues, was independently associated with CVD events and all-cause mortality in HD patients [37]. Together, these findings indicate that a better energy metabolism in the muscle tissues of HD patients is important to maintaining whole body nutritional state and increasing survival, supporting the importance of muscle mass/strength for maintaining nutritional status and thus a better survival rate in HD patients.

6. DM and Sarcopenia in HD Patients

In addition to aging and malnutrition, sarcopenia is known to preferentially occur in HD patients with osteoporosis and DM [38]. Additionally, the rates for the co-existence of sarcopenia, osteoporosis, and DM are known to be higher in HD patients and increase with aging. Although each disease is known to independently affect physical activity and mortality in HD patients, it is possible that DM and osteoporosis, both independently and together with sarcopenia, might reduce longevity and survival rates in these patients. Furthermore, the interaction between these three diseases is important to mention.

The number of DM patients in aged populations is increasing [39]. In Asia, the prevalence of sarcopenia in type 2 (T2) DM has been shown to progressively increase with age (17.4%, 28.1%, 52.4%, and 60% in individuals aged 65–69, 70–74, 75–80, and >80 years, respectively) [40]. Additionally, a study conducted in Japan showed the prevalence of sarcopenia in T2DM patients who were ≥80 years old to be over 40% [41]. Since nearly all DM patients suffer from T2DM, but not T1DM, in Japan, DM patients who we previously examined exclusively had T2DM. A recent meta-analysis confirmed that the prevalence of sarcopenia is significantly higher in T2DM than non-DM patients [42]. It is known that serum creatinine levels are significantly lower in DM as compared to non-DM HD patients without residual renal function, which is consistent with our finding that DM HD patients exhibit significantly lower muscle mass and strength than their non-DM counterparts [31,33,34], and that lower handgrip strength is significantly associated with the presence of T2DM in HD patients [33]. To avoid the confounding effect of DM on the association between lower muscle quality and higher mortality rate, we examined the association between these two parameters separately in HD patients with and without DM [31], and those with lower muscle quality (both non-DM and DM patients) exhibited significantly higher mortality rates, indicating poor muscle quality as a significant and independent factor contributing to the higher mortality both in DM and non-DM HD patients. This may also suggest that the mechanism of increased mortality in HD patients with DM is due, at least in part, to poor muscle quality induced by a sustained DM state.

To elucidate the association between DM alone with muscle strength independent of CKD, we measured handgrip strength in female T2DM patients without clinically overt DM complications in our DM outpatient clinic, and compared the results with those of a non-DM normal female control group of the same age [38]. Figure 2 shows the changes in handgrip strength with age in those female subjects. While non-DM female normal controls exhibited a characteristic decline in handgrip strength after menopause because of loss of estrogen, which has a protective effect on muscle [43], handgrip strength was significantly weaker in female DM patients in their 40 s than in their non-DM counterparts, which supports our finding in HD patients that DM is an independent risk factor for the development of sarcopenia in HD patients [31].

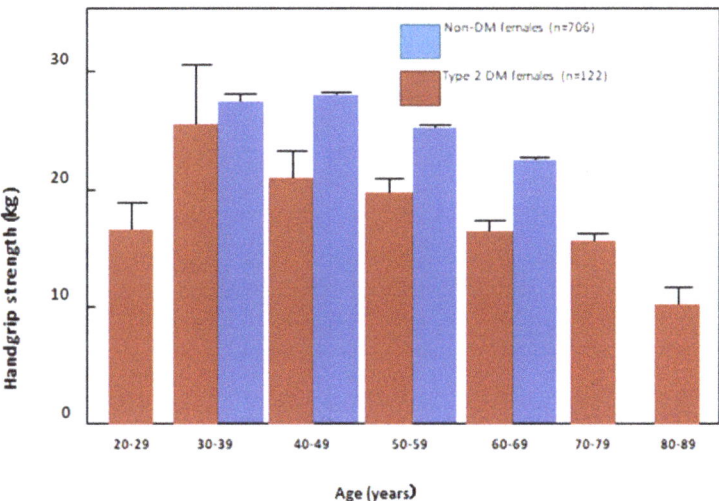

Figure 2. Age-stratified handgrip strength in normal female subjects and type 2 DM patients without overt DM complications. Although handgrip strength started to decrease significantly during the postmenopausal period as compared to normal female subjects, female type 2 diabetes patients exhibited a significant decrease in handgrip strength by their 40 s, supporting the notion that type 2 DM is a risk factor for the early development of muscle strength reduction.

A DM state has been shown to be associated with sarcopenia via several different mechanisms, including malnutrition, insulin/IGF-1 deficiency, and a sustained hyperglycemia condition, while it has been speculated that sarcopenia might exacerbate the DM condition because of reduced muscle tissue, against which insulin treatment protects by stimulating transport plasma glucose into muscle tissue. A study found that the energy intake of DM patients with sarcopenia, often observed in elderly DM patients, is significantly lower than that in sarcopenia-free DM patients [44]. Furthermore, energy intake in DM patients in that study was independently and negatively associated with sarcopenia, after adjustments for age, gender, exercise, smoking habit, HbA1c, and BMI. Since physical activity determines the metabolic rate associated with food intake, it is possible that DM HD patients with sarcopenia undertake less physical activity. In fact, DM prevalence in HD patients with a history of falling was significantly greater compared to those without such a history. The former group of patients also had lower serum levels of albumin and creatinine, and lower physical function test scores [45], suggesting an association between low physical performance and poor nutrition with prevalence of DM in HD patients. Additionally, the postprandial secretion of insulin has been shown to stimulate muscle/adipose tissue blood flow and have a musculotrophic effect that stimulates the cellular uptake of amino acids to induce de novo protein synthesis in muscle tissue [46]. Conversely, in individuals with relative or absolute insulin/IGF-1 deficiency, amino acids are lost from the muscle. Other major mechanisms of muscle injury are a sustained high-glucose condition [47] and broad glucose fluctuation [48]. Since glucose fluctuation is mainly induced by postprandial glucose excursion, which is suppressed by postprandial insulin secretion to enhance glucose entry into muscle tissue, sarcopenia alone presumably induces a greater increase in plasma glucose after consumption of a meal, which might further deteriorate muscle tissue given the increased oxidative stress generated by the increase in postprandial glucose. Indeed, the plasma glucose area under the curve during the 2 h oral glucose test of DM HD patients, which represents the increase in postprandial glucose (evidenced by a significant correlation with glycoalbumin, a clinically reliable marker for postprandial hyperglycemia [49]), exhibited a tendency towards inverse correlation with BMI, although this was not significant (Figure 3). These data also suggest that the maintenance of BMI, which is particularly affected by lean mass in HD patients, might protect postprandial glucose excursion in such patients.

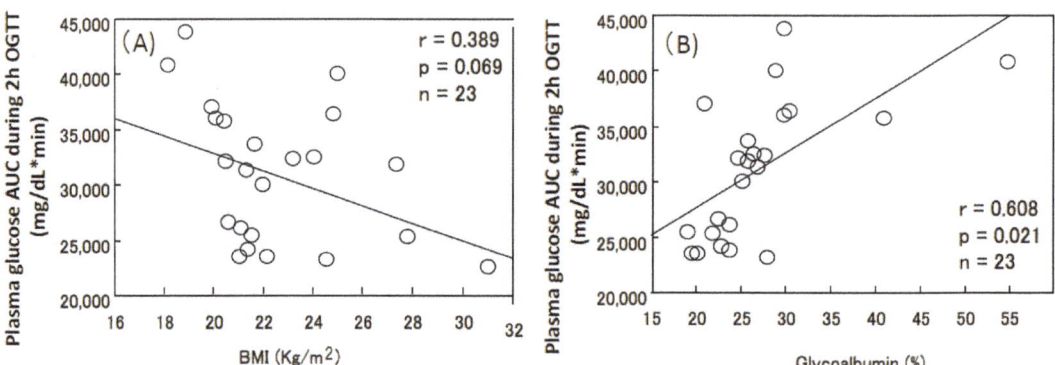

Figure 3. Correlation between area under curve (AUC) of plasma glucose during 2 h oral glucose tolerance test with BMI (**A**) and glycoalbumin (**B**) in hemodialysis patients. Oral glucose (75 g) tolerance test was performed in 23 Japanese hemodialysis patients after an overnight fast. The plasma glucose AUC during the 2 h oral glucose tolerance test exhibited a significant negative correlation with BMI (**A**) and a positive correlation with glycoalbumin (**B**).

Furthermore, hyperglycemia is a result of cellular malnutrition, given the incapability of glucose to enter muscle cells, leading to loss of muscle mass and the development of sarcopenia. DM complications, such as CVD, visual dysfunction, and dementia, can restrict physical activity, leading to loss of muscle tissue. Peripheral arterial disease, another complication often observed in DM HD patients, might also cause loss of muscle tissue by limiting the blood flow to the muscle tissue in the lower limbs [50].

7. Osteoporosis and Sarcopenia in HD Patients

We recently reported that pre-dialysis CKD patients with a fracture exhibited a greater creatinine-based eGFR/cystatin C-based eGFR ratio than those without a fracture [51]. Creatinine-based eGFR is known to overestimate true GFR in aged CKD patients, apparently because of the lower levels of serum creatinine resulting from reduced muscle mass, as observed in HD patients, and it has been shown that cystatin C-based eGFR reflects true GFR more effectively than creatinine-based eGFR in aged CKD patients [52]. Additionally, our results indicate that the fracture rate in pre-dialysis CKD patients is greater in those with than without sarcopenia [51]. Due to the high prevalence of sarcopenia in HD patients in Japan [30], it is reasonable to consider the importance of sarcopenia in the development of osteoporosis and osteoporosis-based fragility fractures. Fall trauma and fracture are amongst the main causes of changes in the conditions of elderly HD patients, from independent living to the requirement of physical support or nursing care. It is known that mechanical force to bone tissue stimulates bone formation, resulting in increased bone mineral density. We reported an association of handgrip strength with cortical thickness, but not with trabecular bone mineral density, at the 5.5% distal radius in both normal and type 2 DM subjects [38]. Thus, mechanical force generated by muscle contractions might exert a preferential effect on cortical bone components, a major determinant of bone strength in appendicular bones such as the femur [53]. Furthermore, sarcopenia is known to be a risk factor for femoral neck fracture because of the increased risk of falling [54,55] and the greater impact on the femur bone during a fall caused by the loss of cushioning provided by the gluteus maximus muscle [56]. Furthermore, HD patients with sarcopenia exhibit a higher risk of falling-induced fragility fractures [45,57]. Therefore, CKD should be regarded as a condition that increases the risk of femoral fracture due to the frequent occurrence of sarcopenia in affected individuals.

Although mechanical loading is a key mechanism that links bone and muscle, as mentioned above, the effects of muscle–bone interactions between two organs via secretome secretion have recently been emphasized [58]. Skeletal muscle tissues secrete chemical substances that have effects on bone metabolism, such as insulin, IGF-1, myostatin [59], basic fibroblast growth factor 2, IL-6, IL-15, osteoglycin, and osteoactivin. Additionally, the chemokines expressed by bone tissues potentially affect muscle metabolism, since osteocytes secrete prostaglandin E2 and Wnt3a, osteoblasts secrete osteocalcin and IGF-1, and both cell types produce sclerostin.

Since phosphate exists in bones as a form of hydroxylapatite, the stimulation of bone resorption via secondary hyperparathyroidism increases the degree of phosphate release from bones into the circulation in CKD patients. It is widely recognized that too much phosphate induces premature aging by stimulating atherosclerotic changes, renal damage, and osteoporosis [60], suggesting premature aging in CKD patients via stimulation of bone resorption. Indeed, previous studies have demonstrated an accelerated increase in acute myocardial infarction and cerebral infarction in postmenopausal women [61,62], and increased intima-media thickness of the common carotid artery and atherosclerotic plaque in middle-aged postmenopausal women compared to premenopausal women of the same age [63]. Furthermore, it was reported that coronary arterial calcification in postmenopausal women was advanced in those with osteoporosis as compared to those without [64], and that postmenopausal women with higher bone turnover exhibited higher mortality than those with lower bone turnover [65]. Other reports also demonstrated that higher serum phosphate may promote CKD progression, and attenuate the renoprotective effects of a low-protein diet and angiotensin-converting enzyme inhibitors in CKD patients [66,67]. We previously reported that higher bone turnover was correlated in a positive manner with higher urinary albumin excretion in postmenopausal women, but not in premenopausal women [68], which suggests the importance of the greater rate of phosphate release from bones caused by increased bone resorption during the development of renal damage in postmenopausal women. Additionally, a series of studies, including ours, confirmed the notion that the increased phosphate released from bones into the circulation, as a result of stimulated bone resorption, causes cardiovascular and renal damage in postmenopausal osteoporotic patients, given the protective effects of bone anti-resorptive drugs, such as denosumab [69] and bazedoxifene [70], on renal function in female osteoporotic patients. Furthermore, it was shown that, in osteoporotic patients with and without bone anti-resorptive drug treatment, those with increased bone mineral density exhibited improved pulse wave velocity (an early marker of arterial wall sclerosis) and carotid artery intima-media thickness (an early marker of arterial wall thickening) [71].

Finally, the administration of bisphosphonate, a potent anti-resorptive agent, was demonstrated to suppress the incidence of acute myocardial infarction in osteoporotic patients [72]. Together, these findings clearly demonstrate that enhanced osteoporosis-associated bone resorption enhances premature aging in vessels and kidneys by increasing the phosphate release from bones.

8. Sarcopenia as a Risk for Mortality and Impaired QOL in HD Patients

In our study that examined the effects of muscle quality on mortality in HD patients in Japan, Kaplan–Meier analysis showed that those with higher muscle quality had a lower mortality rate than those with lower muscle quality [31]. Additionally, Cox regression hazards analysis identified greater muscle quality as a significant independent predictor for better survival in our Japanese HD patients (HR: 0.889, 95% CI 0.814–0.971; $p < 0.05$) after adjustments for age, sex, and prevalence of DM. Previous findings also demonstrate the association between lower muscle quality and impaired physical performance [54]. We consider that the maintenance of muscle quality should be recognized as a clinically important target to elongate the life span and maintain the QOL of HD patients.

9. Importance of Sarcopenia as a Treatment Target to Elongate Longevity of HD Patients in the Era of 100-Year Life

As written above, it seems that various co-morbidities preferentially existing in HD patients, such as diabetes, pretexting CVD, fracture, and malnutrition, can impair longevity and life quality in older HD patients, in part via sarcopenia. Although the main cause of sarcopenia might differ between HD patients, it is now increasingly being identified as an early symptomatic indicator of ill health in elderly people, and thus is a definite target for prevention and treatment in order to elongate longevity in HD patients in the era of 100-year lives. HD patients with sarcopenia, which is often accompanied with malnutrition, are strongly encouraged to maintain sufficient calorie and protein intakes so as to enjoy a satisfactory quality of life, which includes maintaining the activities of daily living that will help to avoid and or reverse emaciation and sarcopenia. However, efforts to increase food intake in HD patients with sarcopenia/emaciation often are not successful due to persistent anorexia resulting from sarcopenia-associated inflammatory status [73]. The first step to stop this vicious cycle should be physical therapy. It is possible that physical therapy might increase appetite by lifting the patient's mood in the short term, and increasing the metabolic rate via activated muscle metabolism/mass in the long term. Since the Japanese Ministry of Health, Labour and Welfare recommends a high-calorie and high-protein diet to increase longevity in the elderly population, this food policy should be extended to elderly HD patients, after encouraging them to undertake physical therapy.

Author Contributions: Investigation; M.I., S.O.; resources; S.O., Y.O.; writing—review and editing M.I., supervision, Y.O. All authors have read and agreed to the published version of the manuscript.

Funding: This research received no external funding.

Conflicts of Interest: M.I. received lecturing fee from Kyowa-Kirin Co. S.O. and Y.O. declare no conflict of interest.

References

1. Masakane, I.; Hasegawa, T.; Ogata, S.; Kimata, N.; Nakai, S.; Hanafusa, N.; Hamano, T.; Wakai, K.; Wada, A.; Nitta, K. Annual peritoneal dialysis report 2014, the peritoneal dialysis registry. *Ren. Replace. Ther.* **2017**, *21*, 119. [CrossRef]
2. Aikawa, A. Current status and future aspects of kidney transplantation in Japan. *Ren. Replace. Ther.* **2018**, *36*, 50. [CrossRef]
3. Nitta, K.; on behalf of Japanese Society for Dialysis Therapy Renal Data Regdistry Committee; Masakane, I.; Hanafusa, N.; Taniguchi, M.; Hasegawa, T.; Nakai, S.; Goto, S.; Wada, A.; Hamano, T.; et al. Annual dialysis data report 2017, JSDT Renal Data Registry. *Ren. Replace. Ther.* **2019**, *5*, 53. [CrossRef]
4. Nitta, K.; Goto, S.; Masakane, I.; Hanafusa, N.; Taniguchi, M.; Hasegawa, T.; Nakai, S.; Wada, A.; Hamano, T.; Hoshino, J.; et al. Annual dialysis data report for 2018, JSDT Renal Data Registry: Survey methods, facility data, incidence, prevalence, and mortality. *Ren. Replace. Ther.* **2020**, *6*, 41. [CrossRef]

5. Uy, M.C.; Hospital, C.G.; Lim-Uy, R.; Chua, E. Association of Dialysis Malnutrition Score with Hypoglycemia and Quality of Life Among Patients with Diabetes on Maintenance Hemodialysis. *J. ASEAN Fed. Endocr. Soc.* **2018**, *33*, 137–145. [CrossRef] [PubMed]
6. Dai, L.; Mukai, H.; Lindholm, B.; Heimbürger, O.; Barany, P.; Stenvinkel, P.; Qureshi, A.R. Clinical global assessment of nutritional status as predictor of mortality in chronic kidney disease patients. *PLoS ONE* **2017**, *12*, e0186659. [CrossRef] [PubMed]
7. Carrero, J.J.; Aguilera, A.; Stenvinkel, P.; Gil, F.; Selgas, R.; Lindholm, B. Appetite Disorders in Uremia. *J. Ren. Nutr.* **2008**, *18*, 107–113. [CrossRef]
8. Sahathevan, S.; Khor, B.H.; Ng, H.M.; Gafor, A.H.A.; Mat Daud, Z.A.; Mafra, D.; Karupaiah, T. Understanding Development of Mal-nutrition in Hemodialysis Patients: A Narrative Review. *Nutrients* **2020**, *12*, 3147. [CrossRef]
9. Darmon, P.; Kaiser, M.J.; Bauer, J.M.; Sieber, C.C.; Pichard, C. Restrictive diets in the elderly: Never say never again? *Clin. Nutr.* **2010**, *29*, 170–174. [CrossRef] [PubMed]
10. Eustace, J.A.; Coresh, J.; Kutchey, C.; Te, P.L.; Gimenez, L.F.; Scheel, P.J.; Walser, M. Randomized double-blind trial of oral essential amino acids for dialysis-associated hypoalbuminemia. *Kidney Int.* **2000**, *57*, 2527–2538. [CrossRef]
11. Kalantar-Zadeh, K.; Kopple, J.D.; Block, G.; Humphreys, M.H. A malnutrition-inflammation score is correlated with morbidity and mortality in maintenance hemodialysis patients. *Am. J. Kidney Dis.* **2001**, *38*, 1251–1263. [CrossRef] [PubMed]
12. Carrero, J.J.; Stenvinkel, P.; Cuppari, L.; Ikizler, T.A.; Kalantar-Zadeh, K.; Kaysen, G.; Mitch, W.E.; Price, S.R.; Wanner, C.; Wang, A.Y.; et al. Etiology of the Protein-Energy Wasting Syndrome in Chronic Kidney Disease: A Consensus Statement from the International Society of Renal Nutrition and Metabolism (ISRNM). *J. Ren. Nutr.* **2013**, *23*, 77–90. [CrossRef] [PubMed]
13. Van de Luijtgaarden, M.W.M.; Noordzij, M.; Wanner, C.; Jager, K.J. Renal replacement therapy in Europe-a summary of the 2009 ERA-EDTA Registry Annual Report. *Clin. Kidney J.* **2012**, *5*, 109–119. [CrossRef] [PubMed]
14. Therrien, M.; Byham-Gray, L.; Beto, J. A Review of Dietary Intake Studies in Maintenance Dialysis Patients. *J. Ren. Nutr.* **2015**, *25*, 329–338. [CrossRef]
15. Fujino, Y.; Ishimura, E.; Okuno, S.; Tsuboniwa, N.; Maekawa, K.; Izumotani, T.; Yamakawa, T.; Inaba, M.; Nishizawa, Y. Annual fat mass change is a significant predictor of mortality in female hemodialysis patients. *Biomed. Pharmacother.* **2006**, *60*, 253–257. [CrossRef]
16. Raja, R.M.; Ijelu, C.; Goldstein, M. Influence of Kt/V and protein catabolic rate on hemodialysis morbidity. A long-term study. *ASAIO J.* **1992**, *38*, M179–M180. [CrossRef]
17. Bergström, J. Metabolic acidosis and nutrition in dialysis patients. *Blood Purif.* **1995**, *13*, 361–367. [CrossRef] [PubMed]
18. Hishida, M.; Imaizumi, T.; Nishiyama, T.; Okazaki, M.; Kaihan, A.B.; Kato, S.; Kubo, Y.; Ando, M.; Kaneda, H.; Maruyama, S. Survival benefit of maintained or increased body mass index in patients under-going extended-hours hemodialysis without dietary restrictions. *J. Ren. Nutr.* **2019**, *30*, 154–162. [CrossRef]
19. Ikizler, T.; Flakoll, P.J.; Parker, R.A.; Hakim, R.M. Amino acid and albumin losses during hemodialysis. *Kidney Int.* **1994**, *46*, 830–837. [CrossRef]
20. Yamada, K.; Furuya, R.; Takita, T.; Maruyama, Y.; Yamaguchi, Y.; Ohkawa, S.; Kumagai, H. Simplifed nutritional screening tools for patients on maintenance hemodialysis. *Am. J. Clin. Nutr.* **2008**, *87*, 106–113. [CrossRef]
21. Kwon, Y.E.; Yoon, C.Y.; Han, I.M.; Han, S.G.; Park, K.S.; Lee, M.J.; Park, J.T.; Han, S.H.; Yoo, T.H.; Kim, Y.L.; et al. Change of Nutritional Status Assessed Using Subjective Global Assessment Is Associated with All-Cause Mortality in Incident Dialysis Patients. *Medicine* **2016**, *95*, e2714. [CrossRef]
22. Bradbury, B.D.; Fissell, R.B.; Albert, J.M.; Anthony, M.S.; Critchlow, C.W.; Pisoni, R.L.; Port, F.K.; Gillespie, B.W. Predictors of Early Mortality among Incident US Hemodialysis Patients in the Dialysis Outcomes and Practice Patterns Study (DOPPS). *Clin. J. Am. Soc. Nephrol.* **2007**, *2*, 89–99. [CrossRef]
23. Murray, D.P.; Young, L.; Waller, J.; Wright, S.; Colombo, R.; Baer, S.; Spearman, V.; Garcia-Torres, R.; Williams, K.; Kheda, M.; et al. Is Dietary Protein Intake Predictive of One-Year Mortality in Dialysis Patients? *Am. J. Med. Sci.* **2018**, *356*, 234–243. [CrossRef]
24. Kobayashi, I.; Ishimura, E.; Kato, Y.; Okuno, S.; Yamamoto, T.; Yamakawa, T.; Mori, K.; Inaba, M.; Nishizawa, Y. Geriatric Nutritional Risk Index, a simplified nutritional screening index, is a significant predictor of mortality in chronic dialysis patients. *Nephrol. Dial. Transplant.* **2010**, *25*, 3361–3365. [CrossRef]
25. Ishimura, E.; Okuno, S.; Kim, M.; Yamamoto, T.; Izumotani, T.; Otoshi, T.; Shoji, T.; Inaba, M.; Nishizawa, Y. Increasing body fat mass in the first year of hemodialysis. *J. Am. Soc. Nephrol.* **2001**, *12*, 1921–1926. [CrossRef]
26. Lacson, E., Jr.; Wang, W.; Zebrowski, B.; Wingard, R.; Hakim, R.M. Outcomes associated with intradialytic oral nutritional supple-ments in patients undergoing maintenance hemodialysis: A quality improvement report. *Am. J. Kidney Dis.* **2012**, *60*, 591–600. [CrossRef]
27. Rosenberg, I.H. Sarcopenia: Origins and Clinical Relevance. *J. Nutr.* **1997**, *127*, 990S–991S. [CrossRef] [PubMed]
28. Chen, L.-K.; Liu, L.-K.; Woo, J.; Assantachai, P.; Auyeung, T.-W.; Bahyah, K.S.; Chou, M.-Y.; Chen, L.-Y.; Hsu, P.-S.; Krairit, O.; et al. Sarcopenia in Asia: Consensus Report of the Asian Working Group for Sarcopenia. *J. Am. Med. Dir. Assoc.* **2014**, *15*, 95–101. [CrossRef] [PubMed]
29. Yamada, S.; Yamamoto, S.; Fukuma, S.; Nakano, T.; Tsuruya, K.; Inaba, M. Geriatric Nutritional Risk Index (GNRI) and Creatinine Index Equally Predict the Risk of Mortality in Hemodialysis Patients: J-DOPPS. *Sci. Rep.* **2020**, *10*, 5756. [CrossRef] [PubMed]
30. Mori, K.; Nishide, K.; Okuno, S.; Shoji, T.; Emoto, M.; Tsuda, A.; Nakatani, S.; Imanishi, Y.; Ishimura, E.; Yamakawa, T.; et al. Impact of diabetes on sarcopenia and mortality in patients undergoing hemodialysis. *BMC Nephrol.* **2019**, *20*, 105. [CrossRef]

31. Yoda, M.; Inaba, M.; Okuno, S.; Yoda, K.; Yamada, S.; Imanishi, Y.; Mori, K.; Shoji, T.; Ishimura, E.; Yamakawa, T.; et al. Poor muscle quality as a predictor of high mortality independent of diabetes in hemodialysis patients. *Biomed. Pharmacother.* **2012**, *66*, 266–270. [CrossRef]
32. Inaba, M.; Kurajoh, M.; Okuno, S.; Imanishi, Y.; Yamada, S.; Mori, K.; Ishimura, E.; Yamakawa, T.; Nishizawa, Y. Poor muscle quality rather than reduced lean body mass is responsible for the lower serum creatinine level in hemodialysis patients with diabetes mellitus. *Clin. Nephrol.* **2010**, *74*, 266–272. [PubMed]
33. Nakagawa, C.; Inaba, M.; Ishimura, E.; Yamakawa, T.; Shoji, S.; Okuno, S. Association of Increased Serum Ferritin With Impaired Muscle Strength/Quality in Hemodialysis Patients. *J. Ren. Nutr.* **2016**, *26*, 253–257. [CrossRef]
34. Inaba, M.; Kumeda, Y.; Yamada, S.; Toi, N.; Hamai, C.; Noguchi, K.; Yasuda, E.; Furumitsu, Y.; Emoto, M.; Ohno, Y. Association of higher arterial ketone body ratio (acetoacetate/β-hydroxybutyrate) with relevant nutritional marker in hemodialysis patients. *BMC Nephrol.* **2020**, *21*, 510. [CrossRef] [PubMed]
35. Shoji, T.; Niihata, K.; Fukuma, S.; Fukuhara, S.; Akizawa, T.; Inaba, M. Both low and high serum ferritin levels predict mortality risk in hemodialysis patients without inflammation. *Clin. Exp. Nephrol.* **2017**, *21*, 685–693. [CrossRef]
36. Bae, E.; Cho, H.; Shin, N.; Kim, S.M.; Yang, S.H.; Kim, D.K.; Kim, Y.-L.; Kang, S.-W.; Yang, C.W.; Kim, N.H.; et al. Lower serum uric acid level predicts mortality in dialysis patients. *Medical (Baltim.)* **2016**, *95*, e3701. [CrossRef] [PubMed]
37. Obokata, M.; Negishi, K.; Sunaga, H.; Ishida, H.; Ito, K.; Ogawa, T.; Iso, T.; Ando, Y.; Kurabayashi, M. Association Between Circulating Ketone Bodies and Worse Outcomes in Hemodialysis Patients. *J. Am. Hear. Assoc.* **2017**, *6*, e006885. [CrossRef] [PubMed]
38. Nakamura, M.; Inaba, M.; Yamada, S.; Ozaki, E.; Maruo, S.; Okuno, S.; Imanishi, Y.; Kuriyama, N.; Watanabe, Y.; Emoto, M.; et al. Association of Decreased Handgrip Strength with Reduced Cortical Thickness in Japanese Female Patients with Type 2 Diabetes Mellitus. *Sci. Rep.* **2018**, *8*, 10767. [CrossRef] [PubMed]
39. Umegaki, H. Sarcopenia and frailty in older patients with diabetes mellitus. *Geriatr. Gerontol. Int.* **2016**, *16*, 293–299. [CrossRef]
40. Cui, M.; Gang, X.; Wang, G.; Xiao, X.; Li, Z.; Jiang, Z.; Wang, G. A cross-sectional study: Associations between sarcopenia and clinical characteristics of patients with type 2 diabetes. *Medicine* **2020**, *99*, e18708. [CrossRef] [PubMed]
41. Murata, Y.; Kadoya, Y.; Yamada, S.; Sanke, T. Sarcopenia in elderly patients with type 2 diabetes mellitus: Prevalence and related clinical factors. *Diabetol. Int.* **2017**, *9*, 136–142. [CrossRef]
42. Anagnostis, P.; Gkekas, N.K.; Achilla, C.; Pananastasiou, G.; Taouxidou, P.; Mitsiou, M.; Kenanidis, E.; Potoupnis, M.; Tsiridis, E.; Goulis, D.G. Type 2 Diabetes Mellitus is Associated with Increased Risk of Sarcopenia: A Systematic Review and Meta-analysis. *Calcif. Tissue Int.* **2020**, *107*, 453–463. [CrossRef] [PubMed]
43. Rolland, Y.M.; Perry, H.M., 3rd; Patrick, P.; Banks, W.A.; Morley, J.E. Loss of appendicular muscle mass and loss of muscle strength in young postmenopausal women. *J. Gerontol. A Biol. Sci. Med. Sci.* **2007**, *62*, 330–335. [CrossRef] [PubMed]
44. Okamura, T.; Miki, A.; Hashimoto, Y.; Kaji, A.; Sakai, R.; Osaka, T.; Hamaguchi, M.; Yamazaki, M.; Fukui, M. Shortage of energy in-take rather than protein intake is associated with sarcopenia in elderly patients with type 2 diabetes: A cross-sectional study of the KAMOGAWA-DM cohort. *J. Diabetes* **2019**, *11*, 477–483. [CrossRef] [PubMed]
45. Desmet, C.; Beguin, C.; Swine, C.; Jadoul, M. Falls in hemodialysis patients: Prospective study of incidence, risk factors, and complications. *Am. J. Kidney Dis.* **2005**, *45*, 148–153. [CrossRef] [PubMed]
46. Garlick, P.J.; Grant, I. Amino acid infusion increases the sensitivity of muscle protein synthesis in vivo to insulin. Effect of branched-chain amino acids. *Biochem. J.* **1988**, *254*, 579–584. [CrossRef] [PubMed]
47. Kalyani, R.R.; Metter, E.J.; Egan, J.; Golden, S.H.; Ferrucci, L. Hyperglycemia predicts persistently lower muscle strength with aging. *Diabetes Care* **2015**, *38*, 82–90. [CrossRef]
48. Ogama, N.; Sakurai, T.; Kawashima, S.; Tanikawa, T.; Tokuda, H.; Satake, S.; Miura, H.; Shimizu, A.; Kokubo, M.; Niida, S.; et al. Association of Glucose Fluctuations with Sarcopenia in Older Adults with Type 2 Diabetes Mellitus. *J. Clin. Med.* **2019**, *8*, 319. [CrossRef]
49. Saisho, Y.; Tanaka, K.; Abe, T.; Shimada, A.; Kawai, T.; Itoh, H. Glycated albumin to glycated hemoglobin ratio reflects post-prandial glucose excursion and relates to beta cell function in both type 1 and type 2 diabetes. *Diabetol. Int.* **2011**, *2*, 146–153. [CrossRef]
50. Abbatecola, A.M.; for the Health ABC Study; Chiodini, P.; Gallo, C.; Lakatta, E.; Sutton-Tyrrell, K.; Tylavsky, F.A.; Goodpaster, B.; De Rekeneire, N.; Schwartz, A.V.; et al. Pulse wave velocity is associated with muscle mass decline: Health ABC study. *AGE* **2011**, *34*, 469–478. [CrossRef] [PubMed]
51. Kurajoh, M.; Inaba, M.; Nagata, Y.; Yamada, S.; Imanishi, Y.; Emoto, M. Association of cystatin C- and creatinine-based eGFR with osteoporotic fracture in Japanese postmenopausal women with osteoporosis: Sarcopenia as risk for fracture. *J. Bone Miner. Metab.* **2019**, *37*, 282–291. [CrossRef] [PubMed]
52. Dharnidharka, V.R.; Kwon, C.; Stevens, G. Serum cystatin C is superior to serum creatinine as a marker of kidney function: A meta-analysis. *Am. J. Kidney Dis.* **2002**, *40*, 221–226. [CrossRef]
53. Holzer, G.; von Skrbensky, G.; Holzer, L.A.; Pichl, W. Hip fractures and the contribution of cortical versus trabecular bone to femoral neck strength. *J. Bone Min. Res.* **2009**, *24*, 468–474. [CrossRef] [PubMed]
54. Lim, S.-K.; Beom, J.; Lee, S.Y.; Kim, B.R.; Chun, S.-W.; Lim, J.-Y.; Lee, E.S. Association between sarcopenia and fall characteristics in older adults with fragility hip fracture. *Injury* **2020**, *51*, 2640–2647. [CrossRef] [PubMed]

55. Zhang, X.; Huang, P.; Dou, Q.; Wang, C.; Zhang, W.; Yang, Y.; Wang, J.; Xie, X.; Zhou, J.; Zeng, Y. Falls among older adults with sarcopenia dwelling in nursing home or community: A meta-analysis. *Clin. Nutr.* **2020**, *39*, 33–39. [CrossRef] [PubMed]
56. Turkmen, I.; Ozcan, C. Osteosarcopenia increases hip fracture risk: A case-controlled study in the elderly. *J. Back Musculoskelet. Rehabil.* **2019**, *32*, 613–618. [CrossRef] [PubMed]
57. Harvey, N.C.; Orwoll, E.; Kwok, T.; Karlsson, M.K.; Rosengren, B.E.; Ribom, E.; Cauley, J.A.; Cawthon, P.M.; Ensrud, K.; Liu, E.; et al. Sar-copenia Definitions as Predictors of Fracture Risk Independent of FRAX®, Falls, and BMD in the Osteoporotic Fractures in Men (MrOS) Study: A Meta-Analysis. *J. Bone Min. Res.* **2021**, in press. [CrossRef]
58. Tagliaferri, C.; Wittrant, Y.; Davicco, M.-J.; Walrand, S.; Coxam, V. Muscle and bone, two interconnected tissues. *Ageing Res. Rev.* **2015**, *21*, 55–70. [CrossRef]
59. Kuriyama, N.; Ozaki, E.; Koyama, T.; Matsui, D.; Watanabe, I.; Tomida, S.; Nagamitsu, R.; Hashiguchi, K.; Inaba, M.; Yamada, S.; et al. Evaluation of myostatin as a possible regulator and marker of skeletal muscle–cortical bone interaction in adults. *J. Bone Miner. Metab.* **2020**. [CrossRef]
60. Burger, D.; Levin, A. 'Shedding' light on mechanisms of hyperphosphatemic vascular dysfunction. *Kidney Int.* **2013**, *83*, 187–189. [CrossRef]
61. Rumana, N.; Kita, Y.; Turin, T.C.; Murakami, Y.; Sugihara, H.; Morita, Y.; Tomioka, N.; Okayama, A.; Nakamura, Y.; Ueshima, H. Sea-sonal pattern of incidence and case fatality of acute myocardial infarction in a Japanese population (from the Takashima AMI Registry, 1988 to 2003). *Am. J. Cardiol.* **2008**, *102*, 1307–1311. [CrossRef] [PubMed]
62. Kita, Y.; Turin, T.; Ichikawa, M.; Sugihara, H.; Morita, Y.; Tomioka, N.; Rumana, N.; Okayama, A.; Nakamura, Y.; Abbott, R.D.; et al. Trend of Stroke Incidence in a Japanese Population: Takashima Stroke Registry, 1990–2001. *Int. J. Stroke* **2009**, *4*, 241–249. [CrossRef]
63. Sutton-Tyrrell, K.; Lassila, H.C.; Meilahn, E.; Bunker, C.; Matthews, K.A.; Kuller, L.H. Carotid Atherosclerosis in Premenopausal and Postmenopausal Women and Its Association With Risk Factors Measured after Menopause. *Stroke* **1998**, *29*, 1116–1121. [CrossRef]
64. Barengolts, E.I.; Berman, M.; Kukreja, S.C.; Kouznetsova, T.; Lin, C.; Chomka, E.V. Osteoporosis and Coronary Atherosclerosis in Asymptomatic Postmenopausal Women. *Calcif. Tissue Int.* **1998**, *62*, 209–213. [CrossRef]
65. Sambrook, P.N.; Chen, C.J.; March, L.; Cameron, I.D.; Cumming, R.; Lord, S.R.; Simpson, J.M.; Seibel, M. High Bone Turnover Is an Independent Predictor of Mortality in the Frail Elderly. *J. Bone Miner. Res.* **2006**, *21*, 549–555. [CrossRef] [PubMed]
66. Zoccali, C.; Ruggenenti, P.; Perna, A.; Leonardis, D.; Tripepi, R.; Tripepi, G.; Mallamaci, F.; Remuzzi, G.; REIN Study Group. Phos-phate may promote CKD progression and attenuate renoprotective effect of ACE inhibition. *J. Am. Soc. Nephrol.* **2011**, *22*, 1923–1930. [CrossRef] [PubMed]
67. Di Iorio, B.R.; Bellizzi, V.; Bellasi, A.; Torraca, S.; D'Arrigo, G.; Tripepi, G.; Zoccali, C. Phosphate attenuates the anti-proteinuric effect of very low-protein diet in CKD patients. *Nephrol. Dial. Transplant.* **2013**, *28*, 632–640. [CrossRef]
68. Ozaki, E.; Yamada, S.; Kuriyama, N.; Matsui, D.; Watanabe, I.; Koyama, T.; Imanishi, Y.; Inaba, M.; Watanabe, Y. Association of BAP with urinary albumin excretion in postmenopausal, but not premenopausal, non-CKD Japanese women. *Sci. Rep.* **2018**, *8*, 82. [CrossRef] [PubMed]
69. Miyaoka, D.; Inaba, M.; Imanishi, Y.; Hayashi, N.; Ohara, M.; Nagata, Y.; Kurajoh, M.; Yamada, S.; Mori, K.; Emoto, M. Denosumab Improves Glomerular Filtration Rate in Osteoporotic Patients With Normal Kidney Function by Lowering Serum Phosphorus. *J. Bone Miner. Res.* **2019**, *34*, 2028–2035. [CrossRef]
70. Masaki, H.; Imanishi, Y.; Naka, H.; Nagata, Y.; Kurajoh, M.; Mori, K.; Emoto, M.; Miki, T.; Inaba, M. Bazedoxifene improves renal function and increases renal phosphate excretion in patients with postmenopausal osteoporosis. *J. Bone Miner. Metab.* **2020**, *38*, 405–411. [CrossRef] [PubMed]
71. Okamoto, K.; Inaba, M.; Furumitsu, Y.; Ban, A.; Mori, N.; Yukioka, K.; Imanishi, Y.; Nishizawa, Y. Beneficial effect of risedronate on arterial thickening and stiffening with a reciprocal relationship to its effect on bone mass in female osteoporosis patients: A longitudinal study. *Life Sci.* **2010**, *87*, 686–691. [CrossRef] [PubMed]
72. Kang, J.-H.; Keller, J.J.; Lin, H.-C. Bisphosphonates reduced the risk of acute myocardial infarction: A 2-year follow-up study. *Osteoporos. Int.* **2013**, *24*, 271–277. [CrossRef] [PubMed]
73. Pourhassan, M.; Babel, N.; Sieske, L.; Westhoff, T.H.; Wirth, R. Inflammatory cytokines and appetite in old-er hospitalized patients. *Appetite* **2021**, *166*, 105470. [CrossRef] [PubMed]

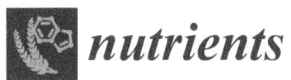

Review

Optimal Protein Intake in Pre-Dialysis Chronic Kidney Disease Patients with Sarcopenia: An Overview

Yoshitaka Isaka

Department of Nephrology, Osaka University Graduate School of Medicine, Suita 565-0871, Japan; isaka@kid.med.osaka-u.ac.jp; Tel.: +81-6-6879-3857; Fax: +81-6-6879-3230

Abstract: Multi-factors, such as anorexia, activation of renin-angiotensin system, inflammation, and metabolic acidosis, contribute to malnutrition in chronic kidney disease (CKD) patients. Most of these factors, contributing to the progression of malnutrition, worsen as CKD progresses. Protein restriction, used as a treatment for CKD, can reduce the risk of CKD progression, but may worsen the sarcopenia, a syndrome characterized by a progressive and systemic loss of muscle mass and strength. The concomitant rate of sarcopenia is higher in CKD patients than in the general population. Sarcopenia is also associated with mortality risk in CKD patients. Thus, it is important to determine whether protein restriction should be continued or loosened in CKD patients with sarcopenia. We may prioritize protein restriction in CKD patients with a high risk of end-stage kidney disease (ESKD), classified to stage G4 to G5, but may loosen protein restriction in ESKD-low risk CKD stage G3 patients with proteinuria <0.5 g/day, and rate of eGFR decline <3.0 mL/min/1.73 m^2/year. However, the effect of increasing protein intake alone without exercise therapy may be limited in CKD patients with sarcopenia. The combination of exercise therapy and increased protein intake is effective in improving muscle mass and strength in CKD patients with sarcopenia. In the case of loosening protein restriction, it is safe to avoid protein intake of more than 1.5 g/kgBW/day. In CKD patients with high risk in ESKD, 0.8 g/kgBW/day may be a critical point of protein intake.

Keywords: malnutrition; protein energy wasting (PEW); sarcopenia

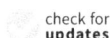

Citation: Isaka, Y. Optimal Protein Intake in Pre-Dialysis Chronic Kidney Disease Patients with Sarcopenia: An Overview. *Nutrients* 2021, 13, 1205. https://doi.org/10.3390/nu13041205

Academic Editors: Masaaki Inaba and Vassilios Liakopoulos

Received: 25 February 2021
Accepted: 4 April 2021
Published: 6 April 2021

Publisher's Note: MDPI stays neutral with regard to jurisdictional claims in published maps and institutional affiliations.

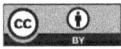

Copyright: © 2021 by the author. Licensee MDPI, Basel, Switzerland. This article is an open access article distributed under the terms and conditions of the Creative Commons Attribution (CC BY) license (https://creativecommons.org/licenses/by/4.0/).

1. Introduction

Nutritional adverse derangement is often observed in patients with chronic kidney disease (CKD), and common in advanced CKD and dialysis patients. The International Society of Renal Nutrition and Metabolism (ISRNM) defines protein energy wasting (PEW) as a "the state of decreased body protein and fat masses" [1]. The pathogenesis of PEW in CKD is multifaceted. Decreased protein and energy intake due to dietary restriction or anorexia, increased protein catabolism due to activation of renin-angiotensin system or hyperparathyroidism, decreased anabolism due to insulin resistance, chronic inflammation, metabolic acidosis, and hormonal imbalances have been reported to be associated with PEW [2] as well as sarcopenia [3] (Figure 1). These two concepts share the same criteria and have similar causes and outcomes, but they are defined differently [4]. PEW focuses on protein and energy loss associated with inflammation, whereas sarcopenia focuses on muscle mass and strength loss associated with aging. CKD patients often belong to both conditions to varying degrees.

Dietary protein intake gradually decreases during the progression of kidney injury, even in the CKD patients with minimal dietary intervention [5]. This trend was similarly observed for urinary creatinine excretion, a marker of muscle mass [5]. Food intake progressively and spontaneously decreases with decline of renal function [6]. Infusion of angiotensin II in rats was shown to induce skeletal muscle wasting via proteolysis [7,8], and in turn, angiotensin converting enzyme inhibitor [9] or angiotensin receptor blocker [10] preserved muscle strength. Parathyroid hormone (PTH) was reported to drive adipose tissue browning and malnutrition via PTH receptor in fat tissue [10]. Systemic inflammation, including elevated cytokines, such as tumor necrosis factor (TNF)-α, interleukin (IL)-6, IL-8, and so on, is often observed in CKD patients, and this tendency becomes more pronounced as the CKD stage progresses [11]. The inflammation in uremic milieu induces cardiovascular diseases and malnutrition [12,13]. Metabolic acidosis increases protein catabolism via up-regulation of ubiquitin-proteasome system in CKD patients [14,15]. Anemic patients were more frequently malnourished or at risk of malnutrition, and albumin levels are strongly associated with anemia in the elderly [16]. Vitamin D is associated with muscle weakness in older people [17], and pre-dialysis CKD patients [18].

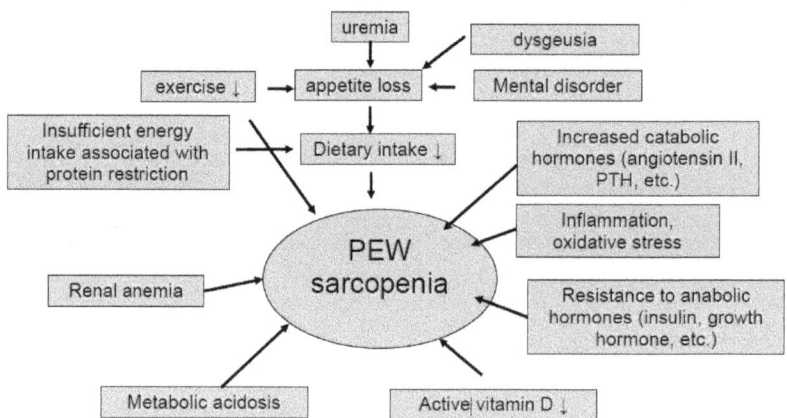

Figure 1. Potential causes of protein-energy wasting and sarcopenia. PEW; protein energy wasting, PTH; parathyroid hormone.

As mentioned above, many factors contribute to malnutrition in CKD. Most of these factors, such as hyperparathyroidism, activation of renin-angiotensin system, metabolic acidosis, and insulin resistance, worsen as CKD progresses. Thus, nutritional condition in CKD patients deteriorates as CKD progresses. In fact, protein energy wasting (PEW) assessed by clinical global assessment was observed in 2% of CKD stage G1-2, 16% of CKD G3-4, 31% of CKD G5 without dialysis, and 44% of CKD G5D [19]. On the other hand, protein restriction is used as a treatment for CKD, but it may lead to sarcopenia, assessed by loss of muscle strength or mass [20]. Energy-adjusted protein intake was associated with three-year changes in lean mass body. Participants in the highest quintile of protein intake lost approximately 40% less lean mass than did those in the lowest quintile of protein intake [20].

As mentioned above, the more advanced CKD becomes, the more severe the malnutrition becomes. Inflammation and other conditions that cause PEW become more serious as CKD progresses. On the other hand, protein intake and exercise therapy are factors that can intervene in CKD patients with sarcopenia. In CKD patients with sarcopenia, increasing protein intake may prevent worsening of sarcopenia and improve life expectancy. On the other hand, increased protein intake may accelerate the progression of CKD. Considering these two opposing effects, it is important to consider the appropriate protein intake for CKD patients with sarcopenia. As the other section in this issue describes the pathogenesis of malnutrition in dialysis patients, this paper will focus on the optimal protein intake and exercise on pre-dialysis CKD patients with sarcopenia.

2. Definition and Epidemiology of Sarcopenia in CKD

Sarcopenia is a syndrome characterized by a progressive and systemic loss of muscle mass and strength, which is associated with physical dysfunction, poor quality of life, and risk of death. It is diagnosed when the loss of muscle mass is accompanied by a loss of muscle strength or physical performance [21]. In addition to common risk factors such as aging and physical inactivity, inadequate protein intake as well as energy deficiency is thought to play a major role in the development and progression of sarcopenia in CKD patients. Furthermore, various factors, such as inflammation [22], metabolic acidosis [23], natural vitamin D deficiency [24], or diuretics treatment [25,26] may contribute to the development and progression of sarcopenia in CKD patients [3]. There are multiple diagnostic criteria for sarcopenia, which are not standardized internationally. The European Working Group on Sarcopenia in Older People (EWGSOP) definition is often used in Western countries [21], while the Asian Working Group on Sarcopenia in Older People (AWGS) [27] is recommended in Asian countries. Recently, the consensus of EWGSOP [27] and AWGS [28] was updated. Both consensus guidelines emphasize muscle strength by grip strength, allowing for diagnosis by family physicians and community health care settings that lack equipment to measure skeletal muscle mass, because low muscle strength can predict a worse outcome than low muscle mass [29]. For the assessment of skeletal muscle mass, many of the cutoffs are based on Dual Energy X-ray Absorptiometry (DEXA), while others are based on the bioelectrical impedance analysis (BIA) method. There have been reports comparing the incidence of sarcopenia in CKD patients according to each cutoff value by using BIA, central upper arm circumference and subcutaneous fat, and subjective global assessment, and it has been reported that the incidence varies depending on the assessment method [25,30–32]. Reports on the epidemiological frequency of complications are currently scarce for any of the diagnostic criteria, and there is a wide range among reports for the same diagnostic criteria. Therefore, we need to choose the diagnostic criteria by considering the body size or race to diagnose sarcopenia.

According to the National Health and Nutrition Examination Survey (NHANES III, 1994–1998), CKD patients have a high incidence of muscle mass loss [33]. In addition, a cohort study showed that walking speed and muscle strength decreases as the CKD stage progressed from creatinine clearance (Ccr) of 90 mL/min or more to 60–89 mL/min and less than 60 mL/min [34]. In a study of CKD patients with minimal dietary guidance, patients with lower Ccr had lower protein intake and lower urinary creatinine excretion, suggesting that appetite decreases and muscle mass decreases as CKD progresses [5]. According to the Korea National Health and Nutrition Examination Survey, the frequency of sarcopenia increases with CKD stage, with 2.6%, 5.6%, and 18.1% of men and 5.3%, 7.1%, and 12.6% of women in CKD stages 1, 2, and 3–5, respectively [30]. Thus, the frequency of sarcopenia is higher in CKD patients than in the general population, and it increases with the progression of CKD stage.

The prognosis of CKD complicated by sarcopenia is worse than that of uncomplicated CKD in terms of mortality and length of hospital stay. In a report examining creatinine excretion and mortality risk, the risk of mortality increases with decreasing creatinine excretion and decreasing muscle mass [35]. In patients with stage 3–5 CKD diagnosed with sarcopenia assessed by BIA, by central upper arm circumference and subcutaneous fat, and by subjective comprehensive assessment, sarcopenia is associated with poor prognosis regardless of the diagnostic method [31]. Furthermore, in hemodialysis patients, the diagnosis of sarcopenia by grip weakness or definition of EWGSOP is associated with mortality risk [32]. In a report on hemodialysis patients from Japan, the modified creatinine (Cr) index using pre-dialysis serum Cr, which is correlated with muscle mass, was assessed by the BIA method, and the lower this value is, the higher the risk of fracture [36].

3. CKD with Sarcopenia and Protein Restriction

End-stage kidney disease (ESKD) and death/cardiovascular death (mortality) are both important as the outcomes of CKD patients, and protein restriction is mainly used to improve the outcome of the former. In elderly CKD patients, the mortality risk is higher than the risk of ESKD [37]. Many of CKD patients with sarcopenia have been treated with protein restriction as a standard therapy. Kidney Disease Quality Initiative—National Kidney Foundation (KDOQI-NKF) guidelines for nutrition in CKD recommends a protein intake of 0.6 to 0.8 g/kg/day for patients with CKD in stages 3 to 5 with an energy intake of 30 kcal/kg/day [38]. The PROT-AGE Study Group recommends a protein intake of 0.8 g/kg/day and >0.8 g/kg/day for the elderly CKD patients with GFR < 30 mL/min and 30 to 60 mL/min, respectively [39]. However, in the case of muscle wasting such as sarcopenia, sufficient energy (30 kcal/kg/day) and protein (0.8–1.0 g/kg/day) are recommended for nutritional needs [4]. Some CKD patients with sarcopenia are at high risk for CKD progression to end-stage renal failure, while others have worsening sarcopenia and are at high risk of shortened life expectancy. In CKD patients with sarcopenia, different decisions (protein intake or protein restriction) need to be made against the dual outcomes of the progression of renal damage and the progression of sarcopenia. If the risk of end-stage renal failure is high, protein restriction is necessary, and if the risk of worsening sarcopenia is high, protein restriction should be loosened. However, such criteria are not clear. Thus, it is important to decide whether protein restriction should be continued or loosened in CKD patients with sarcopenia. CKD patients classified to stage G4 to G5 are belong to the extremely high risk group of renal replacement therapy, and prone to complications such as accumulation of uremic toxins, electrolyte abnormalities, and metabolic disorders [40,41]. Protein restriction can reduce the risk of ESKD in CKD, especially in patients with a GFR < 30 mL/min/1.73 m^2, but does not increase the risk of death [42], suggesting that protein restriction should be considered a priority for patients with CKD stage G4 to G5.

The relative risk of ESKD for CKD patients with stage G3 varies greatly depending on the urinary protein level and rate of eGFR decline. Therefore, the risk of ESKD should be assessed in each individual case to determine whether protein restriction should be continued or loosened in CKD patients with stage G3. It has been reported that the risk of ESKD is low in CKD patients with A1 and A2 severity categories, and the mortality risk is higher than the risk of ESKD in cases with urinary protein levels <0.5 g/day [43]. On the contrary, it has been reported that proteinuria >1.0 g/gCr [44] or albuminuria > 1.0 g/gCr [45] is associated with a higher risk of ESKD.

With regard to the rate of eGFR decline, it has been reported that CKD patients with an eGFR decline >3.0 mL/min/1.73 m^2/year have a higher risk of ESKD than those with a lower eGFR decline [46,47]. In a meta-analysis showing that protein restriction suppresses the rate of GFR decline [48], 12 of the 15 studies showed that the rate of GFR decline was greater than 3.0 mL/min/1.73 m^2/year, suggesting that protein restriction may be effective in patients with a faster rate of eGFR decline. Thus, it is reasonable to consider prioritizing protein restriction in CKD patients with stage G4 to G5, but loosening protein restriction in CKD stage G3 patients with proteinuria <0.5 g/day, and rate of eGFR decline <3.0 mL/min/1.73 m^2/year.

4. Effect of Increased Protein Intake for CKD Patients with Sarcopenia

The supplementation of vitamin D and leucine-enriched diet in elderly patients with sarcopenia for 13 weeks improved the chair-rise test and limb muscle mass compared with controls, but there was no difference in grip strength or short physical performance battery (SPPB) [49]. On the other hand, in a study of sarcopenic older adults using nutritional supplements with different amounts of protein, lower extremity muscle strength, muscle quality, grip strength, and walking speed increased in high protein intake groups after 24 weeks [50]. In addition, in a randomized controlled trial (RCT) of protein loading in elderly people with frailty, protein intake improved short physical performance battery (SPPB) but not lean mass [51]. As described above, there are a number of RCTs showing the efficacy of dietary therapy alone, but none of them reported that dietary therapy was effective for skeletal muscle mass, physical function, or muscle strength. In a meta-analysis of five RCTs of elderly people diagnosed with sarcopenia, there was no clear effect on skeletal muscle mass, lean mass, grip strength, knee extensor strength, walking speed, or Timed Up and Go test at three months [52]. Thus, the effect of increasing protein intake alone without exercise therapy may be limited in CKD patients with sarcopenia.

5. Increased Protein Intake and Exercise for CKD Patients with Sarcopenia

In a systematic review and meta-analysis of three RCTs of elderly people with sarcopenia, exercise therapy improves limb skeletal muscle mass, normal walking speed, maximal walking speed, and knee extension muscle strength compared with dietary intervention or health education [52], suggesting that exercise therapy is effective in improving sarcopenia. In addition, there are several reports that exercise therapy, including resistance exercise, prolonged six-minute walking distance [53], increases thigh cross-sectional area, volume, and knee extension muscle strength [54], and increases muscle fiber area and upper and lower limb muscle strength [55,56]. Furthermore, in a 12-week RCT in CKD patients with stages G3b to G5, including frailty patients, the combination of resistance exercise and aerobic exercise increases muscle mass and strength compared with aerobic exercise alone [57], and it is important to note that there are no significant changes in renal function in both groups. These results suggest that exercise therapy is effective in improving muscle mass and strength in elderly patients with sarcopenia, and that the combination of exercise therapy and diet therapy is more effective than exercise therapy alone in improving sarcopenia in elderly patients. On the other hand, a large increase in protein intake may worsen the renal function in CKD patients. Therefore, it is considered safer to increase protein intake gradually in CKD. Although the amount of energy consumed during exercise therapy varies widely among individuals, total energy requirements are also expected to increase, so energy intake should be adjusted accordingly.

6. Excessive Protein Intake in CKD Patients

The GFR increases physiologically and transiently with protein intake. In the elderly, especially those over 70 years of age, potential glomerular hyperfiltration occurs due to age-related nephron loss [58], and hypertension, diabetes mellitus, and obesity further reduce renal reserve [59]. It has been reported that short-term protein loading (average of 2.0 g/kgBW/day) increases GFR in healthy young adults, but decreases GFR in older adults (average of 1.8 g/kgBW/day for 10 days) [60]. In a report from the United States on healthy subjects with an eGFR > 60 mL/min/1.73 m^2 without cardiovascular disease or diabetes for a median of 23 years [61], a report from the Netherlands on healthy subjects with a mean eGFR of 80 mL/min/1.73 m^2 for a mean of 6.4 years [62], and a report from the United States on healthy women with an eGFR > 80 mL/min/1.73 m^2 for 11 years [63], protein intake was not associated with decreased renal function. Thus, in terms of risk of renal function decline, CKD stage G1 to G2 patients with sarcopenia may benefit from adequate dietary protein intake. On the other hand, an association between high protein intake and cardiovascular mortality has been reported in elderly people at risk for cardiovascular disease [64]. In a Spanish report of elderly subjects at high risk for cardiovascular disease, the risk of cardiovascular and all-cause mortality was higher in the group with a protein intake >1.5 g/kgBW/day compared with the group with a protein intake of 1.0–1.5 g/kgBW/day at a median observation period of 4.8 years [64], suggesting that protein intake may be an independent risk factor for cardiovascular disease risk. Therefore, it is safe to avoid protein intake of more than 1.5 g/kgBW/day at least in elderly people at risk for cardiovascular disease.

In the MDRD (Modification of Diet in Renal Disease) Study A, there was no difference in glomerular filtration rate (GFR) reduction between usual-protein diet group (1.3 g/kg body weight (BW)/day) and low-protein diet group (0.58 g/kgBW/day) among CKD patients (eGFR 25–55 mL/min/1.73 m^2) over the entire three-year analysis [65]. In a subsequent analysis, the rate of GFR decline in the 0.58 g/kgBW/day group was faster than that in the 1.3 g/kgBW/day group up to four months after the start of the study, and the rate of GFR decline was slower in the 0.58 g/kgBW/day group after four months, suggesting the possibility of a long-term renoprotective effect of a low-protein diet [66]. In an RCT of 89 patients with CKD stage G3 and hypertension [67], the GFR decline at 12 months was faster in the unrestricted group (actual intake: 1.54 ± 0.39 g/kgBW/day) compared with the patients with a protein intake instruction of 0.6 g/kgBW/day (actual intake: 0.67 ± 0.21), suggesting that the actual intake of 1.5 g/kgBW/day of protein worsens the rate of renal function decline compared with 0.6 g/kgBW/day. In this report, serum albumin and prealbumin levels did not change in the 0.6 g/kgBW/day group, but energy intake, body weight, and BMI decreased, compared with the unrestricted group. A French report of CKD (stage G3: 50%) with a median follow-up of 5.6 years showed that an increase in protein intake of 0.1 g/kgBW/day increased the risk of ESKD by 1.05 (95% CI, 1.01–1.10) [68]. However, the hazard ratio was even higher in the group with GFR < 30 mL/min/1.73 m^2, but the significance disappeared in the group with GFR ≥ 30 mL/min/1.73 m^2, suggesting that the effect of protein restriction in stage G3 is not high [68]. Furthermore, the risk of ESKD increases linearly with increasing protein intake, but there is no threshold for protein intake [68]. Thus, the upper limit of protein intake for CKD patients who are not at high risk for ESKD is 1.3 g/kgBW/day under the presence of sarcopenia.

On the other hand, protein restriction should be prioritized in CKD patients at high risk for ESKD. CKD patients prioritizing protein restriction are considered to be stage G4-G5 patients and stage G3 patients with proteinuria >0.5 g/day. However, excessive protein restriction may exacerbate sarcopenia. A systematic review and meta-analysis of RCTs in stage G3 to G5 CKD reported that protein restriction of <0.8 g/kgBW/day was associated with a reduced risk of progression to ESKD compared with >0.8 g/kgBW/day, with no change in the risk of total mortality [69]. In an RCT of CKD in stages G4 to G5 with strict protein restriction (0.55 g/kgBW/day) versus usual protein restriction (0.8 g/kgBW/day), there was no difference in survival, non-induction of dialysis, or their combined outcomes [70], suggesting that protein restriction of 0.8 g/kgBW/day does not further worsen renal dysfunction compared to 0.55 g/kgBW/day. Thus, 0.8 g/kgBW/day is considered to be a critical point of protein intake in CKD patients with high risk in ESKD.

7. Conclusions

Reflecting the aging of CKD patients in recent years, malnutrition and sarcopenia have been the focus of much attention. Although many factors are thought to be involved in the development of these pathogenesis, inadequate protein intake may contribute to the progression of sarcopenia. Protein restriction has been used to treat CKD patients for many years, and protein intake for CKD patients with sarcopenia may improve sarcopenia and improve life expectancy. On the other hand, excessive protein intake may accelerate the progression of CKD. For CKD patients with sarcopenia, urinary protein excretion and the rate of eGFR decline should be evaluated to determine whether protein restriction should be continued or loosened.

Author Contributions: The author contributed to this review/manuscript. The conceptualization of the review, the literature search was done by Y.I. The draft and revision of the manuscript was written by Y.I. The author has read and agreed to the published version of the manuscript.

Funding: This research received no external funding.

Conflicts of Interest: The author declares no conflict of interest.

References

1. Fouque, D.; Kalantar-Zadeh, K.; Kopple, J.; Cano, N.; Chauveau, P.; Cuppari, L.; Franch, H.; Guarnieri, G.; Ikizler, T.; Kaysen, G.; et al. A proposed nomenclature and diagnostic criteria for protein–energy wasting in acute and chronic kidney disease. *Kidney Int.* **2008**, *73*, 391–398. [CrossRef]
2. Carrero, J.J.; Stenvinkel, P.; Cuppari, L.; Ikizler, T.A.; Kalantar-Zadeh, K.; Kaysen, G.; Mitch, W.E.; Price, S.R.; Wanner, C.; Wang, A.Y.; et al. Etiology of the Protein-Energy Wasting Syndrome in Chronic Kidney Disease: A Consensus Statement From the International Society of Renal Nutrition and Metabolism (ISRNM). *J. Ren. Nutr.* **2013**, *23*, 77–90. [CrossRef] [PubMed]
3. Moorthi, R.N.; Avin, K.G. Clinical relevance of sarcopenia in chronic kidney disease. *Curr. Opin. Nephrol. Hypertens.* **2017**, *26*, 219–228. [CrossRef] [PubMed]
4. Sabatino, A.; Cuppari, L.; Stenvinkel, P.; Lindholm, B.; Avesani, C.M. Sarcopenia in chronic kidney disease: What have we learned so far? *J. Nephrol.* **2020**, 1–26. [CrossRef] [PubMed]

5. Ikizler, T.A.; Greene, J.H.; Wingard, R.L.; Parker, R.A.; Hakim, R.M. Spontaneous dietary protein intake during progression of chronic renal failure. *J. Am. Soc. Nephrol.* **1995**, *6*, 1386–1391.
6. Duenhas, M.R.; Draibe, S.A.; Avesani, C.M.; Sesso, R.; Cuppari, L. Influence of renal function on spontaneous dietary intake and on nutritional status of chronic renal insufficiency patients. *Eur. J. Clin. Nutr.* **2003**, *57*, 1473–1478. [CrossRef]
7. Rajan, V.; Mitch, W.E. Ubiquitin, proteasomes and proteolytic mechanisms activated by kidney disease. *Biochim. Biophys. Acta Mol. Basis Dis.* **2008**, *1782*, 795–799. [CrossRef]
8. Song, Y.-H.; Li, Y.; Du, J.; Mitch, W.E.; Rosenthal, N.; Delafontaine, P. Muscle-specific expression of IGF-1 blocks angiotensin II–induced skeletal muscle wasting. *J. Clin. Investig.* **2005**, *115*, 451–458. [CrossRef]
9. Onder, G.; Penninx, B.W.J.H.; Balkrishnan, R.; Fried, L.P.; Chaves, P.H.M.; Williamson, J.; Carter, C.; Di Bari, M.; Guralnik, J.M.; Pahor, M. Relation between use of angiotensin-converting enzyme inhibitors and muscle strength and physical function in older women: An observational study. *Lancet* **2002**, *359*, 926–930. [CrossRef]
10. Lin, Y.-L.; Chen, S.-Y.; Lai, Y.-H.; Wang, C.-H.; Kuo, C.-H.; Liou, H.-H.; Hsu, B.-G. Angiotensin II receptor blockade is associated with preserved muscle strength in chronic hemodialysis patients. *BMC Nephrol.* **2019**, *20*, 54. [CrossRef]
11. Nakanishi, I.; Moutabarrik, A.; Okada, N.; Kitamura, E.; Hayashi, A.; Syouji, T.; Namiki, M.; Ishibashi, M.; Zaid, D.; Tsubakihara, Y. Interleukin-8 in chronic renal failure and dialysis patients. *Nephrol. Dial. Transplant.* **1994**, *9*, 1435–1442.
12. Meuwese, C.L.; Carrero, J.J.; Stenvinkel, P. Recent Insights in Inflammation-Associated Wasting in Patients with Chronic Kidney Disease. *Contrib. Nephrol.* **2011**, *171*, 120–126. [CrossRef]
13. Utaka, S.; Avesani, C.M.; Draibe, S.A.; Kamimura, M.A.; Andreoni, S.; Cuppari, L. Inflammation is associated with increased energy expenditure in patients with chronic kidney disease. *Am. J. Clin. Nutr.* **2005**, *82*, 801–805. [CrossRef] [PubMed]
14. Boirie, Y.; Broyer, M.; Gagnadoux, M.F.; Niaudet, P.; Bresson, J.-L. Alterations of protein metabolism by metabolic acidosis in children with chronic renal failure. *Kidney Int.* **2000**, *58*, 236–241. [CrossRef] [PubMed]
15. Pickering, W.P.; Price, S.R.; Bircher, G.; Marinovic, A.C.; Mitch, W.E.; Walls, J. Nutrition in CAPD: Serum bicarbonate and the ubiquitin-proteasome system in muscle. *Kidney Int.* **2002**, *61*, 1286–1292. [CrossRef] [PubMed]
16. Frangos, E.; Trombetti, A.; Graf, C.E.; Lachat, V.; Samaras, N.; Vischer, U.M.; Zekry, D.; Rizzoli, R.; Herrmann, F.R. Malnutrition in very old hospitalized patients: A new etiologic factor of anemia? *J. Nutr. Health Aging* **2016**, *20*, 705–713. [CrossRef]
17. Visser, M.; Deeg, D.J.H.; Lips, P. Low Vitamin D and High Parathyroid Hormone Levels as Determinants of Loss of Muscle Strength and Muscle Mass (Sarcopenia): The Longitudinal Aging Study Amsterdam. *J. Clin. Endocrinol. Metab.* **2003**, *88*, 5766–5772. [CrossRef]
18. Saito, A.; Hiraki, K.; Otobe, Y.; Izawa, K.P.; Sakurada, T.; Shibagaki, Y. Relationship between Serum Vitamin D and Leg Strength in Older Adults with Pre-Dialysis Chronic Kidney Disease: A Preliminary Study. *Int. J. Environ. Res. Public Health* **2020**, *17*, 1433. [CrossRef]
19. Dai, L.; Mukai, H.; Lindholm, B.; Heimbürger, O.; Barany, P.; Stenvinkel, P.; Qureshi, A.R. Clinical global assessment of nutritional status as predictor of mortality in chronic kidney disease patients. *PLoS ONE* **2017**, *12*, e0186659. [CrossRef]
20. Houston, D.K.; Nicklas, B.J.; Ding, J.; Harris, T.B.; Tylavsky, F.A.; Newman, A.B.; Lee, J.S.; Sahyoun, N.R.; Visser, M.; Kritchevsky, S.B.; et al. Dietary protein intake is associated with lean mass change in older, community-dwelling adults: The Health, Aging, and Body Composition (Health ABC) Study. *Am. J. Clin. Nutr.* **2008**, *87*, 150–155. [CrossRef]
21. Cruz-Jentoft, A.J.; Baeyens, J.P.; Bauer, J.M.; Boirie, Y.; Cederholm, T.; Landi, F.; Martin, F.C.; Michel, J.-P.; Rolland, Y.; Schneider, S.M.; et al. Sarcopenia: European consensus on definition and diagnosis: Report of the European Working Group on Sarcopenia in Older People. *Age Ageing* **2010**, *39*, 412–423. [CrossRef]
22. Tuttle, C.S.; Thang, L.A.; Maier, A.B. Markers of inflammation and their association with muscle strength and mass: A systematic review and meta-analysis. *Ageing Res. Rev.* **2020**, *64*, 101185. [CrossRef]
23. Jehle, S.; Krapf, R. Effects of acidogenic diet forms on musculoskeletal function. *J. Nephrol.* **2010**, *23*, 77–84.
24. Tajar, A.; Lee, D.M.; Pye, S.R.; O'Connell, M.D.L.; Ravindrarajah, R.; Gielen, E.; Boonen, S.; Vanderschueren, D.; Pendleton, N.; Finn, J.D.; et al. The association of frailty with serum 25-hydroxyvitamin D and parathyroid hormone levels in older European men. *Age Ageing* **2013**, *42*, 352–359. [CrossRef] [PubMed]
25. Ishikawa, S.; Naito, S.; Iimori, S.; Takahashi, D.; Zeniya, M.; Sato, H.; Nomura, N.; Sohara, E.; Okado, T.; Uchida, S.; et al. Loop diuretics are associated with greater risk of sarcopenia in patients with non-dialysis-dependent chronic kidney disease. *PLoS ONE* **2018**, *13*, e0192990. [CrossRef] [PubMed]
26. Mandai, S.; Furukawa, S.; Kodaka, M.; Hata, Y.; Mori, T.; Nomura, N.; Ando, F.; Mori, Y.; Takahashi, D.; Yoshizaki, Y.; et al. Loop diuretics affect skeletal myoblast differentiation and exercise-induced muscle hypertrophy. *Sci. Rep.* **2017**, *7*, 46369. [CrossRef]
27. Chen, L.-K.; Liu, L.-K.; Woo, J.; Assantachai, P.; Auyeung, T.-W.; Bahyah, K.S.; Chou, M.-Y.; Hsu, P.-S.; Krairit, O.; Lee, J.S.; et al. Sarcopenia in Asia: Consensus Report of the Asian Working Group for Sarcopenia. *J. Am. Med. Dir. Assoc.* **2014**, *15*, 95–101. [CrossRef] [PubMed]
28. Chen, L.-K.; Woo, J.; Assantachai, P.; Auyeung, T.-W.; Chou, M.-Y.; Iijima, K.; Jang, H.C.; Kang, L.; Kim, M.; Kim, S.; et al. Asian Working Group for Sarcopenia: 2019 Consensus Update on Sarcopenia Diagnosis and Treatment. *J. Am. Med. Dir. Assoc.* **2020**, *21*, 300–307.e2. [CrossRef]
29. Leong, D.P.; Teo, K.K.; Rangarajan, S.; Lopez-Jaramillo, P.; Avezum, A.; Orlandini, A.; Seron, P.; Ahmed, S.H.; Rosengren, A.; Kelishadi, R.; et al. Prognostic value of grip strength: Findings from the Prospective Urban Rural Epidemiology (PURE) study. *Lancet* **2015**, *386*, 266–273. [CrossRef]

30. Moon, S.J.; Kim, T.H.; Yoon, S.Y.; Chung, J.H.; Hwang, H.-J. Relationship between Stage of Chronic Kidney Disease and Sarcopenia in Korean Aged 40 Years and Older Using the Korea National Health and Nutrition Examination Surveys (KNHANES IV-2, 3, and V-1, 2), 2008–2011. *PLoS ONE* **2015**, *10*, e0130740. [CrossRef]
31. Pereira, R.A.; Cordeiro, A.C.; Avesani, C.M.; Carrero, J.J.; Lindholm, B.; Amparo, F.C.; Amodeo, C.; Cuppari, L.; Kamimura, M.A. Sarcopenia in chronic kidney disease on conservative therapy: Prevalence and association with mortality. *Nephrol. Dial. Transplant.* **2015**, *30*, 1718–1725. [CrossRef] [PubMed]
32. Ren, H.; Gong, D.; Jia, F.; Xu, B.; Liu, Z. Sarcopenia in patients undergoing maintenance hemodialysis: Incidence rate, risk factors and its effect on survival risk. *Ren. Fail.* **2016**, *38*, 364–371. [CrossRef]
33. Foley, R.N.; Wang, C.; Ishani, A.; Collins, A.J.; Murray, A.M. Kidney Function and Sarcopenia in the United States General Population: NHANES III. *Am. J. Nephrol.* **2007**, *27*, 279–286. [CrossRef] [PubMed]
34. Roshanravan, B.; Patel, K.V.; Robinson-Cohen, C.; De Boer, I.H.; O'Hare, A.M.; Ferrucci, L.; Himmelfarb, J.; Kestenbaum, B. Creatinine Clearance, Walking Speed, and Muscle Atrophy: A Cohort Study. *Am. J. Kidney Dis.* **2015**, *65*, 737–747. [CrossRef] [PubMed]
35. Sinkeler, S.J.; Kwakernaak, A.J.; Bakker, S.J.; Shahinfar, S.; Esmatjes, E.; De Zeeuw, D.; Navis, G.; Heerspink, H.J.L. Creatinine Excretion Rate and Mortality in Type 2 Diabetes and Nephropathy. *Diabetes Care* **2013**, *36*, 1489–1494. [CrossRef]
36. Yamada, S.; Taniguchi, M.; Tokumoto, M.; Yoshitomi, R.; Yoshida, H.; Tatsumoto, N.; Hirakata, H.; Fujimi, S.; Kitazono, T.; Tsuruya, K. Modified Creatinine Index and the Risk of Bone Fracture in Patients Undergoing Hemodialysis: The Q-Cohort Study. *Am. J. Kidney Dis.* **2017**, *70*, 270–280. [CrossRef] [PubMed]
37. O'Hare, A.M.; Choi, A.I.; Bertenthal, D.; Bacchetti, P.; Garg, A.X.; Kaufman, J.S.; Walter, L.C.; Mehta, K.M.; Steinman, M.A.; Allon, M.; et al. Age Affects Outcomes in Chronic Kidney Disease. *J. Am. Soc. Nephrol.* **2007**, *18*, 2758–2765. [CrossRef]
38. Ikizler, T.A.; Burrowes, J.D.; Byham-Gray, L.D.; Campbell, K.L.; Carrero, J.-J.; Chan, W.; Fouque, D.; Friedman, A.N.; Ghaddar, S.; Goldstein-Fuchs, D.J.; et al. KDOQI Clinical Practice Guideline for Nutrition in CKD: 2020 Update. *Am. J. Kidney Dis.* **2020**, *76*, S1–S107. [CrossRef]
39. Bauer, J.; Biolo, G.; Cederholm, T.; Cesari, M.; Cruz-Jentoft, A.J.; Morley, J.E.; Phillips, S.; Sieber, C.; Stehle, P.; Teta, D.; et al. Evidence-Based Recommendations for Optimal Dietary Protein Intake in Older People: A Position Paper From the PROT-AGE Study Group. *J. Am. Med. Dir. Assoc.* **2013**, *14*, 542–559. [CrossRef]
40. Cianciaruso, B.; Pota, A.; Pisani, A.; Torraca, S.; Annecchini, R.; Lombardi, P.; Capuano, A.; Nazzaro, P.; Bellizzi, V.; Sabbatini, M. Metabolic effects of two low protein diets in chronic kidney disease stage 4–5—A randomized controlled trial. *Nephrol. Dial. Transplant.* **2007**, *23*, 636–644. [CrossRef]
41. Mircescu, G.; Gârneaţă, L.; Stancu, S.H.; Căpuşă, C. Effects of a Supplemented Hypoproteic Diet in Chronic Kidney Disease. *J. Ren. Nutr.* **2007**, *17*, 179–188. [CrossRef]
42. Yan, B.; Su, X.; Xu, B.; Qiao, X.; Wang, L. Effect of diet protein restriction on progression of chronic kidney disease: A systematic review and meta-analysis. *PLoS ONE* **2018**, *13*, e0206134. [CrossRef]
43. De Nicola, L.; Provenzano, M.; Chiodini, P.; Borrelli, S.; Russo, L.; Bellasi, A.; Santoro, D.; Conte, G.; Minutolo, R. Epidemiology of low-proteinuric chronic kidney disease in renal clinics. *PLoS ONE* **2017**, *12*, e0172241. [CrossRef]
44. Obi, Y.; Kimura, T.; Nagasawa, Y.; Yamamoto, R.; Yasuda, K.; Sasaki, K.; Kitamura, H.; Imai, E.; Rakugi, H.; Isaka, Y.; et al. Impact of Age and Overt Proteinuria on Outcomes of Stage 3 to 5 Chronic Kidney Disease in a Referred Cohort. *Clin. J. Am. Soc. Nephrol.* **2010**, *5*, 1558–1565. [CrossRef]
45. Inaguma, D.; For The Chronic Kidney Disease Japan Cohort Study Group; Imai, E.; Takeuchi, A.; Ohashi, Y.; Watanabe, T.; Nitta, K.; Akizawa, T.; Matsuo, S.; Makino, H.; et al. Risk factors for CKD progression in Japanese patients: Findings from the Chronic Kidney Disease Japan Cohort (CKD-JAC) study. *Clin. Exp. Nephrol.* **2017**, *21*, 446–456. [CrossRef]
46. Coresh, J.; Turin, T.C.; Matsushita, K.; Sang, Y.; Ballew, S.H.; Appel, L.J.; Arima, H.; Chadban, S.J.; Cirillo, M.; Djurdjev, O.; et al. Decline in Estimated Glomerular Filtration Rate and Subsequent Risk of End-Stage Renal Disease and Mortality. *JAMA* **2014**, *311*, 2518–2531. [CrossRef] [PubMed]
47. Kovesdy, C.P.; Coresh, J.; Ballew, S.H.; Woodward, M.; Levin, A.; Naimark, D.M.J.; Nally, J.; Rothenbacher, D.; Stengel, B.; Iseki, K.; et al. Past Decline Versus Current eGFR and Subsequent ESRD Risk. *J. Am. Soc. Nephrol.* **2015**, *27*, 2447–2455. [CrossRef] [PubMed]
48. Rughooputh, M.S.; Zeng, R.; Yao, Y. Protein Diet Restriction Slows Chronic Kidney Disease Progression in Non-Diabetic and in Type 1 Diabetic Patients, but Not in Type 2 Diabetic Patients: A Meta-Analysis of Randomized Controlled Trials Using Glomerular Filtration Rate as a Surrogate. *PLoS ONE* **2015**, *10*, e0145505. [CrossRef] [PubMed]
49. Bauer, J.M.; Verlaan, S.; Bautmans, I.; Brandt, K.; Donini, L.M.; Maggio, M.; McMurdo, M.E.; Mets, T.; Seal, C.; Wijers, S.L.; et al. Effects of a Vitamin D and Leucine-Enriched Whey Protein Nutritional Supplement on Measures of Sarcopenia in Older Adults, the PROVIDE Study: A Randomized, Double-Blind, Placebo-Controlled Trial. *J. Am. Med. Dir. Assoc.* **2015**, *16*, 740–747. [CrossRef] [PubMed]
50. Cramer, J.T.; Cruz-Jentoft, A.J.; Landi, F.; Hickson, M.; Zamboni, M.; Pereira, S.L.; Hustead, D.S.; Mustad, V.A. Impacts of High-Protein Oral Nutritional Supplements Among Malnourished Men and Women with Sarcopenia: A Multicenter, Randomized, Double-Blinded, Controlled Trial. *J. Am. Med. Dir. Assoc.* **2016**, *17*, 1044–1055. [CrossRef]

51. Tieland, M.; van de Rest, O.; Dirks, M.L.; van der Zwaluw, N.; Mensink, M.; van Loon, L.J.; de Groot, L.C. Protein Supplementation Improves Physical Performance in Frail Elderly People: A Randomized, Double-Blind, Placebo-Controlled Trial. *J. Am. Med. Dir. Assoc.* **2012**, *13*, 720–726. [CrossRef] [PubMed]
52. Yoshimura, Y.; Wakabayashi, H.; Yamada, M.; Kim, H.; Harada, A.; Arai, H. Interventions for Treating Sarcopenia: A Systematic Review and Meta-Analysis of Randomized Controlled Studies. *J. Am. Med. Dir. Assoc.* **2017**, *18*, 553.e1–553.e16. [CrossRef]
53. Rossi, A.P.; Burris, D.D.; Lucas, F.L.; Crocker, G.A.; Wasserman, J.C. Effects of a Renal Rehabilitation Exercise Program in Patients with CKD: A Randomized, Controlled Trial. *Clin. J. Am. Soc. Nephrol.* **2014**, *9*, 2052–2058. [CrossRef] [PubMed]
54. Watson, E.L.; Greening, N.J.; Viana, J.L.; Aulakh, J.; Bodicoat, D.H.; Barratt, J.; Feehally, J.; Smith, A.C. Progressive Resistance Exercise Training in CKD: A Feasibility Study. *Am. J. Kidney Dis.* **2015**, *66*, 249–257. [CrossRef] [PubMed]
55. Castaneda, C.; Gordon, P.L.; Parker, R.C.; Uhlin, K.L.; Roubenoff, R.; Levey, A.S. Resistance training to reduce the malnutrition-inflammation complex syndrome of chronic kidney disease. *Am. J. Kidney Dis.* **2004**, *43*, 607–616. [CrossRef] [PubMed]
56. Castaneda, C.; Gordon, P.L.; Uhlin, K.L.; Levey, A.S.; Kehayias, J.J.; Dwyer, J.T.; Fielding, R.A.; Roubenoff, R.; Singh, M.F. Resistance Training To Counteract the Catabolism of a Low-Protein Diet in Patients with Chronic Renal Insufficiency. *Ann. Intern. Med.* **2001**, *135*, 965–976. [CrossRef] [PubMed]
57. Watson, E.L.; Gould, D.W.; Wilkinson, T.J.; Xenophontos, S.; Clarke, A.L.; Vogt, B.P.; Viana, J.L.; Smith, A.C. Twelve-week combined resistance and aerobic training confers greater benefits than aerobic training alone in nondialysis CKD. *Am. J. Physiol. Physiol.* **2018**, *314*, F1188–F1196. [CrossRef]
58. Denic, A.; Mathew, J.; Lerman, L.O.; Lieske, J.C.; Larson, J.J.; Alexander, M.P.; Poggio, E.; Glassock, R.J.; Rule, A.D. Single-Nephron Glomerular Filtration Rate in Healthy Adults. *N. Engl. J. Med.* **2017**, *376*, 2349–2357. [CrossRef]
59. Hommos, M.S.; Glassock, R.J.; Rule, A.D. Structural and Functional Changes in Human Kidneys with Healthy Aging. *J. Am. Soc. Nephrol.* **2017**, *28*, 2838–2844. [CrossRef]
60. Walrand, S.; Short, K.R.; Bigelow, M.L.; Sweatt, A.J.; Hutson, S.M.; Nair, K.S. Functional impact of high protein intake on healthy elderly people. *Am. J. Physiol. Metab.* **2008**, *295*, E921–E928. [CrossRef]
61. Haring, B.; Selvin, E.; Liang, M.; Coresh, J.; Grams, M.E.; Petruski-Ivleva, N.; Steffen, L.M.; Rebholz, C.M. Dietary Protein Sources and Risk for Incident Chronic Kidney Disease: Results From the Atherosclerosis Risk in Communities (ARIC) Study. *J. Ren. Nutr.* **2017**, *27*, 233–242. [CrossRef]
62. Halbesma, N.; Bakker, S.J.L.; Jansen, D.F.; Stolk, R.P.; De Zeeuw, D.; De Jong, P.E.; Gansevoort, R.T.; for The PREVEND Study Group. High Protein Intake Associates with Cardiovascular Events but not with Loss of Renal Function. *J. Am. Soc. Nephrol.* **2009**, *20*, 1797–1804. [CrossRef] [PubMed]
63. Knight, E.L.; Stampfer, M.J.; Hankinson, S.E.; Spiegelman, D.; Curhan, G.C. The Impact of Protein Intake on Renal Function Decline in Women with Normal Renal Function or Mild Renal Insufficiency. *Ann. Intern. Med.* **2003**, *138*, 460–467. [CrossRef] [PubMed]
64. Hernández-Alonso, P.; Salas-Salvadó, J.; Ruiz-Canela, M.; Corella, D.; Estruch, R.; Fitó, M.; Arós, F.; Gómez-Gracia, E.; Fiol, M.; Lapetra, J.; et al. High dietary protein intake is associated with an increased body weight and total death risk. *Clin. Nutr.* **2016**, *35*, 496–506. [CrossRef] [PubMed]
65. Klahr, S.; Levey, A.S.; Beck, G.J.; Caggiula, A.W.; Hunsicker, L.; Kusek, J.W.; Striker, G. The Effects of Dietary Protein Restriction and Blood-Pressure Control on the Progression of Chronic Renal Disease. *N. Engl. J. Med.* **1994**, *330*, 877–884. [CrossRef] [PubMed]
66. Levey, A.S.; Greene, T.; Beck, G.J.; Caggiula, A.W.; Kusek, J.W.; Hunsicker, L.G.; Klahr, S. Dietary protein restriction and the progression of chronic renal disease: What have all of the results of the MDRD study shown? Modification of Diet in Renal Disease Study group. *J. Am. Soc. Nephrol.* **1999**, *10*, 2426–2439.
67. Meloni, C.; Tatangelo, P.; Cipriani, S.; Rossi, V.; Suraci, C.; Tozzo, C.; Rossini, B.; Cecilia, A.; Di Franco, D.; Straccialano, E.; et al. Adequate protein dietary restriction in diabetic and nondiabetic patients with chronic renal failure. *J. Ren. Nutr.* **2004**, *14*, 208–213. [CrossRef]
68. Metzger, M.; Yuan, W.L.; Haymann, J.-P.; Flamant, M.; Houillier, P.; Thervet, E.; Boffa, J.-J.; Vrtovsnik, F.; Froissart, M.; Bankir, L.; et al. Association of a Low-Protein Diet with Slower Progression of CKD. *Kidney Int. Rep.* **2018**, *3*, 105–114. [CrossRef]
69. Rhee, C.M.; Ahmadi, S.-F.; Kovesdy, C.P.; Kalantar-Zadeh, K. Low-protein diet for conservative management of chronic kidney disease: A systematic review and meta-analysis of controlled trials. *J. Cachex Sarcopenia Muscle* **2017**, *9*, 235–245. [CrossRef]
70. Cianciaruso, B.; Pota, A.; Bellizzi, V.; Di Giuseppe, D.; Di Micco, L.; Minutolo, R.; Pisani, A.; Sabbatini, M.; Ravani, P. Effect of a Low Moderate-Protein Diet on Progression of CKD: Follow-up of a Randomized Controlled Trial. *Am. J. Kidney Dis.* **2009**, *54*, 1052–1061. [CrossRef]

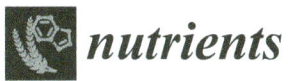

Review

Maintenance of Skeletal Muscle to Counteract Sarcopenia in Patients with Advanced Chronic Kidney Disease and Especially Those Undergoing Hemodialysis

Katsuhito Mori

Department of Nephrology, Osaka City University Graduate School of Medicine 1-4-3, Asahi-Machi, Abeno-ku, Osaka 545-8585, Japan; ktmori@med.osaka-cu.ac.jp; Tel.: +81-6-6645-3806; Fax: +81-6-6645-3808

Abstract: Life extension in modern society has introduced new concepts regarding such disorders as frailty and sarcopenia, which has been recognized in various studies. At the same time, cutting-edge technology methods, e.g., renal replacement therapy for conditions such as hemodialysis (HD), have made it possible to protect patients from advanced lethal chronic kidney disease (CKD). Loss of muscle and fat mass, termed protein energy wasting (PEW), has been recognized as prognostic factor and, along with the increasing rate of HD introduction in elderly individuals in Japan, appropriate countermeasures are necessary. Although their origins differ, frailty, sarcopenia, and PEW share common components, among which skeletal muscle plays a central role in their etiologies. The nearest concept may be sarcopenia, for which diagnosis techniques have recently been reported. The focus of this review is on maintenance of skeletal muscle against aging and CKD/HD, based on muscle physiology and pathology. Clinically relevant and topical factors related to muscle wasting including sarcopenia, such as vitamin D, myostatin, insulin (related to diabetes), insulin-like growth factor I, mitochondria, and physical inactivity, are discussed. Findings presented thus far indicate that in addition to modulation of the aforementioned factors, exercise combined with nutritional supplementation may be a useful approach to overcome muscle wasting and sarcopenia in elderly patients undergoing HD treatments.

Keywords: skeletal muscle; sarcopenia; hemodialysis; aging; chronic kidney disease; diabetes

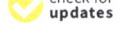

Citation: Mori, K. Maintenance of Skeletal Muscle to Counteract Sarcopenia in Patients with Advanced Chronic Kidney Disease and Especially Those Undergoing Hemodialysis. *Nutrients* **2021**, *13*, 1538. https://doi.org/10.3390/nu13051538

Academic Editor: R. Andrew Shanely

Received: 31 March 2021
Accepted: 30 April 2021
Published: 2 May 2021

Publisher's Note: MDPI stays neutral with regard to jurisdictional claims in published maps and institutional affiliations.

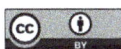

Copyright: © 2021 by the author. Licensee MDPI, Basel, Switzerland. This article is an open access article distributed under the terms and conditions of the Creative Commons Attribution (CC BY) license (https://creativecommons.org/licenses/by/4.0/).

1. Introduction

Most societies, especially those in developed countries, have shown increased longevity over the past few generations and interest has now shifted to how to extend healthy life expectancy. Aging is profoundly associated with changes related to human organs and tissues, and recently 'frailty' has become recognized as a key term related to age-related decline [1]. A sedentary lifestyle, commonly seen in modern society settings, also accelerates deterioration of motor functions. Skeletal muscle, which constitutes the largest type of tissue mass and accounts for 40–45% of total body weight [2], has a core role in maintenance of a healthy life. Its functional failure leads to physical impairment, resulting in poor outcomes, especially in elderly individuals. Thus, much attention has been given to 'sarcopenia', which is generally defined as loss of skeletal muscle mass and function [3].

In addition to aging, other chronic disorders are known to exacerbate frailty and/or sarcopenia, with advanced chronic kidney disease (CKD), especially end-stage kidney disease including hemodialysis (HD), a representative condition [4]. 'Protein-energy wasting (PEW)' is characterized by adverse changes in nutrition and body composition in advanced CKD/HD patients [5]. Historically, frailty and sarcopenia have been considered to originate from aging-related derangement, and PEW has been proposed to express the wasting that occurs in association with kidney dysfunction [6]. As a result, there is considerable overlapping among frailty, sarcopenia, and PEW in elderly patients with advanced CKD/HD.

The aim of this report is not to provide a systematic review of sarcopenia in advanced CKD/HD cases, but rather to examine the wide range of related fields in an easily understood manner in order to facilitate research regarding skeletal muscle maintenance and healthy life expectancy. Specifically, the author would like to focus on the decline and dysfunction of skeletal muscle, along with countermeasures from the viewpoint of aging and advanced CKD/HD as common key components of PEW, sarcopenia, and frailty (Figure 1).

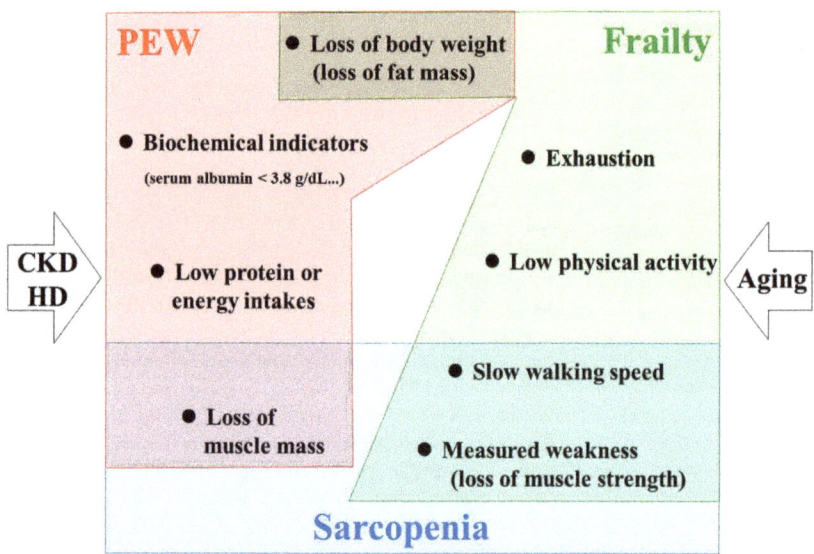

Figure 1. Conceptual overlapping among frailty, sarcopenia, and PEW. Aging accelerates frailty and sarcopenia. Advanced CKD/HD is profoundly associated with PEW. Elderly HD patients have the highest risk for these pathological conditions. Among these conditions, skeletal muscle derangement is a common component. CKD, chronic kidney disease; HD, hemodialysis; PEW, protein-energy wasting.

2. Conceptual Overlapping among Frailty, Sarcopenia, and PEW

The concept of frailty is considered acceptable to describe the condition of an individual. Generally, it is used to explain the state resulting from an age-related decrease in physiological reserve and increase in vulnerability to stressors, resulting in disability, hospitalization, institutionalization, and finally death [4,7]. Fried et al. defined frailty as a clinical syndrome in which three or more of the following abnormalities were combined; unintentional weight loss, self-reported exhaustion, weakness (grip strength), slow walking speed, and low physical activity [1]. In contrast to that phenotype model, Rockwood et al. proposed a frailty index based on accumulation of such deficits as age-associated diseases, non-specific vulnerability, and disabilities (accumulated deficit model) [8]. Nevertheless, no universal standard for diagnosis of frailty has been established.

The term 'sarcopenia' was first proposed by Irwin Rosenberg to describe loss of muscle mass (i.e., *sarx* meaning flesh and *penia* loss in Greek) [9]. However, the concept of sarcopenia has changed over time and later included related dysfunctions, such as loss of muscle strength. The European Working Group on Sarcopenia in Older People (EWGSOP) provided a definition along with diagnostic criteria [10], an objective assessment based on measurements of gait speed, grip strength, and muscle mass that has greatly contributed to progress in research of sarcopenia. Recently, a revised consensus (EWGSOP2) was released to promote early detection and treatment of affected patients [3].

In addition to age-related frailty and sarcopenia, the presence of advanced CKD is independently associated with malnutrition and inflammation. Previously, these conditions were expressed by various terms such as uremic malnutrition [11], uremic cachexia [12], protein-energy malnutrition [13], and malnutrition-inflammation complex syndrome [14] as well as others. Since CKD is commonly associated with atherosclerosis, the term, malnutrition-inflammation atherosclerosis (MIA) syndrome, was also proposed [15]. However, malnutrition includes both under- and overnutrition, and some CKD patients are underweight even with adequate intake. To avoid confusion, the International Society of Renal Nutrition and Metabolism (ISRNM) proposed the nomenclature protein-energy wasting (PEW) for loss of muscle and fat tissues (wasting), or the presence of malnutrition and/or inflammation [5]. For diagnosis of PEW, four categories including biochemical criteria; low body weight, reduced total body fat, or weight loss; decreased muscle mass; and low protein or energy intake, are evaluated [5]. Although useful, an evaluation of chronic inflammation is not necessary for determining a diagnosis. Among those categories, decreased muscle mass is considered to be the most valid criterion for PEW determination [5].

Frailty, sarcopenia, and PEW share common components in elderly patients undergoing HD (Figure 1). Following, this report will mainly focus on sarcopenia in HD patients, including consideration of the physiology and pathology of skeletal muscle.

3. Diagnosis of Sarcopenia in Asians Including Japanese

As noted above, the definition of sarcopenia and criteria used for diagnosis presented by EWGSOP were epoch-making. However, many problems remain to be solved. To develop appropriate measures against sarcopenia, it is necessary to obtain an accurate understanding of its prevalence, as various reports have shown a wide range from 4 to 63% of CKD patients [16], with those findings largely dependent on the methods, cut-off values, and criteria employed. Furthermore, it is also important to consider age- and/or CKD-related muscle histological modifications such as myosteatosis and myofibrosis [17,18], which are described later. Clinically, evaluation of muscle mass is more problematic than that of muscle strength, which is usually assessed based on handgrip strength [3,10,19,20]. For measuring muscle quantity, various methods, including dual-energy X-ray absorptiometry (DXA), bioimpedance analysis (BIA), mid-arm muscle circumference (MAC), and sum of skinfold thickness (SKF), are available. DXA is useful for evaluating body composition [21], while on the other hand the precision of BIA, MAC, and SKF remains controversial, though those are non-invasive and inexpensive [19]. In fact, the prevalence of low muscle mass evaluated by different methods (DXA, BIA, MAC, SKF) showed a wide range of variation from 4.0 to 73.5% [22]. Another problem is related to the different normalizing methods used for muscle mass. For example, muscle mass can be indexed by height squared, percentage of body weight, body surface area, and BMI. Those four different normalization methods were compared in 645 patients undergoing HD [23], with the presence of low muscle mass defined as two standard deviation (SD) below the normal mean of young adults. Intriguingly, the prevalence rate of low muscle mass ranged from 8.1 to 32.4%, even when muscle mass was the same [23]. Thus, a standard definition for sarcopenia is necessary for accurate evaluation of affected individuals. Another problem may be that the adaptation of EWGSOP criteria for Asian patients can be problematic because of anthropometric as well as cultural and/or life-style-related differences as compared with Europeans. As a result, the Asian Working Group on Sarcopenia (AWGS) established criteria for Asian populations in 2014 [19].

Using the AWGS criteria, we carefully evaluated sarcopenia in 308 Japanese patients receiving HD, and determined muscle strength using handgrip strength and muscle mass measurements by DXA. That study reported a sarcopenia prevalence rate (40%) in Japanese HD patients based on the AWGS criteria 2014 [24]. More importantly, the results showed that the presence of sarcopenia was a significant predictor of all-cause mortality in older patients. Thus far, studies regarding sarcopenia according to those criteria are limited, though reports showing prevalence rates in CKD [25] and peritoneal dialysis [26], and kidney transplant recipients [27] of 25.0%, 10.9%, and 11.8%, respectively, have been presented. For interpreting results, age distribution should also be considered. Very recently, the AWGS consensus has been revised and the current version is AWGS 2019 [28]. More careful methods for diagnosis and appropriate intervention are expected.

4. Which Component, Muscle Mass or Muscle Strength, Is Critical for Prognosis?

Although loss of muscle mass and reduced muscle strength are both related to aging, they do not always occur in parallel. In longitudinal observational studies of older healthy adults, a decline in muscle strength appeared to precede muscle loss [29,30], thus suggesting a dissociation between them. Such a dissociation between was observed in 111 HD patients [31], in whom the prevalence of low muscle strength and low muscle mass based on cut-off values in EWGSOP criteria was 88.3% and 33.3%, respectively. Although 31.5% of those was finally diagnosed as sarcopenia, that was largely dependent on low muscle mass, since the majority of the patients (88.3%) showed low muscle strength. Previously, we focused on muscle quality in Japanese patients on HD [32]. Some in the population, such as those affected by diabetes, showed a lower serum creatinine level, possibly reflecting reduced muscle mass, thus we adopted handgrip strength per unit of arm muscle mass determined using DXA to show muscle quality [32]. With this approach, muscle quality was demonstrated to be a predictor of high mortality in Japanese patients undergoing HD independent of age, serum albumin, and presence of diabetes [33]. A later study also showed that handgrip strength was a predictor of all-cause mortality in patients on HD, though muscle mass was not evaluated [34]. Similarly, in an observational retrospective cohort study, the usefulness of handgrip strength as a survival predictor was confirmed in patients receiving HD and peritoneal dialysis [35]. A simple question to determine is which component, muscle mass or muscle strength, can better predict mortality in HD patients. Along that line, both muscle strength and muscle mass were measured at the baseline in incident dialysis patients, then their impact on mortality was examined [36]. The results demonstrated that patients with low muscle strength but not those with low muscle mass were at increased risk of mortality. Similarly, an independent work revealed that muscle strength was a more relevant predictor of survival in patients on HD as compared with low muscle mass [23]. As well as handgrip strength, decreased muscle strength in the lower extremities was also found to be strongly associated with increased mortality in HD patients [37]. Although evaluation of muscle mass is necessary for assessing nutritional status (wasting) in advanced CKD/HD cases, handgrip strength measurement should be incorporated to evaluate physical performance in clinical practice, as it is easy to perform and inexpensive [16].

5. Physiology of Skeletal Muscle

Recently, detailed studies have provided advanced knowledge regarding the association of CKD and/or aging-related factors with pathological and functional changes of skeletal muscle. At the same time, the abundant information available can be confusing for non-experts. Therefore, relevant summaries showing the basic morphology and physiology of skeletal muscle for understanding pathophysiology are important. The availability of such materials can help with deep communication among specialists in each field.

5.1. Development and Regeneration of Skeletal Muscle

Skeletal muscle consists of muscle fibers, or myofibers, which function as a syncytium originating from the fusion of myoblasts [2]. During development, myoblasts, mononucleated muscle precursor cells, fuse together to generate nascent myotubes that exhibit central nucleation. The nuclei are located in the central portion of nascent myotubes. When muscle fibers become mature, they migrate to the periphery of the myofibers [2]. Satellite cells, stem cells of skeletal muscle, are located between the basal lamina and plasma membrane of muscle fibers, where they proliferate and differentiate into myoblasts in response to diverse stimuli, such as injury, exercise, stretching, and denervation [38]. Upon stimulation, some satellite cells differentiate into myoblasts and subsequently fuse with exiting fibers (regeneration). During this process, another small proportion returns to quiescence to form a new pool of myoblasts (self-renewal) (Figure 2) [39]. Although the mechanisms of self-renewal are poorly understood, one of the postulated models shows that asymmetric cell division can produce two types of daughter cells, those committed as myogenic precursor cells for regeneration and other uncommitted pluripotent cells involved in self-renewal [38].

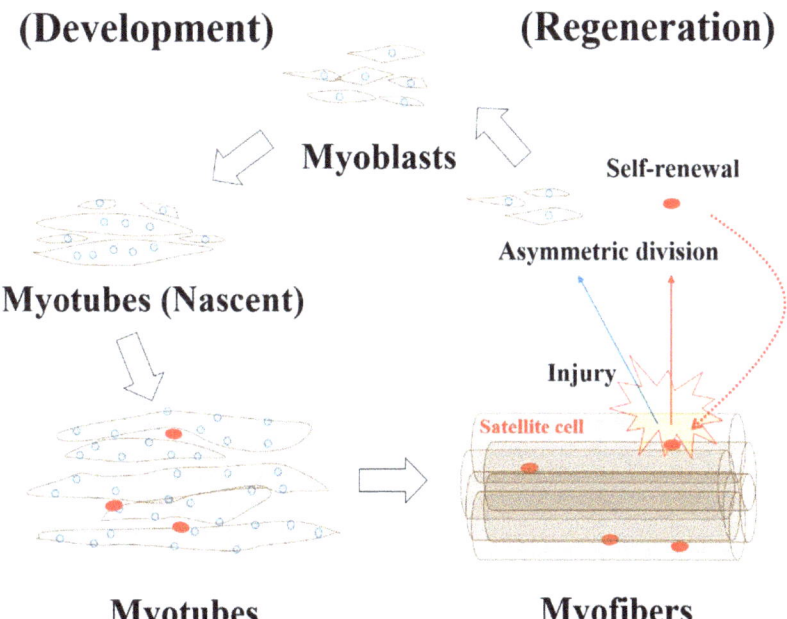

Figure 2. Muscle development and regeneration. During the early stage of development, myoblasts fuse to form multinucleated nascent myotubes that show central nucleation. In a later stage, nuclei migrate to the periphery of mature myotubes, resulting in formation of myofibers. Satellite cells are located between the basal lamina and plasma membrane. For muscle regeneration, satellite cells have a key role. Diverse stimuli including injury activate those cells, which is followed by asymmetric division to conserve the satellite cell pool (self-renewal) and generation of committed myogenic precursors (myoblasts) for regeneration via a process equivalent to development.

As satellite cell markers, paired domain transcription factors such as Pax7 and Pax3, and the myogenic factor 5 (Myf5) are well known. Among those, Pax7 is expressed in all quiescent and proliferating satellite cells in various species including humans [40]. During development, myogenic regulatory factors are required for myoblast commitment and differentiation, and the primary factors Myf5 and MyoD are necessary for determination of myoblasts. Subsequently, secondary factors, myogenin and myogenic regulatory factor 4 (MRF4), regulate terminal differentiation [38].

5.2. Classification of Skeletal Muscle Fiber Types

By 1873, Ranvier had already categorized muscle into red muscle, with slow contraction, and white muscle, which shows fast contraction. In the 1970s, the classification of type I (slow-twitch red) and type II (fast-twitch white) was proposed based on contractile properties and oxidative capacity. Mitochondria have a critical role in oxidative phosphorylation. The higher density of mitochondria in muscle is correlated with its red color. Some type II fibers possess a faster contractile property than type I, though type I has a higher oxidative capacity. Therefore, type II was subsequently divided into type IIA (fast-twitch red) and type IIB (fast-twitch white). Later, a correlation of myosin heavy chain

(MHC) isoform expression and contractile property with myofibrillar ATPase activity was identified. The new type IIx MHC protein was also found. Type IIb MHC is not typically expressed in human skeletal muscle. Currently, fiber types are classified based on MHC isoforms into type I (slow-red), type IIA (fast-red), type IIB (fast-white in rodents), and type IIX (fast-white in humans) (Table 1) [41–44].

Table 1. Classification of skeletal muscle fiber types.

	Type I	Type IIA	Type IIX (Human)	Type IIB (Mouse, Rat)
Anatomical color	Red	Red	White	White
Contractile speed	Slow-twitch	Fast-twitch	Fast-twitch	Fast-twitch
Myosin heavy chain isoform	Type I	Type IIa	Type IIx	Type IIb
Metabolic	Oxidative	Oxidative	Glycolytic	Glycolytic
Myofibrillar ATPase activity	Low	High	High	High
Mitochondrial density	High	High	Medium	Low
Fatigue	Resistant	Resistant	Fast	Fast

Presently, skeletal muscle fiber types are classified using histochemical methods and based on metabolic differences. Most skeletal muscle tissues consist of heterogenous fiber types that show a mosaic pattern. In response to various stimuli and circumstances, muscle fiber types are transformed.

Basically, human skeletal muscles consist of a mixture of muscle fiber types. Some are characterized as type I fiber-dominant (soleus muscle) or type II fiber-dominant (triceps brachii muscle) [43]. The distribution of muscle fiber types in an individual may change with various stimuli such as exercise. For example, muscle-biopsy specimens from elite sprinters were found have an increased number of type II myofibers, in contrast to an increased number of type I myofibers in those from distance runners [2].

Although this classification and nomenclature for skeletal muscle may be insufficient, it is very convenient to use when communicating and sharing findings with other researchers in various fields [42].

6. Skeletal Muscle Changes Related to Aging and Damage by CKD

6.1. Age-Related Changes of Skeletal Muscle

Aging is a well-known risk factor for loss of skeletal muscle mass. Using magnetic resonance imaging (MRI), skeletal muscle mass and distribution were evaluated in 268 men and 200 women aged 18–88 years [45]. Findings of that quantitative approach showed an apparent decrease in skeletal muscle mass in healthy subjects 60 years of age and older, while notable results indicated a prominent age-related decline in muscle mass in the lower limbs [45]. Aging atrophy seems to be associated with reductions in both number and size of muscle fibers, though that is not well understood [46]. To examine the influence of aging on muscle fiber number and size, quadriceps muscle biopsies, as well as DXA and computed tomography (CT) examinations were performed in healthy young and older males and females [47]. Skeletal muscle mass in the males was significantly greater as compared to that in the females. Furthermore, lean leg mass was significantly lower in the elderly than the young group, while whole-body lean mass did not differ between them. In line with those findings, cross-sectional area (CSA), evaluated based on the quadriceps muscle biopsy results, was smaller in the older as compared to the young group. Especially, type II muscle fiber size was substantially smaller in the older subjects, with a tendency for smaller type I muscle fibers. The calculated number of fibers in the quadriceps did not differ between the groups examined in that study. Therefore, it was concluded that age-related decline in skeletal muscle is mainly due to a reduction in type II muscle fiber size [47]. A contrasting example may be changes in skeletal muscle after a spinal cord injury (SCI), which can cause a fiber-type transformation. In patients treated for SCI, fiber-type shifts from type I or type IIA to type IIX were observed [43]. Interestingly, the transformation pattern in individuals with an SCI is opposite of that induced by aging.

Satellite cells have critical roles for repair and hypertrophy of skeletal muscle, and fiber characteristics and fiber type-specific content related to those cells were examined in young and elderly males [48]. As noted in the report mentioned above [47], biopsy specimens in the vastus lateralis showed that type II, but not type I, muscle fiber CSA was significantly smaller in the older as compared with the young subjects. Satellite cell content determined based on Pax 7-positive cells was also examined, with no difference found between the young and older groups for that content in type I muscle fibers. In contrast, satellite cell content in the type II muscle fibers was significantly lower in the older subjects. These findings suggest that an age-related decline in satellite cell content may be associated with type II muscle fiber atrophy and loss of skeletal muscle mass in older individuals [48].

6.2. Histopathological Changes of Skeletal Muscle in Advanced CKD/HD Cases

It seems that skeletal muscle atrophy should be expected in patients with advanced CKD/HD. However, in a study of 13 patients with advanced CKD, type II fiber areas tended to be smaller as compared to the control group, though the difference was not significant [49]. In another study, mean sizes of type I and II fibers in eight patients on dialysis or with kidney transplantation were not different from those in the controls [50], while a different report noted that while type II fibers were slightly but not significantly smaller in 12 dialysis patients as compared to the controls [51]. Rather unexpectedly, no clear findings have yet been presented to support greater muscle atrophy in patients with advanced CKD/HD as compared to control subjects.

A precise muscle biopsy (vastus lateralis)-based study was performed with relatively large groups of subjects (60 patients on HD, 21 controls) [52]. Surprisingly, the mean CSA values for type I, IIA, and IIX fibers were 33%, 26%, and 28%, respectively, greater in the HD patients as compared with the controls [52]. Since those muscle biopsy-specimens were obtained from patients one day after undergoing HD, the greater CSA size might be explained by interstitial edema of skeletal muscle. Another interesting finding in that study showed that the activity of succinate dehydrogenase, a mitochondrial oxidative enzyme, was decreased in muscle fibers of patients undergoing HD. Ultrastructural analysis also revealed swollen mitochondria in the HD patients. In addition, capillary density, evaluated by the number of capillaries per square millimeter of muscle area, was significantly reduced by 34% in the HD patients as compared with the control group [52]. Although interpretation of their results showing impaired oxidative capacity and reduced capillary density in the skeletal muscle of HD patients is difficult, except for enlargement of muscle fibers possibly due to edema, they seem to indicate that impaired energy production together with reduced oxygen supply and substrates may lead to skeletal muscle dysfunction.

Nevertheless, it is also important to note that qualitative changes may veil actual quantity of skeletal muscle. Histopathological findings showing substitution of contractile muscle fibers because of fat infiltration and/or fibrosis may indicate muscle dysfunction, even when muscle mass is similar. Especially, myosteatosis, equivalent to intermuscular adipose tissue, has attracted much attention [17]. Since skeletal muscle attenuation determined using CT is significantly associated with muscle lipid content based on histological findings with oil red O staining and muscle triglyceride measurements in biopsy specimens [53], myosteatosis was previously evaluated indirectly with CT or MRI results. Myofibrosis, pathological fibrosis in skeletal muscle, is thought to accompany myosteatosis and may be the result of various events including injury, inflammation, and degeneration. Recent technological innovations have made it possible to determine myosteatosis and/or myofibrosis using ultrasound. With this method, it has been reported that myosteatosis and/or myofibrosis were negatively correlated with physiological performance in CKD patients [18]. Furthermore, since those might be involved in systemic metabolic and inflammatory disorders, as well as subsequent mortality, additional investigations are required to confirm the impact of myosteatosis and myofibrosis on sarcopenia in advanced CKD/HD.

7. Aging Kidneys in CKD Patients

Various organs including the kidneys are involved in its onset and development of sarcopenia [3,10,19,28]. When lifespans were short, kidney failure might not have been a major issue, as most humans experienced mortality first. However, the recent super-aging society is faced with new disorders such as CKD.

The prevalence of CKD throughout the world including Japan increases with age. It has been reported that 13% of the Japanese general population (13.3 million people) has CKD when that is defined as glomerular filtration rate (GFR) < 60 mL/min/1.73 m^2) [54]. Along with aging, the prevalence of CKD gradually increases, with four out of ten individuals aged 80 and older affected. Although it seems to be a natural occurrence, age-related structural changes in kidneys have not been clarified. Recent studies have reported macroanatomical changes based on results obtained with imaging modalities such as CT [55] and microanatomical changes based on kidney biopsy findings [56,57] in living kidney donors who had no obvious kidney disease.

Contrast-enhanced CT imaging can be used to measure not only total kidney volume, but also cortical and medullary volumes separately. Cortical volume seems to decrease with age, whereas medullary volume increases until age 60, which may be compensatory, and then remains unchanged thereafter [55]. Thus, total kidney volume does not change until age 60 and then subsequently decreases [55]. Since the cortex includes nephron and proximal tubules, it would be interesting to know whether age-related loss of cortical volume reflects nephron loss and/or decrease in GFR, though those have yet to be clarified [58].

Using renal biopsy samples obtained from living kidney donors, anatomical changes were examined [56,57]. Nephrosclerosis, a major age-related change, includes glomerulosclerosis, tubular atrophy, interstitial fibrosis, and arteriosclerosis. Sclerosis score was determined as the total number of abnormalities, including any type of global glomerulosclerosis, tubular atrophy, and arteriosclerosis, and interstitial fibrosis > 5%. When nephrosclerosis was defined as two or more of the total four, an increasing prevalence of nephrosclerosis associated with aging was observed in 2.7% of the subjects younger than 29 years and in 73% of those aged greater than 70 [57]. Decreased glomerular density, calculated based on the number of glomeruli divided by the area of the cortex, was also associated with older age in living donors [56]. These findings suggest that conditions related to aging kidneys and consequent CKD-related sarcopenia are inevitable in super-aging societies.

8. Factors Possibly Affecting Muscle Wasting in Advanced CKD/HD

Large numbers of different factors and/or mechanisms including persistent inflammation are considered to be involved with age-related muscle derangement (sarcopenia) in CKD/HD patients, with both expected and unexpected findings reported [4,16,59,60] [61], and new information presented even in the last few years. For example, uremic toxins such as indoxyl sulfate and p-cresol were shown to impair myogenic differentiation of cultured C2C12 skeletal muscle cells [62]. Inorganic phosphate (Pi) was also found to decrease myogenic differentiation in vitro and promoted muscle atrophy in CKD mice [63]. In a randomized controlled study of pre-dialysis CKD patients, oral sodium bicarbonate achieved a serum level of ~24 mEq/L for preserved muscle mass [64]. These recent reports have provided new insights in this field. Nevertheless, systematic and comprehensive classifications of cause and etiology are still required, though currently very difficult to establish. In the following, clinically relevant and topical factors that have been relatively well investigated and established to some extent in this field will be discussed (Figure 3).

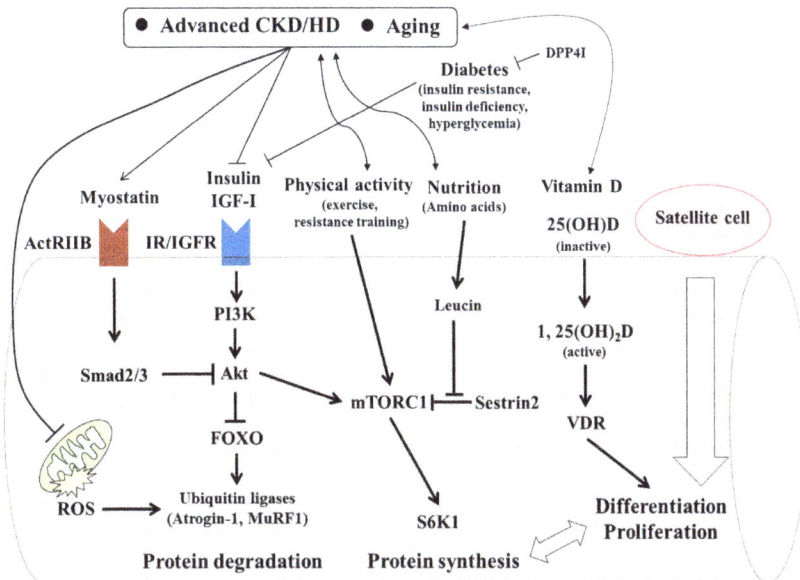

Figure 3. Various factors affecting skeletal muscle maintenance in aged patients with advanced CKD/HD. In aged patients with advanced CKD/HD, various factors have interaction with and transduce their effects intracellularly, thus affecting skeletal muscle maintenance. Insulin and IGF-I positively regulate skeletal muscle maintenance via binding of their cognate receptors. Subsequent activation of mTORC1 through PI3K/Akt is necessary for protein synthesis. Simultaneously, insulin-stimulated PI3K/Akt increases FOXO phosphorylation and subsequent inhibition of its translocation into the nucleus. On the other hand, myostatin, a negative regulator, binds to ActRIIB. Subsequent phosphorylation of Smad2/3 reduces Akt activation and decreases FOXO phosphorylation. Intranuclear translocated FOXO activates transcription of MuRF1 and Atrogin-1, which accelerates protein degradation via the ubiquitin-proteasome pathway. Defective mitochondrial quality control (derangements in fusion-fission) leads to ROS production and results in muscle protein degradation. Vitamin D is involved in muscle differentiation and proliferation by binding VDR, which is accompanied by interaction with muscle protein metabolism. Among amino acids, leucin activates mTORC1 by binding to Sestrin2, leading to protein synthesis. In addition, satellite cells, which can be modulated by the various aforementioned factors, may contribute to muscle maintenance. CKD, chronic kidney disease; HD, hemodialysis; ActRIIB, activin type II B receptor; IGF-I, insulin-like growth factor I; mTORC1, mammalian target of rapamycin complex 1; PI3K, phosphatidylinositol-3-kinase; FOXO, forkhead box O; MuRF1, muscle ring finger 1; ROS, reactive oxygen species; VDR, vitamin D receptor; DPP4-I; dipeptidyl peptidase 4 inhibitors.

8.1. Vitamin D

Vitamin D is one of the critical components in CKD-mineral and bone disorder (CKD-MBD) [65]. It regulates not only calcium homeostasis and bone metabolism, but also skeletal muscle metabolism [66,67]. Furthermore, the active form of 1α,25-dihydroxyvitamin D [1,25(OH)$_2$D] binds to vitamin D receptor (VDR), and can exert diverse biological effects through genomic and non-genomic activities, while expression of VDR in both animal and human muscle tissues was identified [66,67]. Another investigation showed that though synthesis of 1,25(OH)$_2$D from 25(OH)D is mediated by mitochondrial 1α-hydroxylase encoded by the *Cyp27b1* gene, predominantly expressed in the kidneys, C2C12 myoblasts and myotubes expressed both VDR and CYP27B1 [68]. Therefore, skeletal muscle cells seem to possess machinery for response to vitamin D. In fact, addition of 1,25(OH)$_2$D to C2C12 myoblasts increased VDR expression, decreased cell proliferation, and promoted myogenic differentiation [69]. Those authors also showed that 1,25(OH)$_2$D increased expression of MyoD and subsequently suppressed myostatin in a time-dependent manner, and finally increased the diameter and size of MHC type II-positive cells. Findings obtained in mice with deletion of the vitamin D receptor (VDRKO) also support the role of vitamin D in skeletal muscle maintenance. The VDRKO group showed smaller muscle mass and weaker grip strength as compared with the controls [70]. Another study reported that mice following VDRKO had smaller diameter muscle fibers with an aberrant reversed higher expression of myogenic differentiation factors as compared to wild-type mice, suggesting a physiological role of vitamin D through temporal up-regulation of myogenic transcription factors [71]. In this context, vitamin D (calcitriol) also seems to antagonize CKD-induced skeletal muscle changes [72]. That study reported that high-phosphate diet accelerated skeletal muscle changes in CKD rats (5/6 nephrectomy) as compared with a standard diet. Furthermore, low dose calcitriol attenuated adverse skeletal muscle changes in CKD rats that received a high phosphate diet. Interestingly, calcitriol improved the number of capillaries in contact with muscle fibers. Although the precise mechanisms are still unclear, vitamin D may have pleiotropic effects on skeletal muscle maintenance in patients with CKD.

A link between vitamin D and skeletal muscle is probable in rodents, while related effects on and mechanisms in human skeletal muscle remain to be established. It has been reported that a vitamin D system was detected in human muscle precursor cells, though was low in adult skeletal muscle [73]. They also noted that vitamin D seems to promote myoblast self-renewal and maintain the satellite stem cell pool through modulation of the forkhead box O (FOXO) 3 and Notch signaling pathways. In contrast to rodents, how vitamin D can affect skeletal muscle maintenance in humans remains to be elucidated.

Vitamin D deficiency in humans is evaluated based on the storage form of vitamin D, 25(OH)D, and a strong association of vitamin D deficiency with muscle dysfunction has been shown [74]. Generally, optimal musculoskeletal benefits occur at 25(OH)D levels above 30 ng/mL. In contrast, in evaluated biopsy specimens, vitamin D deficiency was found to be correlated with skeletal muscle dysfunction and predominantly associated with type II muscle fiber atrophy [66]. More directly, an examination of the correlation between vitamin D deficiency and sarcopenia, defined based on appendicular skeletal muscle mass divided by body weight less than two standard deviation (SD) below the sex-specific mean for young adults, performed in 3169 Korean participants showed that the mean 25(OH)D concentration was significantly lower in those with than without sarcopenia [75].

8.2. Myostatin

Myostatin, also known as growth development factor-8 (GDF-8), has been identified as a negative regulator of skeletal muscle growth [76,77]. This newly established factor is mainly secreted by muscle cells and belongs to the transforming growth factor-β (TGF-β) superfamily. Myostatin binds to its cognate receptor, activin type II B receptor (ActRIIB), and exerts diverse effects. Upon activation of Smad2/Smad3 and dephosphorylation of Akt, muscle protein ubiquitination and degradation by proteasomes and autophagy are induced through Atrogin-1 and muscle ring finger 1 (MuRF1), leading to increased protein degradation [60,78]. Myostatin can also inhibit mammalian target of rapamycin complex 1 (mTORC1), one of the key molecules in protein synthesis, resulting in a decrease in that process [60,78]. Additionally, myostatin-induced apoptosis was shown to occur via activation of the p38-caspase pathway [78].

Although myostatin might be involved in development of sarcopenia in CKD/HD, limited data are available. Cy/+ rats, which develop advanced CKD due to a genetic defect, were reported to show a progressive decline in muscle function [79]. Additionally, as compared to control rats, Cy/+ rats had a significantly higher serum level of myostatin and increased expression of myostatin in skeletal muscle, along with higher indices of oxidative stress [80]. In half-nephrectomized mice, indoxyl sulfate, a uremic toxin, induced skeletal muscle weight loss, which was accompanied by expression of myostatin and atrogin-1 in addition to increased production of inflammatory cytokines in skeletal muscle [81].

In humans, it has been speculated that the plasma or serum concentration of myostatin can be used as a biomarker of muscle wasting. However, inconsistent results have been presented i.e., both positive and negative, or no significant correlation between myostatin and muscle mass and/or muscle strength [82]. Nevertheless, that report noted that emerging evidence suggests that myostatin is influenced by various factors such as age, gender, and physical activity as well as a wide range of disorders including heart failure, metabolic syndrome, CKD, and inflammatory diseases. Another reason for conflicting results may be the different assay techniques utilized. Generally, the level of myostatin in CKD/HD patients seems to be higher than that in healthy controls [78]. A recent study showed that myostatin was positively associated with muscle strength, evaluated by handgrip strength, as well as muscle mass in patients undergoing HD [83]. Moreover, a lower level of myostatin was demonstrated to be a significant predictor of one-year mortality in that study. Additional investigations are needed to confirm whether myostatin is a biomarker for sarcopenia in advanced cases of CKD/HD.

8.3. IGF-I

Insulin-like growth factor-I (IGF-I), well known to be associated with muscle mass and fiber size [84,85], binds to its receptor and exerts biological effects. Although IGF-I shares common intracellular signaling pathway with insulin, it appears to have more growth effects than metabolic effects as compared to insulin, though the mechanisms are unknown [86]. In protein synthesis, IGF-I-induced activation of mTORC1 through phosphatidylinositol-3-kinase (PI3K)/Akt is necessary. At the same time, activation of the PI3K/Akt pathway results in phosphorylation of FOXO proteins. It has also been reported that IGF-I suppressed ubiquitin ligases, such as Atrogin-1 and MuRF1, via Akt-mediated inhibition of FOXO1, suggesting antagonizing effects of IGF-I in skeletal muscle catabolism [87,88].

To examine growth factors including IGF-I, vastus lateralis muscle biopsies were performed in 55 patients undergoing HD and 21 healthy subjects. As expected, mRNA for IGF-I/IGF-I receptor was decreased in skeletal muscle from the HD patients as compared with the healthy controls. However, protein levels for muscle IGF-I and serum IGF-II were increased [89]. Although IGF-I plays a critical role in muscle maintenance, its action mechanisms may be complicated, i.e., transient binding of the IGF-I receptor, degradation of the IGF-I/IGF-I receptor, local concentrations of IGF-I, and the influence of IGF-I binding proteins.

In addition to direct effects on skeletal muscle, IGF-I seems to be involved in CKD-induced dysfunction of satellite cells. It has been reported that isolated Pax-7 positive cells (satellite cells) from CKD mice obtained by use of a subtotal nephrectomy had lower levels of MyoD expression and showed suppressed myotube formation [90]. Additionally, CKD mice showed delayed regeneration of injured muscle, and decreased MyoD and myogenin expression. IGF-I increased the expression of myogenic genes in response to injury in satellite cells from the control group but not in those from CKD mice. Therefore, impaired IGF-I signaling may be associated with satellite cell dysfunction as well as protein catabolism in CKD-related sarcopenia.

8.4. Insulin and Glucose (Hyperglycemia)

Insulin is one of most important hormones in human body and its metabolic disarrangement in skeletal muscle is profoundly associated with the etiology of diabetes [91–94]. In addition to metabolic effects, insulin has also been shown to be involved in protein anabolism in vitro [95], as well as in vivo in rats [96,97], and humans [98]. However, the direct effects of insulin on protein metabolism in human skeletal muscle is poorly understood as compared with glucose and lipid metabolism.

A detailed study provided new insights in regard to insulin-mediated protein synthesis in human skeletal muscle [99]. Insulin was infused within a physiological range in

19 young subjects, then protein synthesis was evaluated in muscle biopsy specimens to determine uptake of isotope-labeled phenylalanine, which was not intracellularly oxidized. At the same time, blood flow was measured using indocyanine green. Insulin can stimulate muscle protein synthesis. Interestingly, increases in blood flow and amino acid delivery to skeletal muscle were found to be critical factors in insulin-induced protein synthesis in that study. Using a similar technique, insulin-stimulated protein synthesis in skeletal muscle was compared between young and older healthy subjects [100]. In the older group, protein synthesis was found to be resistant to insulin, suggesting that aging is a critical risk factor for maintenance of skeletal muscle via age-related insulin resistance.

In addition to insulin, glucose may be involved in skeletal muscle maintenance. A recent study demonstrated suppressed proliferation of satellite cells in high-glucose culture media [101]. In contrast, glucose restriction led to a relative increase in Pax7-positive/MyoD-negative cells, which were equivalent to reserve cells for self-renewal. Those findings suggest that hyperglycemia might inhibit regeneration of skeletal muscles and accelerate sarcopenia in patients with diabetes. To examine whether hyperglycemia is associated with sarcopenia, a multicenter cross-sectional study was performed in 746 patients with type 2 diabetes (T2D) and 2067 other older participants [102]. Hyperglycemia represented as HbA1c was found to be an independent contributor to the presence of sarcopenia, especially in the non-obese subjects. Interestingly, HbA1c level was specifically associated with low skeletal mass index (SMI) rather than weak grip strength or slow gait speed. Therefore, appropriate glycemic control should be considered as a requirement for prevention of sarcopenia, probably in HD patients with diabetes.

8.5. Physical Inactivity and Sedentary Lifestyle in Older Patients with CKD and HD

Physical activity gradually decreases with aging and incidental HD patients show a greater tendency for physical inactivity. The association of physical inactivity with malnutritional status was examined in HD patients and healthy sedentary controls [103]. Both physical activity, measured by a three-dimensional accelerometer, and energy expenditure, evaluated by questionnaire, were lower in the patients and the difference between those groups increased with advancing age. Additionally, physical activity in the HD patients was associated with serum albumin and creatinine levels, as well as phase angle derived from BIA. These findings suggest an association between physical inactivity and malnutritional status including muscle wasting. The benefit of regular physical activity on mortality was examined in a national cohort of new patients with end-stage kidney disease in the United States, which showed that mortality risk was lower in those who exercised 2–3 or 4–5 times a week, suggesting an association of physical activity with survival in dialysis patients [104]. In addition to aging, the presence of advanced CKD/HD may have a strong impact on the skeletal muscle system, leading to significant exercise intolerance [105]. To break the vicious cycle between physical inactivity and mortality, exercise may be one of most promising and hopeful approaches, which will be discussed later.

8.6. Mitochondria

Mitochondria, small membrane-bound organelles, generate a significant amount of energy in the form of ATP. Due to its heavy demand for energy as a motor organ, skeletal muscle has a large number of mitochondria. Mitochondrial dynamics are regulated by fine balance between fusion and fission [106,107]. For mitochondrial fusion, the mitofusins Mfn1 and Mfn2, mitochondrial GTPases, are essential [108], while on the other hand, fission protein 1 (Fis1) and dynamin-related protein 1 (DRP-1) maintain mitochondrial homeostasis through appropriate fission (fragmentation) [106]. Mitochondrial quality control is necessary for structural and functional integrity [109]. A critical contributing factor to mitochondrial decay, closely linked to sarcopenia, is aging, which has been shown to be related to decreases in mitochondrial content, enzyme activities such as cytochrome c oxidase and citrate synthase, and oxidative capacity in human skeletal muscle [110]. Impaired mitochondrial respiration leads to reactive oxygen species (ROS) production and increased mitochondrial DNA mutations. In association with that, defective mitochondrial quality control has also been detected in aged muscle and hyperfusion is known to be associated with the appearance of enlarged mitochondria, which cannot be effectively eliminated and results in increased ROS production [109]. In contrast, hyperfission is also observed during the progression of sarcopenia. ROS production by derangements in fusion-fission results in muscle protein breakdown through ubiquitin ligases such as atrogin-1 and Murf-1 [109].

In addition to aging, CKD appears to be involved in mitochondrial dysfunction. Microarray analysis of CKD patients including those undergoing HD suggested an impaired mitochondrial respiratory system and related oxidative stress [111]. More directly, mitochondrial function was evaluated using ^{31}P magnetic resonance spectroscopy to determine phosphocreatine recovery time constant in patients with CKD and those on HD [112]. In that study, faster phosphocreatine recovery kinetics (shorter time constant) indicated better mitochondrial function, and a prolonged phosphocreatine recovery time was found in HD and CKD patients as compared with controls. Mitochondrial dysfunction is correlated with poor physical performance, increased intermuscular adipose tissue, and increased markers of inflammation and oxidative stress. Interestingly, that study also found that DRP-1, a marker of mitochondrial fission, was up-regulated in skeletal muscle of HD patients as compared to controls. Therefore, correction of mitochondrial dysfunction is an attractive therapeutic approach for elderly patients with advanced CKD/HD.

9. Management of Skeletal Muscle Maintenance in HD Patients

9.1. Vitamin D

Based on findings described above showing a positive correlation of vitamin D deficiency with skeletal muscle dysfunction, supplementation with vitamin D is an attractive interventional approach against sarcopenia. In fact, two meta-analysis reports have suggested the beneficial effects of vitamin D supplementation on muscle strength and function in older individuals with a low serum 25(OH)D level at the baseline (vitamin D deficiency) [113,114]. In the same context, a double-blind randomized placebo-controlled trial was performed to explore the effects of 12 months of vitamin D supplementation on lower-extremity power (primary endpoint) and function in healthy community-dwelling elderly subjects [115]. Unexpectedly, there were no differences for lower-extremity power, strength, or lean mass found between the placebo and vitamin D groups. However, the period of intervention, subject background details, and target level of vitamin D should be considered when interpreting those results. Notably, HD patients tend to show severe abnormal vitamin D metabolism as compared to healthy elderly individuals.

A retrospective cross-sectional study was performed to examine the association of vitamin D treatment with muscle mass and function in HD patients, in which muscle size was evaluated by MRI and strength in the lower limbs was measured, with or without treatment with active vitamin D (calcitriol or paricalcitol) [116]. They found that vitamin D treatment was associated with greater muscle size and strength. Additionally, two double-blind randomized placebo-controlled trial were performed to investigate the pleiotropic effects of vitamin D (cholecalciferol) in HD patients [117,118]. In both, the results of various muscle function tests including muscle strength were examined as clinical endpoints. No significant effect of vitamin D supplementation was found in those tests. Although the studies were well-designed, the sample sizes were small (n = 52, 60, respectively) and the intervention periods short (eight weeks and six months, respectively), which are limitations. Under these conditions, it might be difficult to confirm the effects of vitamin D supplementation on muscle function. In addition, muscle mass was not evaluated. In future, randomized trials with larger sample sizes and longer periods that focus on sarcopenia as the primary endpoint will be needed.

9.2. Myostatin

Myostatin is an attractive therapeutic target for treatment of age- and CKD-related sarcopenia [16,60]. Two strategies to inhibit myostatin pathways are under development, one is a blockade caused by direct binding to myostatin itself and the other is inhibition of the myostatin-ActRIIB complex [78]. One of the candidates is the monoclonal antibody LY2495655, which binds and neutralizes myostatin, and was examined in a phase II study [119]. This antibody was found to have a relationship with lean mass and partially improved functional measures of muscle power in older frail individuals. On the other hand, results of another phase II trial showed no significant effect of LY2495655 on lean body mass in patients undergoing elective total hip arthroplasty [120]. Similarly, the efficacy of bimagrumab, an anti-ActRIIB antibody, was examined in older adults with sarcopenia in a phase II trial [121], and found to increase muscle mass and strength.

Administration of an anti-myostatin peptibody in CKD mice reversed loss of muscle mass and suppressed circulating inflammatory cytokines [122]. Additionally, it has recently been reported that formononetin, a bioactive isoflavone compound, ameliorates muscle atrophy in CKD rats by antagonizing myostatin [123]. If myostatin-mediated treatment is found to be effective in older patients with advanced CKD/HD, important points for consideration will be whether it improves not only muscle mass but also muscle strength.

9.3. Insulin and Anti-Diabetic Treatments

Since insulin deficiency is an independent risk factor for sarcopenia, the next question may be whether insulin treatment can protect against sarcopenia. A retrospective observational study examined the association of insulin treatment with SMI, calculated as appendicular muscle mass using DXA divided by the square of height, in 312 patients with T2D [124]. Insulin treatment was shown to be protective against annual decline in SMI after adjusting for various factors. In a propensity score-matched cohort in the same study, the annual change in SMI was greater in the insulin-treated than non-insulin-treated group. These findings suggest that insulin has a critical role not only in glucose metabolism but also maintenance of skeletal muscle mass in patients with diabetes.

Few studies have investigated the association of oral anti-diabetic drugs with sarcopenia. Considering the possible efficacy of insulin, dipeptidyl peptidase 4 inhibitors (DPP4-I) are good candidates for sarcopenia treatment because they stimulate insulin secretion in a blood glucose-level dependent manner. DPP4-I is preferrable in regard to its efficacy, low risk of hypoglycemia, and good tolerability in elderly patients with T2D. In line with those factors, the association of sarcopenia, diagnosed according to the EWGSOP criteria, with DPP4-I was examined in 80 elderly patients with T2D [125]. The participants were divided into the sulfonylurea (n = 43) and DPP4-I (n = 37) groups, and followed for at least 24 months. The DPP4-I group showed greater muscle mass, as well as better muscle strength and physical performance as compared with sulfonylurea group. Since physical activity and nutritional status of those participants were relatively stable, the authors suggested that the better sarcopenic parameters noted were mainly due to treatment effects. Similarly, the association of use of DPP4-I with loss of muscle mass was examined in a retrospective observational study that included 105 patients with T2D [126]. Propensity-score matching analysis was performed to remove bias. SMI, determined using DXA, was evaluated and its annual change was significantly higher in patients with as compared to those without DPP4-I [126]. On the other hand, there were no significant differences in regard to changes in visceral and subcutaneous fat area between those groups.

Most oral anti-diabetic drugs are contraindicated or restricted in HD patients, as renal dysfunction brings about profound pharmacokinetic abnormalities [127]. Among those drugs, DPP4-I are available for HD patients [128,129]. Although no report of the efficacy of DPP4-I on sarcopenia in HD patients has been presented, those inhibitors may be considered as candidates for preventing age-related loss of muscle mass in patients with T2D.

9.4. Nutrition

Adequate intake of nutrients is necessary to prevent the onset and progression of sarcopenia, PEW, and frailty. In contrast to common agreement regarding adequate energy intake (generally, 30–35 kcal/kg/day), how much dietary protein intake is ideal for CKD and dialysis patients remains controversial. Typically, protein intake of 0.6–0.8 g/kg/day is recommended for advanced pre-dialysis patients from the viewpoint of uremia and kidney protection. On the other hand, that recommendation is usually ~1.2 g/kg/day in dialysis patients to preserve muscle mass [6]. When a standard prevention approach is not enough, nutritional supplementation is considered, with many methods available, including oral supplementation, intradialytic parental nutrition, and tube feeding [4,6,61,130].

When focusing on maintenance of skeletal muscle in CKD patients, especially those undergoing HD, amino acid supplementation is reasonable. Amino acids are not only precursors for muscle protein synthesis but also stimulators of intracellular signaling. Notably, among essential amino acids, leucin has a distinct anabolic action via the mTORC1 pathway [131]. As an intracellular regulator, sestrin2 has received much attention and it has been reported that its leucine-binding capacity is necessary for leucin-induced activation of mTORC1, indicating that sestrin2 functions as a sensor of leucin and inhibitor of mTORC1 [132]. A recent systematic review reported no clear effects of supplementation with essential amino acids on muscle mass, muscle strength, or physical performance, whereas a significant effect of leucine on muscle mass was shown in subjects with sarcopenia as compared with healthy subjects [133].

Another possible supplementation strategy might be use of β-hydroxy-β-methylbutyrate (HMB), a metabolite of leucin [134]. To examine its effects on body composition, bone density, strength, physical function, and other such parameters in HD patients, a double-blind placebo-controlled randomized trial was performed over a period of six months, though no significant effects of HMB supplementation were observed [135]. Based on findings presented to date, leucin may be one of the good candidates for nutritional supplementation to maintain skeletal muscle. As described, following exercise or physical activity, nutritional supplementation should be able to provide synergistic beneficial effects on maintenance of skeletal muscle in HD patients [136].

9.5. Exercise

Skeletal muscle is characterized as a dynamic organ, and muscle contractions may have a special role in homeostasis of skeletal muscle separate from hormones and cytokines [137,138]. Thus, to overcome aging-related sarcopenia, it may be a powerful approach. Especially, aerobic exercise has been shown to improve insulin-stimulated muscle protein synthesis in elderly individuals, though aging dampens the anabolic effects of insulin on skeletal muscle [139]. In patients undergoing HD, aerobic exercise seemed to increase CSA, while an interesting finding also noted was an improvement in exercise-induced capillarization in skeletal muscle [140]. In combination with previous findings [99,139], it is considered that an increase in blood flow in skeletal muscle in response to aerobic exercise and insulin may contribute to maintenance of muscle mass and function.

Exercise may also counteract CKD-induced muscle wasting. Using CKD mice induced by a subtotal nephrectomy, the effects of resistance exercise (muscle overload) and endurance training (treadmill running) on skeletal muscle wasting were examined [141]. Although both types of exercises suppressed CKD-induced muscle protein degradation, the specific effects differed between them, as improved muscle protein synthesis was observed in mice with resistance exercise but not in those with endurance training. Additionally, those results showed that resistance exercise counteracted CKD-induced suppression of phosphorylation of S6K and mTORC1 in muscle, resulting in maintenance of protein synthesis. In these mice, resistance exercise but not endurance training increased the number of muscle progenitor cells. Together, these findings suggest that different types of exercise can provide various effects related to skeletal muscle maintenance.

Muscle biopsy procedures were performed in dialysis patients (18 HD, three peritoneal dialysis) to examine the effects of resistance training on skeletal muscle [142]. The number of satellite cells in type I muscle fibers was increased after 16 weeks of resistance training performed three times a week, whereas those in type II fibers remained unchanged. However, an increase in the myonuclear contents of the type II fibers was observed. Satellite cells may directly differentiate into myonuclei without asymmetric division, though that does not seem likely. Although interpretation of their observations is difficult, one of the most important findings might be increased muscle strength, which can be determined by torque measurements in clinical settings.

In addition to exercise, that in combination with dietary protein supplementation might exert synergistic effects on maintenance of skeletal muscle mass and function in various individuals [143,144]. As described above, leucin may have a key role. To determine the effects of leucin ingestion on muscle protein synthesis after resistance exercise in elderly male subjects, the results of infusion of isotope-labeled phenylalanine with leucin shown in muscle biopsy specimens were examined [145]. At 24 h after exercise, protein synthesis remained elevated in the leucin group as compared with the controls, which indicated a potential impact of leucin in combination with exercise for muscle maintenance in the older individuals. Additionally, it is possible that a combination of exercise with nutritional support, especially leucin, has beneficial effects in HD patients [136], though clear evidence remains lacking.

10. Conclusions

The modernization of society along with progress in medical treatments have led to new disorders, such as frailty, sarcopenia, and PEW, especially in elderly HD patients. The increased risk of those conditions has led to speculation and reservations regarding patient care. On the other hand, intensive investigations have provided abundant new insights in this field. A broad range of communication, from bench to bedside, and the reverse as well, will be required. In clinical practice, incorporation of various therapeutic options should also be considered, as such fusion will result in a much better outcome including extended healthy life expectancy in elderly patients receiving HD treatments.

Funding: This research received no external funding.

Conflicts of Interest: The author has no conflict of interest to declare.

References

1. Fried, L.P.; Tangen, C.M.; Walston, J.; Newman, A.B.; Hirsch, C.; Gottdiener, J.; Seeman, T.; Tracy, R.; Kop, W.J.; Burke, G.; et al. Frailty in older adults: Evidence for a phenotype. *J. Gerontol. A Biol. Sci. Med. Sci.* **2001**, *56*, M146–M156. [CrossRef]
2. Huard, J.; Li, Y.; Fu, F.H. Muscle injuries and repair: Current trends in research. *J. Bone Jt. Surg Am.* **2002**, *84*, 822–832. [CrossRef]
3. Cruz-Jentoft, A.J.; Bahat, G.; Bauer, J.; Boirie, Y.; Bruyere, O.; Cederholm, T.; Cooper, C.; Landi, F.; Rolland, Y.; Sayer, A.A.; et al. Sarcopenia: Revised European consensus on definition and diagnosis. *Age Ageing* **2019**, *48*, 601. [CrossRef] [PubMed]
4. Kim, J.C.; Kalantar-Zadeh, K.; Kopple, J.D. Frailty and protein-energy wasting in elderly patients with end stage kidney disease. *J. Am. Soc. Nephrol.* **2013**, *24*, 337–351. [CrossRef] [PubMed]
5. Fouque, D.; Kalantar-Zadeh, K.; Kopple, J.; Cano, N.; Chauveau, P.; Cuppari, L.; Franch, H.; Guarnieri, G.; Ikizler, T.A.; Kaysen, G.; et al. A proposed nomenclature and diagnostic criteria for protein-energy wasting in acute and chronic kidney disease. *Kidney Int.* **2008**, *73*, 391–398. [CrossRef] [PubMed]
6. Hanna, R.M.; Ghobry, L.; Wassef, O.; Rhee, C.M.; Kalantar-Zadeh, K. A Practical Approach to Nutrition, Protein-Energy Wasting, Sarcopenia, and Cachexia in Patients with Chronic Kidney Disease. *Blood Purif.* **2020**, *49*, 202–211. [CrossRef]
7. Johansen, K.L.; Chertow, G.M.; Jin, C.; Kutner, N.G. Significance of frailty among dialysis patients. *J. Am. Soc. Nephrol.* **2007**, *18*, 2960–2967. [CrossRef] [PubMed]
8. Rockwood, K.; Mitnitski, A. Frailty in relation to the accumulation of deficits. *J. Gerontol. A Biol. Sci. Med. Sci.* **2007**, *62*, 722–727. [CrossRef]
9. Rosenberg, I.H. Sarcopenia: Origins and clinical relevance. *J. Nutr.* **1997**, *127*, 990S–991S. [CrossRef]
10. Cruz-Jentoft, A.J.; Baeyens, J.P.; Bauer, J.M.; Boirie, Y.; Cederholm, T.; Landi, F.; Martin, F.C.; Michel, J.P.; Rolland, Y.; Schneider, S.M.; et al. Sarcopenia: European consensus on definition and diagnosis: Report of the European Working Group on Sarcopenia in Older People. *Age Ageing* **2010**, *39*, 412–423. [CrossRef]

11. Pupim, L.B.; Caglar, K.; Hakim, R.M.; Shyr, Y.; Ikizler, T.A. Uremic malnutrition is a predictor of death independent of inflammatory status. *Kidney Int.* **2004**, *66*, 2054–2060. [CrossRef] [PubMed]
12. Mak, R.H.; Cheung, W.; Cone, R.D.; Marks, D.L. Mechanisms of disease: Cytokine and adipokine signaling in uremic cachexia. *Nat. Clin. Pr. Nephrol.* **2006**, *2*, 527–534. [CrossRef]
13. Herselman, M.; Moosa, M.R.; Kotze, T.J.; Kritzinger, M.; Wuister, S.; Mostert, D. Protein-energy malnutrition as a risk factor for increased morbidity in long-term hemodialysis patients. *J. Ren. Nutr.* **2000**, *10*, 7–15. [CrossRef]
14. Kalantar-Zadeh, K.; Ikizler, T.A.; Block, G.; Avram, M.M.; Kopple, J.D. Malnutrition-inflammation complex syndrome in dialysis patients: Causes and consequences. *Am. J. Kidney Dis.* **2003**, *42*, 864–881. [CrossRef]
15. Pecoits-Filho, R.; Lindholm, B.; Stenvinkel, P. The malnutrition, inflammation, and atherosclerosis (MIA) syndrome—The heart of the matter. *Nephrol. Dial. Transpl.* **2002**, *17*, 28–31. [CrossRef] [PubMed]
16. Sabatino, A.; Cuppari, L.; Stenvinkel, P.; Lindholm, B.; Avesani, C.M. Sarcopenia in chronic kidney disease: What have we learned so far? *J. Nephrol.* **2020**. [CrossRef] [PubMed]
17. McGregor, R.A.; Cameron-Smith, D.; Poppitt, S.D. It is not just muscle mass: A review of muscle quality, composition and metabolism during ageing as determinants of muscle function and mobility in later life. *Longev. Healthspan* **2014**, *3*, 9. [CrossRef]
18. Wilkinson, T.J.; Gould, D.W.; Nixon, D.G.D.; Watson, E.L.; Smith, A.C. Quality over quantity? Association of skeletal muscle myosteatosis and myofibrosis on physical function in chronic kidney disease. *Nephrol. Dial. Transpl.* **2019**, *34*, 1344–1353. [CrossRef] [PubMed]
19. Chen, L.K.; Liu, L.K.; Woo, J.; Assantachai, P.; Auyeung, T.W.; Bahyah, K.S.; Chou, M.Y.; Chen, L.Y.; Hsu, P.S.; Krairit, O.; et al. Sarcopenia in Asia: Consensus report of the Asian Working Group for Sarcopenia. *J. Am. Med. Dir. Assoc.* **2014**, *15*, 95–101. [CrossRef]
20. Cederholm, T.; Jensen, G.L.; Correia, M.; Gonzalez, M.C.; Fukushima, R.; Higashiguchi, T.; Baptista, G.; Barazzoni, R.; Blaauw, R.; Coats, A.; et al. GLIM criteria for the diagnosis of malnutrition—A consensus report from the global clinical nutrition community. *Clin. Nutr.* **2019**, *38*, 1–9. [CrossRef]
21. Shepherd, J.A.; Ng, B.K.; Sommer, M.J.; Heymsfield, S.B. Body composition by DXA. *Bone* **2017**, *104*, 101–105. [CrossRef] [PubMed]
22. Lamarca, F.; Carrero, J.J.; Rodrigues, J.C.; Bigogno, F.G.; Fetter, R.L.; Avesani, C.M. Prevalence of sarcopenia in elderly maintenance hemodialysis patients: The impact of different diagnostic criteria. *J. Nutr. Health Aging* **2014**, *18*, 710–717. [CrossRef] [PubMed]
23. Kittiskulnam, P.; Chertow, G.M.; Carrero, J.J.; Delgado, C.; Kaysen, G.A.; Johansen, K.L. Sarcopenia and its individual criteria are associated, in part, with mortality among patients on hemodialysis. *Kidney Int.* **2017**, *92*, 238–247. [CrossRef]
24. Mori, K.; Nishide, K.; Okuno, S.; Shoji, T.; Emoto, M.; Tsuda, A.; Nakatani, S.; Imanishi, Y.; Ishimura, E.; Yamakawa, T.; et al. Impact of diabetes on sarcopenia and mortality in patients undergoing hemodialysis. *BMC Nephrol.* **2019**, *20*, 105. [CrossRef] [PubMed]
25. Ishikawa, S.; Naito, S.; Iimori, S.; Takahashi, D.; Zeniya, M.; Sato, H.; Nomura, N.; Sohara, E.; Okado, T.; Uchida, S.; et al. Loop diuretics are associated with greater risk of sarcopenia in patients with non-dialysis-dependent chronic kidney disease. *PLoS ONE* **2018**, *13*, e0192990. [CrossRef] [PubMed]
26. Kamijo, Y.; Kanda, E.; Ishibashi, Y.; Yoshida, M. Sarcopenia and Frailty in PD: Impact on Mortality, Malnutrition, and Inflammation. *Perit. Dial. Int.* **2018**, *38*, 447–454. [CrossRef]
27. Yanishi, M.; Kimura, Y.; Tsukaguchi, H.; Koito, Y.; Taniguchi, H.; Mishima, T.; Fukushima, Y.; Sugi, M.; Kinoshita, H.; Matsuda, T. Factors Associated with the Development of Sarcopenia in Kidney Transplant Recipients. *Transpl. Proc.* **2017**, *49*, 288–292. [CrossRef] [PubMed]
28. Chen, L.K.; Woo, J.; Assantachai, P.; Auyeung, T.W.; Chou, M.Y.; Iijima, K.; Jang, H.C.; Kang, L.; Kim, M.; Kim, S.; et al. Asian Working Group for Sarcopenia: 2019 Consensus Update on Sarcopenia Diagnosis and Treatment. *J. Am. Med. Dir. Assoc.* **2020**, *21*, 300–307.e2. [CrossRef] [PubMed]
29. Goodpaster, B.H.; Park, S.W.; Harris, T.B.; Kritchevsky, S.B.; Nevitt, M.; Schwartz, A.V.; Simonsick, E.M.; Tylavsky, F.A.; Visser, M.; Newman, A.B. The loss of skeletal muscle strength, mass, and quality in older adults: The health, aging and body composition study. *J. Gerontol. A Biol. Sci. Med. Sci.* **2006**, *61*, 1059–1064. [CrossRef]
30. Delmonico, M.J.; Harris, T.B.; Visser, M.; Park, S.W.; Conroy, M.B.; Velasquez-Mieyer, P.; Boudreau, R.; Manini, T.M.; Nevitt, M.; Newman, A.B.; et al. Longitudinal study of muscle strength, quality, and adipose tissue infiltration. *Am. J. Clin. Nutr.* **2009**, *90*, 1579–1585. [CrossRef]
31. Bataille, S.; Serveaux, M.; Carreno, E.; Pedinielli, N.; Darmon, P.; Robert, A. The diagnosis of sarcopenia is mainly driven by muscle mass in hemodialysis patients. *Clin. Nutr.* **2017**, *36*, 1654–1660. [CrossRef] [PubMed]
32. Inaba, M.; Kurajoh, M.; Okuno, S.; Imanishi, Y.; Yamada, S.; Mori, K.; Ishimura, E.; Yamakawa, T.; Nishizawa, Y. Poor muscle quality rather than reduced lean body mass is responsible for the lower serum creatinine level in hemodialysis patients with diabetes mellitus. *Clin. Nephrol.* **2010**, *74*, 266–272. [PubMed]
33. Yoda, M.; Inaba, M.; Okuno, S.; Yoda, K.; Yamada, S.; Imanishi, Y.; Mori, K.; Shoji, T.; Ishimura, E.; Yamakawa, T.; et al. Poor muscle quality as a predictor of high mortality independent of diabetes in hemodialysis patients. *Biomed. Pharm.* **2012**, *66*, 266–270. [CrossRef] [PubMed]
34. Matos, C.M.; Silva, L.F.; Santana, L.D.; Santos, L.S.; Protasio, B.M.; Rocha, M.T.; Ferreira, V.L.; Azevedo, M.F.; Martins, M.T.; Lopes, G.B.; et al. Handgrip strength at baseline and mortality risk in a cohort of women and men on hemodialysis: A 4-year study. *J. Ren. Nutr.* **2014**, *24*, 157–162. [CrossRef]

35. Vogt, B.P.; Borges, M.C.C.; Goes, C.R.; Caramori, J.C.T. Handgrip strength is an independent predictor of all-cause mortality in maintenance dialysis patients. *Clin. Nutr.* **2016**, *35*, 1429–1433. [CrossRef] [PubMed]
36. Isoyama, N.; Qureshi, A.R.; Avesani, C.M.; Lindholm, B.; Barany, P.; Heimburger, O.; Cederholm, T.; Stenvinkel, P.; Carrero, J.J. Comparative associations of muscle mass and muscle strength with mortality in dialysis patients. *Clin. J. Am. Soc. Nephrol.* **2014**, *9*, 1720–1728. [CrossRef] [PubMed]
37. Matsuzawa, R.; Matsunaga, A.; Wang, G.; Yamamoto, S.; Kutsuna, T.; Ishii, A.; Abe, Y.; Yoneki, K.; Yoshida, A.; Takahira, N. Relationship between lower extremity muscle strength and all-cause mortality in Japanese patients undergoing dialysis. *Phys. Ther.* **2014**, *94*, 947–956. [CrossRef]
38. Seale, P.; Rudnicki, M.A. A new look at the origin, function, and "stem-cell" status of muscle satellite cells. *Dev. Biol.* **2000**, *218*, 115–124. [CrossRef]
39. Demonbreun, A.R.; Biersmith, B.H.; McNally, E.M. Membrane fusion in muscle development and repair. *Semin. Cell Dev. Biol.* **2015**, *45*, 48–56. [CrossRef]
40. Yin, H.; Price, F.; Rudnicki, M.A. Satellite cells and the muscle stem cell niche. *Physiol. Rev.* **2013**, *93*, 23–67. [CrossRef]
41. Berchtold, M.W.; Brinkmeier, H.; Muntener, M. Calcium ion in skeletal muscle: Its crucial role for muscle function, plasticity, and disease. *Physiol. Rev.* **2000**, *80*, 1215–1265. [CrossRef] [PubMed]
42. Spangenburg, E.E.; Booth, F.W. Molecular regulation of individual skeletal muscle fibre types. *Acta Physiol. Scand.* **2003**, *178*, 413–424. [CrossRef] [PubMed]
43. Biering-Sorensen, B.; Kristensen, I.B.; Kjaer, M.; Biering-Sorensen, F. Muscle after spinal cord injury. *Muscle Nerve* **2009**, *40*, 499–519. [CrossRef] [PubMed]
44. Girgis, C.M.; Clifton-Bligh, R.J.; Hamrick, M.W.; Holick, M.F.; Gunton, J.E. The roles of vitamin D in skeletal muscle: Form, function, and metabolism. *Endocr. Rev.* **2013**, *34*, 33–83. [CrossRef]
45. Janssen, I.; Heymsfield, S.B.; Wang, Z.M.; Ross, R. Skeletal muscle mass and distribution in 468 men and women aged 18-88 yr. *J. Appl. Physiol.* **2000**, *89*, 81–88. [CrossRef]
46. Lexell, J. Human aging, muscle mass, and fiber type composition. *J. Gerontol. A Biol. Sci. Med. Sci.* **1995**, *50*, 11–16. [CrossRef]
47. Nilwik, R.; Snijders, T.; Leenders, M.; Groen, B.B.; van Kranenburg, J.; Verdijk, L.B.; van Loon, L.J. The decline in skeletal muscle mass with aging is mainly attributed to a reduction in type II muscle fiber size. *Exp. Gerontol.* **2013**, *48*, 492–498. [CrossRef]
48. Verdijk, L.B.; Koopman, R.; Schaart, G.; Meijer, K.; Savelberg, H.H.; van Loon, L.J. Satellite cell content is specifically reduced in type II skeletal muscle fibers in the elderly. *Am. J. Physiol. Endocrinol. Metab.* **2007**, *292*, E151–E157. [CrossRef]
49. Clyne, N.; Esbjornsson, M.; Jansson, E.; Jogestrand, T.; Lins, L.E.; Pehrsson, S.K. Effects of renal failure on skeletal muscle. *Nephron* **1993**, *63*, 395–399. [CrossRef]
50. Diesel, W.; Emms, M.; Knight, B.K.; Noakes, T.D.; Swanepoel, C.R.; van Zyl Smit, R.; Kaschula, R.O.; Sinclair-Smith, C.C. Morphologic features of the myopathy associated with chronic renal failure. *Am. J. Kidney Dis.* **1993**, *22*, 677–684. [CrossRef]
51. Fahal, I.H.; Bell, G.M.; Bone, J.M.; Edwards, R.H. Physiological abnormalities of skeletal muscle in dialysis patients. *Nephrol. Dial. Transpl.* **1997**, *12*, 119–127. [CrossRef]
52. Lewis, M.I.; Fournier, M.; Wang, H.; Storer, T.W.; Casaburi, R.; Cohen, A.H.; Kopple, J.D. Metabolic and morphometric profile of muscle fibers in chronic hemodialysis patients. *J. Appl. Physiol.* **2012**, *112*, 72–78. [CrossRef]
53. Goodpaster, B.H.; Kelley, D.E.; Thaete, F.L.; He, J.; Ross, R. Skeletal muscle attenuation determined by computed tomography is associated with skeletal muscle lipid content. *J. Appl. Physiol.* **2000**, *89*, 104–110. [CrossRef]
54. Imai, E.; Horio, M.; Watanabe, T.; Iseki, K.; Yamagata, K.; Hara, S.; Ura, N.; Kiyohara, Y.; Moriyama, T.; Ando, Y.; et al. Prevalence of chronic kidney disease in the Japanese general population. *Clin. Exp. Nephrol.* **2009**, *13*, 621–630. [CrossRef] [PubMed]
55. Wang, X.; Vrtiska, T.J.; Avula, R.T.; Walters, L.R.; Chakkera, H.A.; Kremers, W.K.; Lerman, L.O.; Rule, A.D. Age, kidney function, and risk factors associate differently with cortical and medullary volumes of the kidney. *Kidney Int.* **2014**, *85*, 677–685. [CrossRef] [PubMed]
56. Rule, A.D.; Semret, M.H.; Amer, H.; Cornell, L.D.; Taler, S.J.; Lieske, J.C.; Melton, L.J., 3rd; Stegall, M.D.; Textor, S.C.; Kremers, W.K.; et al. Association of kidney function and metabolic risk factors with density of glomeruli on renal biopsy samples from living donors. *Mayo Clin. Proc.* **2011**, *86*, 282–290. [CrossRef] [PubMed]
57. Denic, A.; Glassock, R.J.; Rule, A.D. Structural and Functional Changes with the Aging Kidney. *Adv. Chronic Kidney Dis.* **2016**, *23*, 19–28. [CrossRef] [PubMed]
58. O'Neill, W.C. Structure, not just function. *Kidney Int.* **2014**, *85*, 503–505. [CrossRef] [PubMed]
59. Machowska, A.; Carrero, J.J.; Lindholm, B.; Stenvinkel, P. Therapeutics targeting persistent inflammation in chronic kidney disease. *Transl. Res.* **2016**, *167*, 204–213. [CrossRef]
60. Wang, X.H.; Mitch, W.E. Mechanisms of muscle wasting in chronic kidney disease. *Nat. Rev. Nephrol.* **2014**, *10*, 504–516. [CrossRef]
61. Oliveira, E.A.; Zheng, R.; Carter, C.E.; Mak, R.H. Cachexia/Protein energy wasting syndrome in CKD: Causation and treatment. *Semin. Dial.* **2019**, *32*, 493–499. [CrossRef]
62. Alcalde-Estevez, E.; Sosa, P.; Asenjo-Bueno, A.; Plaza, P.; Olmos, G.; Naves-Diaz, M.; Rodriguez-Puyol, D.; Lopez-Ongil, S.; Ruiz-Torres, M.P. Uraemic toxins impair skeletal muscle regeneration by inhibiting myoblast proliferation, reducing myogenic differentiation, and promoting muscular fibrosis. *Sci. Rep.* **2021**, *11*, 512. [CrossRef]

63. Chung, L.H.; Liu, S.T.; Huang, S.M.; Salter, D.M.; Lee, H.S.; Hsu, Y.J. High phosphate induces skeletal muscle atrophy and suppresses myogenic differentiation by increasing oxidative stress and activating Nrf2 signaling. *Aging* **2020**, *12*, 21446–21468. [CrossRef]
64. Kittiskulnam, P.; Srijaruneruang, S.; Chulakadabba, A.; Thokanit, N.S.; Praditpornsilpa, K.; Tungsanga, K.; Eiam-Ong, S. Impact of Serum Bicarbonate Levels on Muscle Mass and Kidney Function in Pre-Dialysis Chronic Kidney Disease Patients. *Am. J. Nephrol.* **2020**, *51*, 24–34. [CrossRef] [PubMed]
65. Nigwekar, S.U.; Tamez, H.; Thadhani, R.I. Vitamin D and chronic kidney disease-mineral bone disease (CKD-MBD). *Bonekey Rep.* **2014**, *3*, 498. [CrossRef] [PubMed]
66. Ceglia, L. Vitamin D and its role in skeletal muscle. *Curr. Opin. Clin. Nutr. Metab. Care* **2009**, *12*, 628–633. [CrossRef]
67. Molina, P.; Carrero, J.J.; Bover, J.; Chauveau, P.; Mazzaferro, S.; Torres, P.U.; European Renal, N.; Chronic Kidney, D.-M.; Bone Disorder Working Groups of the European Renal Association-European Dialysis Transplant, A. Vitamin D, a modulator of musculoskeletal health in chronic kidney disease. *J. Cachexia Sarcopenia Muscle* **2017**, *8*, 686–701. [CrossRef] [PubMed]
68. Srikuea, R.; Zhang, X.; Park-Sarge, O.K.; Esser, K.A. VDR and CYP27B1 are expressed in C2C12 cells and regenerating skeletal muscle: Potential role in suppression of myoblast proliferation. *Am. J. Physiol. Cell Physiol.* **2012**, *303*, C396–C405. [CrossRef] [PubMed]
69. Garcia, L.A.; King, K.K.; Ferrini, M.G.; Norris, K.C.; Artaza, J.N. 1,25(OH)2vitamin D3 stimulates myogenic differentiation by inhibiting cell proliferation and modulating the expression of promyogenic growth factors and myostatin in C2C12 skeletal muscle cells. *Endocrinology* **2011**, *152*, 2976–2986. [CrossRef] [PubMed]
70. Girgis, C.M.; Cha, K.M.; Houweling, P.J.; Rao, R.; Mokbel, N.; Lin, M.; Clifton-Bligh, R.J.; Gunton, J.E. Vitamin D Receptor Ablation and Vitamin D Deficiency Result in Reduced Grip Strength, Altered Muscle Fibers, and Increased Myostatin in Mice. *Calcif. Tissue Int.* **2015**, *97*, 602–610. [CrossRef]
71. Endo, I.; Inoue, D.; Mitsui, T.; Umaki, Y.; Akaike, M.; Yoshizawa, T.; Kato, S.; Matsumoto, T. Deletion of vitamin D receptor gene in mice results in abnormal skeletal muscle development with deregulated expression of myoregulatory transcription factors. *Endocrinology* **2003**, *144*, 5138–5144. [CrossRef]
72. Acevedo, L.M.; Lopez, I.; Peralta-Ramirez, A.; Pineda, C.; Chamizo, V.E.; Rodriguez, M.; Aguilera-Tejero, E.; Rivero, J.L. High-phosphorus diet maximizes and low-dose calcitriol attenuates skeletal muscle changes in long-term uremic rats. *J. Appl. Physiol.* **2016**, *120*, 1059–1069. [CrossRef]
73. Olsson, K.; Saini, A.; Stromberg, A.; Alam, S.; Lilja, M.; Rullman, E.; Gustafsson, T. Evidence for Vitamin D Receptor Expression and Direct Effects of 1alpha,25(OH)2D3 in Human Skeletal Muscle Precursor Cells. *Endocrinology* **2016**, *157*, 98–111. [CrossRef]
74. Shuler, F.D.; Wingate, M.K.; Moore, G.H.; Giangarra, C. Sports health benefits of vitamin d. *Sports Health* **2012**, *4*, 496–501. [CrossRef] [PubMed]
75. Kim, M.K.; Baek, K.H.; Song, K.H.; Il Kang, M.; Park, C.Y.; Lee, W.Y.; Oh, K.W. Vitamin D deficiency is associated with sarcopenia in older Koreans, regardless of obesity: The Fourth Korea National Health and Nutrition Examination Surveys (KNHANES IV) 2009. *J. Clin. Endocrinol. Metab.* **2011**, *96*, 3250–3256. [CrossRef] [PubMed]
76. McPherron, A.C.; Lawler, A.M.; Lee, S.J. Regulation of skeletal muscle mass in mice by a new TGF-beta superfamily member. *Nature* **1997**, *387*, 83–90. [CrossRef] [PubMed]
77. Grobet, L.; Martin, L.J.; Poncelet, D.; Pirottin, D.; Brouwers, B.; Riquet, J.; Schoeberlein, A.; Dunner, S.; Menissier, F.; Massabanda, J.; et al. A deletion in the bovine myostatin gene causes the double-muscled phenotype in cattle. *Nat. Genet.* **1997**, *17*, 71–74. [CrossRef] [PubMed]
78. Bataille, S.; Chauveau, P.; Fouque, D.; Aparicio, M.; Koppe, L. Myostatin and muscle atrophy during chronic kidney disease. *Nephrol. Dial. Transpl.* **2020**. [CrossRef]
79. Organ, J.M.; Srisuwananukorn, A.; Price, P.; Joll, J.E.; Biro, K.C.; Rupert, J.E.; Chen, N.X.; Avin, K.G.; Moe, S.M.; Allen, M.R. Reduced skeletal muscle function is associated with decreased fiber cross-sectional area in the Cy/+ rat model of progressive kidney disease. *Nephrol. Dial. Transpl.* **2016**, *31*, 223–230. [CrossRef]
80. Avin, K.G.; Chen, N.X.; Organ, J.M.; Zarse, C.; O'Neill, K.; Conway, R.G.; Konrad, R.J.; Bacallao, R.L.; Allen, M.R.; Moe, S.M. Skeletal Muscle Regeneration and Oxidative Stress Are Altered in Chronic Kidney Disease. *PLoS ONE* **2016**, *11*, e0159411. [CrossRef]
81. Enoki, Y.; Watanabe, H.; Arake, R.; Sugimoto, R.; Imafuku, T.; Tominaga, Y.; Ishima, Y.; Kotani, S.; Nakajima, M.; Tanaka, M.; et al. Indoxyl sulfate potentiates skeletal muscle atrophy by inducing the oxidative stress-mediated expression of myostatin and atrogin-1. *Sci. Rep.* **2016**, *6*, 32084. [CrossRef] [PubMed]
82. Baczek, J.; Silkiewicz, M.; Wojszel, Z.B. Myostatin as a Biomarker of Muscle Wasting and other Pathologies-State of the Art and Knowledge Gaps. *Nutrients* **2020**, *12*, 2401. [CrossRef] [PubMed]
83. Delanaye, P.; Bataille, S.; Quinonez, K.; Buckinx, F.; Warling, X.; Krzesinski, J.M.; Pottel, H.; Burtey, S.; Bruyere, O.; Cavalier, E. Myostatin and Insulin-Like Growth Factor 1 Are Biomarkers of Muscle Strength, Muscle Mass, and Mortality in Patients on Hemodialysis. *J. Ren. Nutr.* **2019**, *29*, 511–520. [CrossRef]
84. DeVol, D.L.; Rotwein, P.; Sadow, J.L.; Novakofski, J.; Bechtel, P.J. Activation of insulin-like growth factor gene expression during work-induced skeletal muscle growth. *Am. J. Physiol.* **1990**, *259*, E89–E95. [CrossRef] [PubMed]

85. Coleman, M.E.; DeMayo, F.; Yin, K.C.; Lee, H.M.; Geske, R.; Montgomery, C.; Schwartz, R.J. Myogenic vector expression of insulin-like growth factor I stimulates muscle cell differentiation and myofiber hypertrophy in transgenic mice. *J. Biol. Chem.* **1995**, *270*, 12109–12116. [CrossRef] [PubMed]
86. Mori, K.; Giovannone, B.; Smith, R.J. Distinct Grb10 domain requirements for effects on glucose uptake and insulin signaling. *Mol. Cell Endocrinol.* **2005**, *230*, 39–50. [CrossRef]
87. Stitt, T.N.; Drujan, D.; Clarke, B.A.; Panaro, F.; Timofeyva, Y.; Kline, W.O.; Gonzalez, M.; Yancopoulos, G.D.; Glass, D.J. The IGF-1/PI3K/Akt pathway prevents expression of muscle atrophy-induced ubiquitin ligases by inhibiting FOXO transcription factors. *Mol. Cell* **2004**, *14*, 395–403. [CrossRef]
88. Sugimoto, K.; Wang, C.-C.; Rakugi, H. Sarcopenia in Diabetes Mellitus. In *Musculoskeletal Disease Associated with Diabetes Mellitus*; Springer: Berlin/Heidelberg, Germany, 2016; pp. 237–252.
89. Wang, H.; Casaburi, R.; Taylor, W.E.; Aboellail, H.; Storer, T.W.; Kopple, J.D. Skeletal muscle mRNA for IGF-IEa, IGF-II, and IGF-I receptor is decreased in sedentary chronic hemodialysis patients. *Kidney Int.* **2005**, *68*, 352–361. [CrossRef]
90. Zhang, L.; Wang, X.H.; Wang, H.; Du, J.; Mitch, W.E. Satellite cell dysfunction and impaired IGF-1 signaling cause CKD-induced muscle atrophy. *J. Am. Soc. Nephrol.* **2010**, *21*, 419–427. [CrossRef]
91. Fujii, N.L. Overview. In *Musculoskeletal Disease Associated with Diabetes Mellitus*; Springer: Berlin/Heidelberg, Germany, 2016; pp. 127–137.
92. Hocking, S.; Samocha-Bonet, D.; Milner, K.L.; Greenfield, J.R.; Chisholm, D.J. Adiposity and insulin resistance in humans: The role of the different tissue and cellular lipid depots. *Endocr. Rev.* **2013**, *34*, 463–500. [CrossRef]
93. Watt, M.J.; Hoy, A.J. Lipid metabolism in skeletal muscle: Generation of adaptive and maladaptive intracellular signals for cellular function. *Am. J. Physiol. Endocrinol Metab.* **2012**, *302*, E1315–E1328. [CrossRef] [PubMed]
94. Mori, K.; Morioka, T.; Motoyama, K.; Emoto, M. Ectopic Fat Accumulation and Glucose Homeostasis: Ectopic Fat Accumulation in Muscle. In *Musculoskeletal Disease Associated with Diabetes Mellitus*; Springer: Berlin/Heidelberg, Germany, 2016; pp. 171–183.
95. Kimball, S.R.; Horetsky, R.L.; Jefferson, L.S. Signal transduction pathways involved in the regulation of protein synthesis by insulin in L6 myoblasts. *Am. J. Physiol.* **1998**, *274*, C221–C228. [CrossRef] [PubMed]
96. Garlick, P.J.; Grant, I. Amino acid infusion increases the sensitivity of muscle protein synthesis in vivo to insulin. Effect of branched-chain amino acids. *Biochem. J.* **1988**, *254*, 579–584. [CrossRef]
97. Lee, S.W.; Dai, G.; Hu, Z.; Wang, X.; Du, J.; Mitch, W.E. Regulation of muscle protein degradation: Coordinated control of apoptotic and ubiquitin-proteasome systems by phosphatidylinositol 3 kinase. *J. Am. Soc. Nephrol.* **2004**, *15*, 1537–1545. [CrossRef]
98. Louard, R.J.; Fryburg, D.A.; Gelfand, R.A.; Barrett, E.J. Insulin sensitivity of protein and glucose metabolism in human forearm skeletal muscle. *J. Clin. Invest.* **1992**, *90*, 2348–2354. [CrossRef] [PubMed]
99. Fujita, S.; Rasmussen, B.B.; Cadenas, J.G.; Grady, J.J.; Volpi, E. Effect of insulin on human skeletal muscle protein synthesis is modulated by insulin-induced changes in muscle blood flow and amino acid availability. *Am. J. Physiol. Endocrinol. Metab.* **2006**, *291*, E745–E754. [CrossRef]
100. Rasmussen, B.B.; Fujita, S.; Wolfe, R.R.; Mittendorfer, B.; Roy, M.; Rowe, V.L.; Volpi, E. Insulin resistance of muscle protein metabolism in aging. *FASEB J.* **2006**, *20*, 768–769. [CrossRef]
101. Furuichi, Y.; Kawabata, Y.; Aoki, M.; Mita, Y.; Fujii, N.L.; Manabe, Y. Excess Glucose Impedes the Proliferation of Skeletal Muscle Satellite Cells Under Adherent Culture Conditions. *Front. Cell Dev. Biol.* **2021**, *9*, 640399. [CrossRef]
102. Sugimoto, K.; Tabara, Y.; Ikegami, H.; Takata, Y.; Kamide, K.; Ikezoe, T.; Kiyoshige, E.; Makutani, Y.; Onuma, H.; Gondo, Y.; et al. Hyperglycemia in non-obese patients with type 2 diabetes is associated with low muscle mass: The Multicenter Study for Clarifying Evidence for Sarcopenia in Patients with Diabetes Mellitus. *J. Diabetes Investig.* **2019**, *10*, 1471–1479. [CrossRef] [PubMed]
103. Johansen, K.L.; Chertow, G.M.; Ng, A.V.; Mulligan, K.; Carey, S.; Schoenfeld, P.Y.; Kent-Braun, J.A. Physical activity levels in patients on hemodialysis and healthy sedentary controls. *Kidney Int.* **2000**, *57*, 2564–2570. [CrossRef]
104. Stack, A.G.; Molony, D.A.; Rives, T.; Tyson, J.; Murthy, B.V. Association of physical activity with mortality in the US dialysis population. *Am. J. Kidney Dis.* **2005**, *45*, 690–701. [CrossRef]
105. Adams, G.R.; Vaziri, N.D. Skeletal muscle dysfunction in chronic renal failure: Effects of exercise. *Am. J. Physiol. Ren. Physiol.* **2006**, *290*, F753–F761. [CrossRef]
106. Dimmer, K.S.; Scorrano, L. (De)constructing mitochondria: What for? *Physiology* **2006**, *21*, 233–241. [CrossRef] [PubMed]
107. Ishihara, N.; Otera, H.; Oka, T.; Mihara, K. Regulation and physiologic functions of GTPases in mitochondrial fusion and fission in mammals. *Antioxid Redox Signal.* **2013**, *19*, 389–399. [CrossRef] [PubMed]
108. Chen, H.; Vermulst, M.; Wang, Y.E.; Chomyn, A.; Prolla, T.A.; McCaffery, J.M.; Chan, D.C. Mitochondrial fusion is required for mtDNA stability in skeletal muscle and tolerance of mtDNA mutations. *Cell* **2010**, *141*, 280–289. [CrossRef] [PubMed]
109. Marzetti, E.; Calvani, R.; Cesari, M.; Buford, T.W.; Lorenzi, M.; Behnke, B.J.; Leeuwenburgh, C. Mitochondrial dysfunction and sarcopenia of aging: From signaling pathways to clinical trials. *Int J. Biochem. Cell Biol.* **2013**, *45*, 2288–2301. [CrossRef]
110. Rooyackers, O.E.; Adey, D.B.; Ades, P.A.; Nair, K.S. Effect of age on in vivo rates of mitochondrial protein synthesis in human skeletal muscle. *Proc. Natl. Acad. Sci. USA* **1996**, *93*, 15364–15369. [CrossRef] [PubMed]
111. Granata, S.; Zaza, G.; Simone, S.; Villani, G.; Latorre, D.; Pontrelli, P.; Carella, M.; Schena, F.P.; Grandaliano, G.; Pertosa, G. Mitochondrial dysregulation and oxidative stress in patients with chronic kidney disease. *BMC Genom.* **2009**, *10*, 388. [CrossRef] [PubMed]

112. Gamboa, J.L.; Roshanravan, B.; Towse, T.; Keller, C.A.; Falck, A.M.; Yu, C.; Frontera, W.R.; Brown, N.J.; Ikizler, T.A. Skeletal Muscle Mitochondrial Dysfunction Is Present in Patients with CKD before Initiation of Maintenance Hemodialysis. *Clin. J. Am. Soc. Nephrol.* **2020**, *15*, 926–936. [CrossRef]
113. Stockton, K.A.; Mengersen, K.; Paratz, J.D.; Kandiah, D.; Bennell, K.L. Effect of vitamin D supplementation on muscle strength: A systematic review and meta-analysis. *Osteoporos Int.* **2011**, *22*, 859–871. [CrossRef]
114. Beaudart, C.; Buckinx, F.; Rabenda, V.; Gillain, S.; Cavalier, E.; Slomian, J.; Petermans, J.; Reginster, J.Y.; Bruyere, O. The effects of vitamin D on skeletal muscle strength, muscle mass, and muscle power: A systematic review and meta-analysis of randomized controlled trials. *J. Clin. Endocrinol. Metab.* **2014**, *99*, 4336–4345. [CrossRef] [PubMed]
115. Shea, M.K.; Fielding, R.A.; Dawson-Hughes, B. The effect of vitamin D supplementation on lower-extremity power and function in older adults: A randomized controlled trial. *Am. J. Clin. Nutr.* **2019**, *109*, 369–379. [CrossRef] [PubMed]
116. Gordon, P.L.; Sakkas, G.K.; Doyle, J.W.; Shubert, T.; Johansen, K.L. Relationship between vitamin D and muscle size and strength in patients on hemodialysis. *J. Ren. Nutr.* **2007**, *17*, 397–407. [CrossRef] [PubMed]
117. Marckmann, P.; Agerskov, H.; Thineshkumar, S.; Bladbjerg, E.M.; Sidelmann, J.J.; Jespersen, J.; Nybo, M.; Rasmussen, L.M.; Hansen, D.; Scholze, A. Randomized controlled trial of cholecalciferol supplementation in chronic kidney disease patients with hypovitaminosis D. *Nephrol. Dial. Transpl.* **2012**, *27*, 3523–3531. [CrossRef] [PubMed]
118. Hewitt, N.A.; O'Connor, A.A.; O'Shaughnessy, D.V.; Elder, G.J. Effects of cholecalciferol on functional, biochemical, vascular, and quality of life outcomes in hemodialysis patients. *Clin. J. Am. Soc. Nephrol.* **2013**, *8*, 1143–1149. [CrossRef] [PubMed]
119. Becker, C.; Lord, S.R.; Studenski, S.A.; Warden, S.J.; Fielding, R.A.; Recknor, C.P.; Hochberg, M.C.; Ferrari, S.L.; Blain, H.; Binder, E.F.; et al. Myostatin antibody (LY2495655) in older weak fallers: A proof-of-concept, randomised, phase 2 trial. *Lancet Diabetes Endocrinol.* **2015**, *3*, 948–957. [CrossRef]
120. Woodhouse, L.; Gandhi, R.; Warden, S.J.; Poiraudeau, S.; Myers, S.L.; Benson, C.T.; Hu, L.; Ahmad, Q.I.; Linnemeier, P.; Gomez, E.V.; et al. A Phase 2 Randomized Study Investigating the Efficacy and Safety of Myostatin Antibody LY2495655 versus Placebo in Patients Undergoing Elective Total Hip Arthroplasty. *J. Frailty Aging* **2016**, *5*, 62–70. [CrossRef]
121. Rooks, D.; Praestgaard, J.; Hariry, S.; Laurent, D.; Petricoul, O.; Perry, R.G.; Lach-Trifilieff, E.; Roubenoff, R. Treatment of Sarcopenia with Bimagrumab: Results from a Phase II, Randomized, Controlled, Proof-of-Concept Study. *J. Am. Geriatr. Soc.* **2017**, *65*, 1988–1995. [CrossRef]
122. Zhang, L.; Rajan, V.; Lin, E.; Hu, Z.; Han, H.Q.; Zhou, X.; Song, Y.; Min, H.; Wang, X.; Du, J.; et al. Pharmacological inhibition of myostatin suppresses systemic inflammation and muscle atrophy in mice with chronic kidney disease. *FASEB J.* **2011**, *25*, 1653–1663. [CrossRef]
123. Liu, L.; Hu, R.; You, H.; Li, J.; Liu, Y.; Li, Q.; Wu, X.; Huang, J.; Cai, X.; Wang, M.; et al. Formononetin ameliorates muscle atrophy by regulating myostatin-mediated PI3K/Akt/FoxO3a pathway and satellite cell function in chronic kidney disease. *J. Cell Mol. Med.* **2021**, *25*, 1493–1506. [CrossRef]
124. Bouchi, R.; Fukuda, T.; Takeuchi, T.; Nakano, Y.; Murakami, M.; Minami, I.; Izumiyama, H.; Hashimoto, K.; Yoshimoto, T.; Ogawa, Y. Insulin Treatment Attenuates Decline of Muscle Mass in Japanese Patients with Type 2 Diabetes. *Calcif. Tissue Int.* **2017**, *101*, 1–8. [CrossRef]
125. Rizzo, M.R.; Barbieri, M.; Fava, I.; Desiderio, M.; Coppola, C.; Marfella, R.; Paolisso, G. Sarcopenia in Elderly Diabetic Patients: Role of Dipeptidyl Peptidase 4 Inhibitors. *J. Am. Med. Dir. Assoc.* **2016**, *17*, 896–901. [CrossRef]
126. Bouchi, R.; Fukuda, T.; Takeuchi, T.; Nakano, Y.; Murakami, M.; Minami, I.; Izumiyama, H.; Hashimoto, K.; Yoshimoto, T.; Ogawa, Y. Dipeptidyl peptidase 4 inhibitors attenuates the decline of skeletal muscle mass in patients with type 2 diabetes. *Diabetes Metab. Res. Rev.* **2018**, *34*. [CrossRef] [PubMed]
127. Mori, K.; Emoto, M.; Abe, M.; Inaba, M. Visualization of Blood Glucose Fluctuations Using Continuous Glucose Monitoring in Patients Undergoing Hemodialysis. *J. Diabetes Sci. Technol.* **2019**, *13*, 413–414. [CrossRef] [PubMed]
128. Wada, N.; Mori, K.; Nakagawa, C.; Sawa, J.; Kumeda, Y.; Shoji, T.; Emoto, M.; Inaba, M. Improved glycemic control with teneligliptin in patients with type 2 diabetes mellitus on hemodialysis: Evaluation by continuous glucose monitoring. *J. Diabetes Complicat.* **2015**, *29*, 1310–1313. [CrossRef] [PubMed]
129. Mori, K.; Emoto, M.; Shoji, T.; Inaba, M. Linagliptin monotherapy compared with voglibose monotherapy in patients with type 2 diabetes undergoing hemodialysis: A 12-week randomized trial. *BMJ Open Diabetes Res. Care* **2016**, *4*, e000265. [CrossRef] [PubMed]
130. Ikizler, T.A.; Cano, N.J.; Franch, H.; Fouque, D.; Himmelfarb, J.; Kalantar-Zadeh, K.; Kuhlmann, M.K.; Stenvinkel, P.; TerWee, P.; Teta, D.; et al. Prevention and treatment of protein energy wasting in chronic kidney disease patients: A consensus statement by the International Society of Renal Nutrition and Metabolism. *Kidney Int.* **2013**, *84*, 1096–1107. [CrossRef] [PubMed]
131. Atherton, P.J.; Smith, K.; Etheridge, T.; Rankin, D.; Rennie, M.J. Distinct anabolic signalling responses to amino acids in C2C12 skeletal muscle cells. *Amino Acids* **2010**, *38*, 1533–1539. [CrossRef] [PubMed]
132. Wolfson, R.L.; Chantranupong, L.; Saxton, R.A.; Shen, K.; Scaria, S.M.; Cantor, J.R.; Sabatini, D.M. Sestrin2 is a leucine sensor for the mTORC1 pathway. *Science* **2016**, *351*, 43–48. [CrossRef] [PubMed]
133. Gielen, E.; Beckwee, D.; Delaere, A.; De Breucker, S.; Vandewoude, M.; Bautmans, I. Sarcopenia Guidelines Development Group of the Belgian Society of, G.; Geriatrics. Nutritional interventions to improve muscle mass, muscle strength, and physical performance in older people: An umbrella review of systematic reviews and meta-analyses. *Nutr. Rev.* **2021**, *79*, 121–147. [CrossRef]

134. Wu, H.; Xia, Y.; Jiang, J.; Du, H.; Guo, X.; Liu, X.; Li, C.; Huang, G.; Niu, K. Effect of beta-hydroxy-beta-methylbutyrate supplementation on muscle loss in older adults: A systematic review and meta-analysis. *Arch. Gerontol. Geriatr.* **2015**, *61*, 168–175. [CrossRef] [PubMed]
135. Fitschen, P.J.; Biruete, A.; Jeong, J.; Wilund, K.R. Efficacy of beta-hydroxy-beta-methylbutyrate supplementation in maintenance hemodialysis patients. *Hemodial. Int.* **2017**, *21*, 107–116. [CrossRef] [PubMed]
136. Hendriks, F.K.; Kooman, J.P.; van Loon, L.J.C. Dietary protein interventions to improve nutritional status in end-stage renal disease patients undergoing hemodialysis. *Curr. Opin. Clin. Nutr. Metab. Care* **2021**, *24*, 79–87. [CrossRef] [PubMed]
137. Manabe, Y. Mechanism of Skeletal Muscle Contraction: Intracellular Signaling in Skeletal Muscle Contraction. In *Musculoskeletal Disease Associated with Diabetes Mellitus*; Springer: Berlin/Heidelberg, Germany, 2016; pp. 139–153.
138. Furuichi, Y. Mechanism of Skeletal Muscle Contraction: Role of Mechanical Muscle Contraction in Glucose Homeostasis. In *Musculoskeletal Disease Associated with Diabetes Mellitus*; Springer: Berlin/Heidelberg, Germany, 2016; pp. 155–169.
139. Fujita, S.; Rasmussen, B.B.; Cadenas, J.G.; Drummond, M.J.; Glynn, E.L.; Sattler, F.R.; Volpi, E. Aerobic exercise overcomes the age-related insulin resistance of muscle protein metabolism by improving endothelial function and Akt/mammalian target of rapamycin signaling. *Diabetes* **2007**, *56*, 1615–1622. [CrossRef]
140. Sakkas, G.K.; Sargeant, A.J.; Mercer, T.H.; Ball, D.; Koufaki, P.; Karatzaferi, C.; Naish, P.F. Changes in muscle morphology in dialysis patients after 6 months of aerobic exercise training. *Nephrol. Dial. Transpl.* **2003**, *18*, 1854–1861. [CrossRef]
141. Wang, X.H.; Du, J.; Klein, J.D.; Bailey, J.L.; Mitch, W.E. Exercise ameliorates chronic kidney disease-induced defects in muscle protein metabolism and progenitor cell function. *Kidney Int.* **2009**, *76*, 751–759. [CrossRef]
142. Molsted, S.; Andersen, J.L.; Harrison, A.P.; Eidemak, I.; Mackey, A.L. Fiber type-specific response of skeletal muscle satellite cells to high-intensity resistance training in dialysis patients. *Muscle Nerve* **2015**, *52*, 736–745. [CrossRef]
143. McKendry, J.; Currier, B.S.; Lim, C.; McLeod, J.C.; Thomas, A.C.Q.; Phillips, S.M. Nutritional Supplements to Support Resistance Exercise in Countering the Sarcopenia of Aging. *Nutrients* **2020**, *12*, 2057. [CrossRef]
144. Ispoglou, T.; Witard, O.C.; Duckworth, L.C.; Lees, M.J. The efficacy of essential amino acid supplementation for augmenting dietary protein intake in older adults: Implications for skeletal muscle mass, strength and function. *Proc. Nutr. Soc.* **2020**, 1–13. [CrossRef]
145. Dickinson, J.M.; Gundermann, D.M.; Walker, D.K.; Reidy, P.T.; Borack, M.S.; Drummond, M.J.; Arora, M.; Volpi, E.; Rasmussen, B.B. Leucine-enriched amino acid ingestion after resistance exercise prolongs myofibrillar protein synthesis and amino acid transporter expression in older men. *J. Nutr.* **2014**, *144*, 1694–1702. [CrossRef] [PubMed]

Renal Rehabilitation: Exercise Intervention and Nutritional Support in Dialysis Patients

Junichi Hoshino

Nephrology Center, Toranomon Hospital, Tokyo 105-8470, Japan; hoshino@toranomon.gr.jp; Tel.: +81-3-3588-1111

Abstract: With the growing number of dialysis patients with frailty, the concept of renal rehabilitation, including exercise intervention and nutrition programs for patients with chronic kidney disease (CKD), has become popular recently. Renal rehabilitation is a comprehensive multidisciplinary program for CKD patients that is led by doctors, rehabilitation therapists, diet nutritionists, nursing specialists, social workers, pharmacists, and therapists. Many observational studies have observed better outcomes in CKD patients with more physical activity. Furthermore, recent systematic reviews have shown the beneficial effects of exercise intervention on exercise tolerance, physical ability, and quality of life in dialysis patients, though the beneficial effect on overall mortality remains unclear. Nutritional support is also fundamental to renal rehabilitation. There are various causes of skeletal muscle loss in CKD patients. To prevent muscle protein catabolism, in addition to exercise, a sufficient supply of energy, including carbohydrates, protein, iron, and vitamins, is needed. Because of decreased digestive function and energy loss due to dialysis treatment, dialysis patients are recommended to ingest 1.2-fold more protein than the regular population. Motivating patients to join in activities is also an important part of renal rehabilitation. It is essential for us to recognize the importance of renal rehabilitation to maximize patient satisfaction.

Keywords: renal rehabilitation; exercise; sarcopenia and frailty; nutritional support; protein synthesis; muscle physiology; dialysis; physical activity; exercise tolerance; quality of life

1. Introduction

An aging society is a worldwide problem, especially in developed countries. For example, more than 28% of Japan's population was over 65 years old in 2018, the highest proportion in the world, and by 2030, one-third of the population will be 65 or older and one-fifth will be 75 or older. One of the main reasons for this phenomenon in the developed countries is the prolonged life expectancy at birth. Fifty years ago, life expectancy at birth in Japan was approximately 72 years, but it has since climbed to 84 years. On the contrary, prolonged life expectancy is not equivalent to a healthier life expectancy at birth (HALE), which is defined by the World Health Organization as the average number of years of full health that a newborn could expect to live if he or she were to pass through life subject to the age-specific death rates and ill-health rates of a given newborn. It has been reported that the difference between HALE and life expectancy is approximately nine years in males and 12 years in females [1]. The difference could be considered as equal to the number of years of life during which one needs the support of nursing and family care, which patients and healthcare providers should work together to minimize.

This phenomenon has also been observed in chronic kidney disease (CKD) patients, including dialysis patients. As patients with the end stage renal disease (ESRD) rates tend to rise with age, the 2018 annual data report by the United States Renal Data System revealed that trends in the incidence rate of treated ESRD patients from 2003 to 2016 have remained high in approximately half of countries [2]. The Japanese Society for Dialysis Therapy Renal Data Registry (JRDR) reported that the number of chronic dialysis patients in Japan has been increasing every year, and reached more than 339,841 patients (the prevalence ratio was 2688 per million population) with the mean age of all dialysis patients was 68.8 years at the end of 2018 [3]. Thanks to great advances in dialysis technologies, the circumstances of dialysis patients have been changing dramatically. For example, the proportion of facilities with ultrapure dialysate (endotoxin level in dialysate lower than 0.001 EU/mL) increased from 43.1% in 2009 to 74.6% in 2018 [3], and the number of patients treated with online hemodiafiltration increased dramatically from 16,853 (5.8% of all maintenance dialysis patients) in 2009 to 144,686 (42.0%) in 2019 in Japan [4]. All of these improvements may contribute to a better quality of life and a lower mortality rate in dialysis patients in the world, however, the Japanese registry data also show that the crude mortality rate in these patients has been almost the same, approximately 10%, in recent years [4]. The reasons for this phenomenon may vary, but an increase in the elderly population and changes in social behaviors are considered important factors associated with an increase in dialysis patients with lower physical activity and frailty, resulting in lower quality of life and higher mortality. In fact, the proportion of dialysis patients who have been on dialysis for more than 20 years increased from less than 1% in 1992 to 8.4% at the end of 2018 [3,5]. As a result, the percentage of patients with multiple disabilities has also increased. In addition, dialysis-related complications, including malnutrition, dialysis-related amyloidosis, and skeletal joint disabilities, are still unsolved problems that significantly decrease patients' quality of life [6–14]. Many clinical workers in dialysis centers in developed countries may recognize the clinical relevance for patients with multiple disabilities, sarcopenia, joint pain, and fatigue, despite advances in dialysis technologies. One solution to resolving this issue is to extend the healthy life expectancy so that everyone can continue to live healthy and autonomous lives. Efforts are underway in countries all over the world to develop new treatment strategies to extend the healthy life expectancy of CKD patients, including those on dialysis. Here, the history and concepts of renal rehabilitation, the current status of the dialysis population, the implementation of renal rehabilitation in this population, and future perspectives are reviewed.

2. History and Conception of Renal Rehabilitation

Previously, rest was considered one of the treatment options for CKD, especially for patients with nephrotic syndrome, because there were reports in the 1990s suggesting that exercise may worsen the level of proteinuria and renal function. As it became clear that exercise-induced proteinuria was temporary and reversible without renal function loss, exercise therapy for CKD patients gradually gained the interest of nephrologists, dialysis health professionals, and rehabilitation therapists. At the same time, there has been an increase in the elderly population and an increase in the rate of frailty in CKD patients in the world. Since frailty is closely associated with higher mortality and lower quality of life, there is an urgent need to clarify the effects of exercise intervention in CKD patients [12,13,15,16]. To address these concerns, the Japanese Society of Renal Rehabilitation (JSRR) was established in 2011. Rehabilitation is defined by the WHO as "all means to alleviate the effects of conditions that may bring about disabilities and social disadvantages and achieve social integration of people with disabilities and social disadvantages." Renal rehabilitation was defined as "a long-term comprehensive program consisting of exercise therapy, diet therapy and water management, drug therapy, education, psychological/mental support, etc., to alleviate physical/mental effects based on kidney disease and dialysis therapy, prolong the life expectancy, and improve psychosocial and occupational circumstances." Rehabilitation in its original form means conducting all possible treatments and exhausting all support options to help kidney disease patients smoothly achieve social rehabilitation instead of simply implementing exercise therapy. Because renal rehabilitation is a comprehensive, multidisciplinary concept for patients with CKD, it is essential that the healthcare professionals associated with CKD treatment, including doctors, rehabilitation therapists, diet nutritionists, nursing specialists, social workers, pharmacists, and therapists, collaborate. All of these health professionals are equally essential components of the program [17]. On the November 2016, a group of international researchers and clinicians first met as the Global Renal Exercise (GREX) Working Group to discuss research priorities related to exercise in CKD at Chicago. They are having regular meetings to foster collaborative research and innovations across multiple disciplines to develop effective and feasible strategies to increase physical activity in CKD patients. Nowadays, many study groups in the world are working for renal rehabilitation.

3. Guidelines for Renal Rehabilitation

While a number of papers and narrative reviews regarding exercise in CKD have been published in the 2010's, there was no comprehensive guidelines related to exercise and physical activity for patients with CKD. The Kidney Disease Improving Global Outcomes (KDIGO) 2012 clinical practice guideline and other guidelines recommended to increase physical activity levels [18]. In 2013 and 2014, both the Exercise and Sports Science Australia position statement and the American Colleges of Sports Medicine guideline recommended aerobic, resistance, and flexibility exercises in CKD patients [19,20]. However, at this point, there was no specific suggestions regarding the types, intensity, and volume of specific types of exercises for CKD patients. The JSRR published the "Guide for Renal Rehabilitation for Predialysis Stage Renal Failure" on their website in 2016 to clarify the recommended exercise menus for CKD patients. Moreover, exercise therapy for diabetic patients with CKD were newly approved by the health insurance system of Japan in 2016.

Through these developments, the clinical practice guidelines for renal rehabilitation by the JSRR were established in 2018 [21]. This was the one of the first sets of clinical practice guidelines for renal rehabilitation based on systematic reviews and body of evidence. Since exercise therapy is the core of a comprehensive renal rehabilitation program, the relatively rich literature about exercise therapy for CKD patients was primarily reviewed. Thereafter, a number of systematic reviews for physical activity, renal function, lifestyle change in CKD including dialysis patients, as well as international surveys and editors' commentary, has been published in recent years [22–32].

4. Physical Activity in Dialysis Patients

Physical activity levels in dialysis patients are drastically reduced compared to the general elderly population, because dialysis patients tend to have sedentary lifestyles on the day of dialysis, probably due to inactivity for the dialysis procedure and postdialysis fatigue syndrome [33–36]. It has been reported that the physical activity of dialysis patients is 17% lower on dialysis days than on nondialysis days [36]. Dialysis patients are often exposed to several factors associated with decreased physical activity, such as catabolic disorders that may cause loss of muscle mass and lead to sarcopenia [37], mitochondrial dysfunction [38,39], and comorbidities such as anemia [40], bone and mineral disorders [41], protein energy wasting, diabetes, neurological dysfunction [15,42], and cardiovascular dysfunction [43]. A recent study of nursing home residents in the United States showed that the initiation of dialysis was associated with a decline in functional status, independently of age, sex, race, and functional status trajectory before the initiation of dialysis [44]. Consequently, the physical function of elderly dialysis patients is reportedly approximately half that of the general population [45]. The prevalence of frailty in the ESRD population in the United States is very high and is strongly associated with mortality and hospitalization, even after adjustment for well-established risk factors across multiple domains [46]. Frailty is a similar but not identical concept to sarcopenia. Frailty includes age-associated declines in lean body mass, strength, endurance, balance, walking performance, low activity, and physiological disorders, and the diagnostic criteria of the Cardiovascular Health Study (CHS), the FRAIL scale, or criteria for domestic populations such as the Japanese version of the CHS criteria (J-CHS) have often been used in clinical practice [47–49]. More importantly, frailty is a concept of reversible physical, cognitive, and/or social disability, which rehabilitation may play an important role to overcome it [50,51].

Physical activity and exercise habits are closely associated with better outcomes. The Dialysis Outcomes and Practice Pattern Study (DOPPS) reported that patients who habitually exercised more than once a week had better outcomes across all DOPPS countries regardless of physical status or social factors [52]. Many observational studies have suggested an association between physical activity and lower mortality in both CKD and dialysis patients [13,26,53,54]. Matsuzawa et al. also reported that dialysis patients with physical activity of more than 50 min per day and who took a median of approximately 4000 steps a day had better outcomes [55]. Even in patients with CKD with multiple disabilities, it was reported that a less sedentary lifestyle was associated with better outcomes [56]. Of course, a higher level of activity is desirable not only in terms of dialysis mortality, but also for general health; however, efforts to avoid a sedentary lifestyle are the first and most important step for dialysis patients with frailty.

On the contrary, there is still a large gap between theoretical knowledge and real-world clinical practice. The JRDR reported that more than 60% of dialysis patients of all ages and dialysis vintages did not have an exercise habit. The proportion of patients without an exercise habit increased with older age and longer dialysis vintage. In Japanese patients older than 75 years and with a dialysis vintage of over 40 years, for example, almost 80% of patients had no exercise habit [3]. A recent study indicated that only 6.9% of CKD patients met the recommended physical activity levels [57].

5. Exercise Tolerance in CKD Patients

Exercise is not only performed by skeletal muscle contraction. The energy supplied by the circulatory and respiratory systems is needed for skeletal muscle contraction. These interactions between metabolic, circulatory, and respiratory functions are called "Wasserman's gear" (Figure 1) [58]. This schematic diagram demonstrates the importance of cooperative work among the skeletal muscle, cardiovascular system, respiratory system, and nervous system to achieve exercise tolerance. The intensity of aerobic exercise training is a key issue in renal rehabilitation, since exercise intensity is directly linked to both the amount of improvement in exercise capacity and the risk of adverse events during exercise. Therefore, although assessing muscle function is an essential part of exercise, we need to undertake a comprehensive assessment of these organs to assess exercise tolerance.

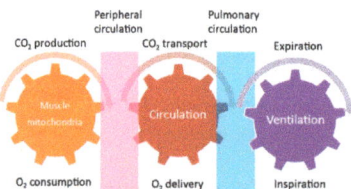

Figure 1. Wasserman's gear.

Exercise tolerance is defined by oxygen-dependent biological systems, the respiratory system, and the circulatory system, and by oxygen consumption by mitochondria in muscular tissue, as described above. Peak oxygen uptake (VO_2) and the first and second ventilatory thresholds (i.e., the physiological descriptors of the O_2 transport and utilization system in response to exercise) are the gold-standard references for the evaluation of aerobic metabolic function and, consequently, for aerobic exercise intensity assessment and prescription [59]. Cardiopulmonary exercise testing (CPX) may be the most widely used method to assess exercise tolerance. The clinician's guidelines for exercise testing, with a comprehensive overview of CPX, are described in detail in the scientific statement paper from the American Heart Association [60]. Modern CPX systems allow for the analysis of gas exchange at rest, during exercise, and during recovery and yield through breath-by-breath measures of oxygen uptake, carbon dioxide output, and ventilation. As a consequence, they also allow for the analysis of the submaximal index of exercise capacity, called the anaerobic threshold (AT) or ventilatory threshold (VT). These parameters are often measured before initiating renal rehabilitation to achieve treatment goals efficiently and safely.

As described above, most CKD patients have very low exercise tolerance because of a decrease in muscle mass due to CKD-related catabolic status, mitochondrial dysfunction, cardiovascular complications, CKD-related mineral bone disorders, and anemia. Exercise tolerance is a strong prognostic factor associated with mortality independent of renal function. In fact, it has been reported in patients with renal transplantation that recovery from physical dysfunction and cardiovascular risks is limited after improvement of renal function [61]. Therefore, increasing or maintaining exercise tolerance is a key factor to improve quality of life in CKD patients.

6. Muscle Energy Metabolism and Nutrients

6.1. Mechanisms of Adenosine Triphosphate (ATP) Production

Skeletal muscle contraction is a movement produced by the free energy extracted by the hydrolysis of adenosine triphosphate (ATP). ATP is produced in the muscle anaerobically and aerobically. The earliest mechanism for ATP production in the muscle is the creatine phosphate pathway, which utilizes the creatine phosphate (PCr) stored in skeletal muscle (Figure 2). This is a kind of reserve mechanism for high-intensity exercise, where energy demand rises rapidly. However, performance is usually maintained for only approximately 10 s. Thereafter, another anaerobic ATP production system, called the glycolysis pathway, produces 2ATP from glycogen, whose metabolic capacity is about one-half to one-seventh that of the PCr pathway. Then, the main body of ATP production is gradually switched from anaerobic to aerobic exercise, which can produce ATP under oxygen supply. Therefore, organs in the Wasserman's gear are very important players in aerobic exercise. In order to produce ATP aerobically, energy sources, including sugars, lipids, and proteins, are needed. Sugars and lipids are preferentially used for ATP production. Thereafter, most of the ATP for exercise is produced through the tricarboxylic acid cycle (TCA cycle or Krebs cycle) and the electron transport chain [62].

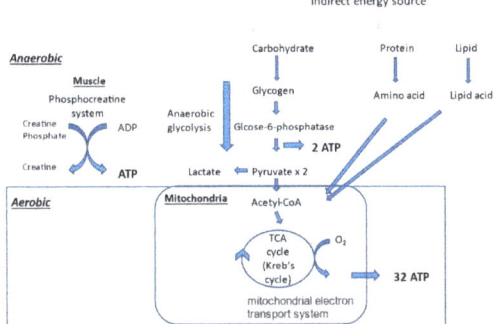

Figure 2. Mechanisms of adenosine triphosphate (ATP) production in muscle. ADP, adenosine diphosphate; TCA, tricarboxylic acid.

6.2. Synthesis of Skeletal Muscle and Its Related Nutrients

Muscle is the most important and largest site of storage of amino acids in the body. After digestion, carbohydrates are broken into glycogen, proteins into amino acids, and lipids into fatty acids. Glycogens and muscle protein formed by amino acids are stored in the muscle. When glycogen is used up and/or malnutrition is present, muscle protein is broken down into amino acids. When performing exercise therapy, it is necessary to supply additional energy to replace the energy burned by exercise, based on METs (metabolic equivalents). The amount of replenishment energy is calculated as 1.05 × METs × time × body weight. In addition, because elderly people have a higher amino acid threshold for anabolic and lower gastrointestinal absorption capacity, more protein is needed to maintain the nitrogen balance.

Ingestion of branched-chain amino acids (BCAAs) such as valine, leucine, and isoleucine, especially leucine and its metabolite 3-hydroxy-3-methylbutanoic acid, is important to promote the synthesis of skeletal muscle protein [63]. BCAAs are abundant in dairy products and animal proteins.

Maintaining high blood amino acid levels after exercise is important for skeletal muscle maintenance and enhancement. BCAA-rich whey protein can relatively rapidly increase the level of blood amino acid concentration after ingestion, while casein and soy protein have a relatively slow digestion and absorption rate. Approximately 20% of milk protein consists of whey protein and 80% of that consists of casein. Therefore, milk protein is expected to both promote and sustain muscle protein synthesis. A recent meta-analysis reported that glycogen synthesis rates are enhanced when carbohydrates and protein are co-ingested after exercise compared to carbohydrates only, when the added energy of protein is consumed in addition to, not in place of, carbohydrates, suggesting the importance of an increase in the energy intake [64]. It is well known that modulating postexercise nutrition is an effective approach to enhance the replenishment of muscle glycogen stores. Considering the absorption time, it may be preferable to ingest protein and carbohydrates before exercise, or just after exercise in the case of fast-absorbing nutrients such as milk protein or amino acids. For athletes, it is recommended to ingest 1.2 g/kg of carbohydrates per hour for 4–6 h postexercise and 0.3 g/kg of a high-quality protein to stimulate muscle protein synthesis and repair [65]. This recommendation for athletes may not be exactly suitable for ESRD patients; however, we need to keep in mind that nutritional support is important for improving muscle functions and physiological performance in ESRD patients.

6.3. Muscle Energy Metabolism and Nutrients in CKD

Skeletal muscle atrophy in renal dysfunction begins in the early stages of CKD and progresses with the progression of renal impairment [66]. Skeletal muscle atrophy is caused by an imbalance between protein synthesis and degradation, but there are various causes of skeletal muscle loss in CKD patients [67]. It was reported that the pathophysiology of muscle wasting and weakness is complex and multifactorial. One or more of (1) insufficient nutritional intake; (2) catabolic effects of dialysis therapy; (3) hormonal abnormalities of anabolic hormones (e.g., testosterone, growth hormone, insulin-like growth factor-1), catabolic hormones (e.g., cortisol), or thyroid hormone; (4) chronic inflammation; (5) metabolic acidosis; and (6) concurrent comorbidities [68]. Patients with CKD have a high prevalence of protein energy malnutrition. In order to avoid extra release of muscle protein and to retain muscle in the body, it is essential to meet one's energy requirements to keep nitrogen balance in CKD patients. For dialysis patients, a 30–35 kcal/kg/day energy intake is recommended, because the estimated energy leak during 4 h of dialysis is approximately 300 kcal. In addition, during the dialysis session, there is a 6–13 g amino acid loss, as well as albumin losses by dialysis circuit absorption and by leakage from the dialysis membrane. Therefore, it is usually recommended to ingest 1.0 to 1.2 g/kg/day of protein, which is 1.2 times higher than recommended for healthy individuals. Furthermore, elderly people should increase their protein intake by 20%.

In addition to protein and energy intake, sufficient intake of vitamins and minerals such as vitamin D and iron is also very important to prevent muscle protein catabolism [69]. Vitamin D deficiency is common phenomenon in CKD patients. It is reported that maintaining appropriate vitamin D levels is crucial to protect muscle from significant atrophy [70]. Moreover, iron deficiency in skeletal muscle metabolism is strongly associated with lower exercise tolerance independent from anemia, since it is an essential component of oxygen uptake, transport, storage, erythropoiesis, the mitochondrial electron transport chain, and antioxidant enzymes [71]. Uremic toxins such as indoxyl sulfate induce oxidative stress and reduce exercise tolerance and mitochondrial function [72]. There is a report suggesting that reducing the level of indoxyl sulfate results in improvement of exercise tolerance and skeletal muscle function [73]. It has also been reported that EPA and DHA have the effect of suppressing skeletal muscle decomposition [74]. Milk contains a lot of vitamin D, which is necessary for maintaining skeletal muscle. Though it is a very promising ingredient, proper serum phosphorus concentration control using a phosphorus binder is also important. It was reported in the USA that higher protein intake and a concurrent decline in serum phosphorus appear to be associated with the lowest mortality, and diligent use of potent phosphorus binders may be helpful in the dialysis population [75]. The risk of controlling serum phosphorus by restricting dietary protein may outweigh the benefits of controlled phosphorus and may lead to greater mortality.

7. Efficacy of Exercise in Dialysis Patients

With the increase in studies and review papers suggesting the benefits of physical exercise for dialysis patients [76–78], scientific societies started to recommend exercise therapy for dialysis patients in the 2010s. In 2012, the KDIGO clinical practice guidelines for CKD encouraged participants to undertake physical activity compatible with cardiovascular health and tolerance, aiming for at least 30 min, five times per week [18]. In 2013, Exercise & Sports Science Australia issued a position statement concerning exercise therapy for CKD patients that describes specific methods of exercise therapy for patients with end-stage kidney disease, both during dialysis and on nondialysis days [19]. It recommends up to 180 min of aerobic exercise with an intensity of 11–13 on the rating of perceived exertion (RPE) scale, 8–12 sessions of resistance exercises with a 60–70% repetition maximum on two nonconsecutive days per week, and 10 min of flexibility exercise 5–7 days per week for dialysis patients. In 2014, the American College of Sports Medicine released its guideline for exercise testing and prescription [20], and specific methods and cautions about exercise therapy for dialysis patients are presented in the latest edition. These guidelines in the 2010s were the standards for exercise therapy in the dialysis population. However, most of these recommendations were based on observational studies, and it was unclear whether exercise intervention was effective for dialysis patients with frailty, until 2018. In 2018, what was, to the best of my knowledge, the first set of evidence-based clinical guidelines for exercise therapy in dialysis patients was published [21,79].

In this systematic review, survival, exercise tolerance, QOL, physical ability (walking ability), physical function (muscle strength), muscle mass, albumin, activity of daily living, Kt/V (a marker of dialysis adequacy), and C-reactive protein (CRP) were selected as outcomes. A meta-analysis of 41 randomized controlled trials demonstrated the significant efficacy of exercise therapy on exercise tolerance (mean difference (MD) in VO_2: 5.25 L/min/kg, 95% confidence interval (CI): 4.30–6.20 L/min/kg), QOL (MD of physical component summary: 7.39, 95% CI: 2.26–12.51; MD of mental component summary: 9.46, 95% CI: 0.26–18.65), physical ability (MD of 6 min walking distance: 30.2 m, 95% CI: 24.22–36.07 m), and Kt/V (MD: 0.07, 95% CI: 0.01–0.14) (Figures 3–6) [21]. Similar results were found in another systematic review [23]. However, no statistically significant difference was noted in terms of muscle strength, muscle mass, albumin, or CRP, although they were all improved. In addition, no significant improvement in survival was observed, perhaps due to the small number of events.

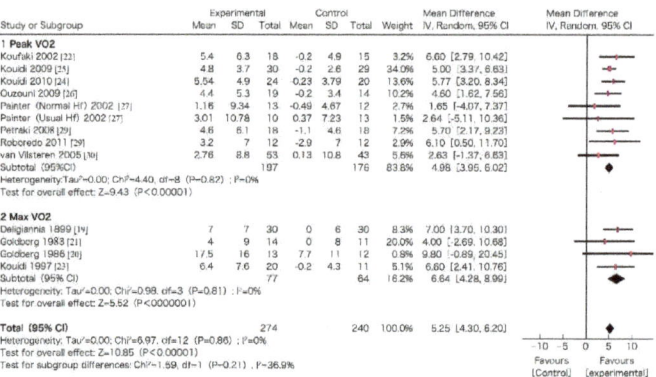

Figure 3. The effects of the exercise intervention on the changes in the exercise tolerance (VO$_2$ peak) of dialysis patients [21,79]. SD, standard deviation; CI, confidential interval; IV, inverse variance; VO2, VO$_2$.

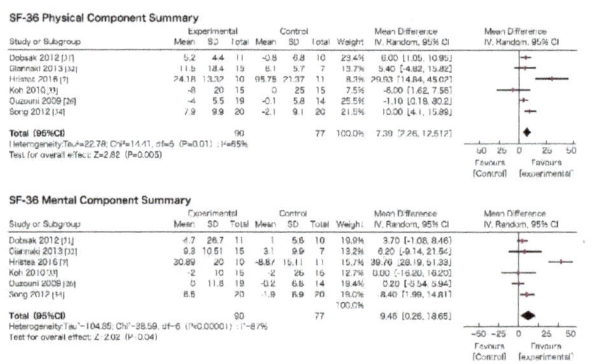

Figure 4. The effects of the exercise intervention on the changes in the quality of life of dialysis patients [21,79]. SD, standard deviation; CI, confidential interval; IV, inverse variance.

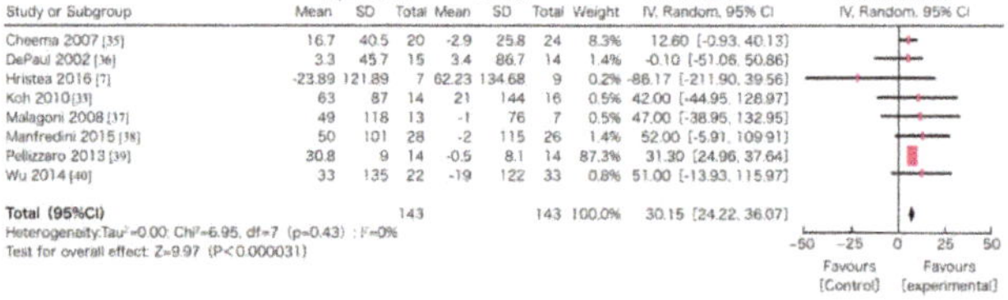

Figure 5. The effects of the exercise intervention on the changes in the 6 min walking distance of dialysis patients [21,79]. SD, standard deviation; CI, confidential interval; IV, inverse variance.

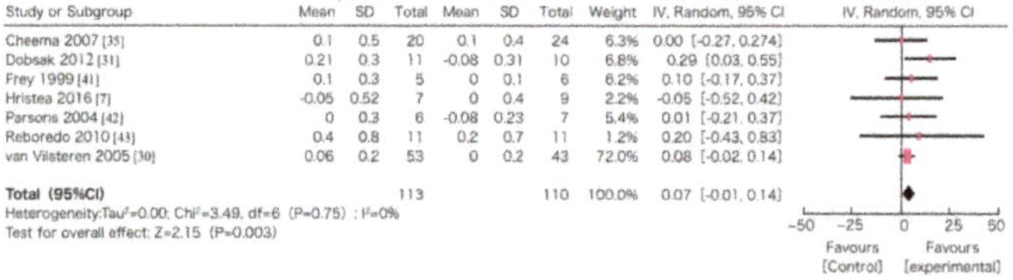

Figure 6. The effects of the exercise intervention on the changes in the 6 min walking distance of dialysis patients [21,79]. SD, standard deviation; CI, confidential interval; IV, inverse variance.

As for the duration and type of exercise, it has been reported that more than six months of intradialytic exercise intervention has significant effects on exercise tolerance (VO_2) [80]. The same meta-analysis showed that the improvement in exercise tolerance was greater in clinical studies using both aerobic exercise therapy and resistance training than in studies using aerobic exercise therapy alone. There has also been a report showing that the improvement in exercise tolerance is greater with exercise therapy under supervision on nondialysis days, despite a larger number of dropouts [81]. In conducting exercise therapy, the relationship between such specific methods and the effectiveness of exercise therapy must be considered. It is highly significant that physical ability and QOL were improved by exercise, as these are two major components of renal rehabilitation. In this respect, renal rehabilitation plays a major role in achieving the goals of dialysis therapy. In the future, it will be necessary to validate the optimal method of exercise therapy for peritoneal dialysis patients and its effectiveness.

In addition, a recent study suggested that exercise may increase the levels of nitric oxide and myokines and decrease the level of activated oxygen, which are associated with improvements in capillary function, insulin resistance, and other aging-related factors [82,83].

8. Implementation of Exercise in Dialysis Patients

The target of exercise therapy is patients with a stable physical condition. The three important steps for exercise therapy in dialysis patients are prior physical evaluation, prescription of an adequate exercise menu, and provision of a continuous support program. Since dialysis patients often have cardiovascular complications, it is essential to promptly assess before prescription whether the patient's cardiovascular functions and laboratory data, including serum potassium and anemia, are amenable to exercise therapy. In diabetic patients, diabetic complications, including retinopathy, neuropathy, and diabetic foot, may affect the target levels of exercise. If some vital changes are observed, it is preferable to stop exercise until the problems are resolved.

8.1. Prior Evaluation

The guidelines for rehabilitation in patients with cardiovascular disease by the Japanese Circulation Society state that, prior to beginning exercise training programs, participants should be assessed for clinical status and should undergo examinations at rest and exercise stress tests to determine the appropriateness of exercise training and to establish the appropriate exercise prescriptions [84]. Acute or uncontrolled cardiovascular diseases are contraindications for exercise. Those with a blood pressure $\geq 180/100$ mmHg, a fasting blood glucose level ≥ 250 mg/dL, and a body mass index ≥ 30.0 are also considered contraindications for exercise. In addition, the goals of rehabilitation should be modified based on the patient's condition. See details in these guidelines or the JSRR renal rehabilitation guidelines.

8.2. Four Components of an Exercise Intervention

There are four main components in an exercise intervention: aerobic exercise, represented by walking and swimming; resistance training, represented by push-ups and squats; flexibility exercise, represented by stretching; balance training, represented by standing on one leg (Figure 7). The examples of four types of exercise can be seen in the National Institute on Aging homepage [85]. At this point, it is still unclear which combination is the best for dialysis patients. Most previous papers chose a combination of aerobic and resistance training with some flexibility training. Recent studies of patients with severe renal impairment comparing the effectiveness of resistance training and balance training concluded that the beneficial effects on physical activity and renal function were similar in both groups [86,87]. Therefore, it is preferable to combine these components in a balanced way or to modify them individually to maximize the treatment effects of exercise in dialysis patients.

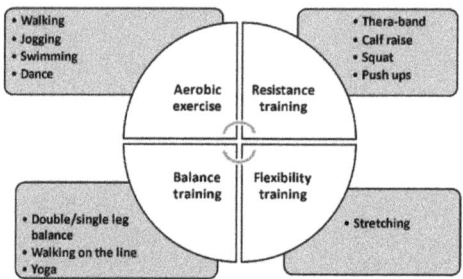

Figure 7. Components in an exercise intervention.

8.3. Menu of Exercise Intervention

The JSRR guidelines recommend that dialysis patients evaluate the causes of walking disability if they have a decreased comfortable walking speed (<1.0 m/s) or short physical performance battery (SPPB) (<12 points) [79]. If patients do not have a walking disability, the first target goal is more than 4000 steps on nondialysis days and walking more than 30 min more than five days per week. In addition, evaluations should be done every six or 12 months. In patients with physical disability, lower-grade center exercise with supervisors should be undertaken.

The exercise prescription should be based on the concept of "FITT": frequency, intensity, time, and type of exercise. On this point, an example of a suitable exercise program for dialysis patients is a combination of aerobic exercise (e.g., walking $\geq$ 30 min, five times per week), resistance training (e.g., Thera-band exercise for 10–20 min with a rating of perceived exertion (RPE) of 13–17), and balance training (e.g., double-/single-leg balancing for 5 min 3–5 times a week) [79]. As described before, the rate of frailty in dialysis patients is very high. Therefore, it is preferable to start with a low intensity and adjust it based on the patient's physical condition.

9. Barriers to CKD-Specific Exercise Behavior

Why are dialysis patients sedentary? There are barriers to exercise that keep real clinical practice from adhering to the evidence. In other words, in addition to exercise prescriptions, continuous support programs are essential to achieve our goals, especially in the dialysis population. What are the factors associated with behavioral change? Everyone hesitates over starting exercise because of bad weather, no time, not feeling like it, etc. A study from the U.K. suggested some key factors associated with behavioral changes in CKD patients. They reported that barriers to exercise included physical factors (frailty, anemia, and aging), mental factors (fear of injury or aggravating their condition), absence of motivational support (familial support, encouraging, enjoyment, adequate goals, and accomplishment), and environmental factors (supervisors, facilities, and weather) [88]. Poor physical condition as a result of both comorbid conditions and CKD-related symptoms (fatigue, joint pain, and shortness of breath) [89] was felt by the participants to be the predominant barrier to exercise. The perceived psychological barriers to exercise included fear of injury. Some concerns about exercise may be partly due to the lack of information patients receive about the benefits of exercise from healthcare professionals [57]. Patients expressed a need for tailored advice and support from their healthcare professionals regarding the specific exercises that are safe and appropriate for renal patients.

The Standardized Outcomes in Nephrology—Hemodialysis (SONG-HD) study group reported that the core outcomes that are critically important for dialysis patients and health professionals to avoid are fatigue, cardiovascular disease, vascular access, and mortality [90]. Additionally, a patient-reported outcome (PRO) study from Canada reported that the major barriers for the remaining patients were fatigue (55%), shortness of breath (50%), and weakness (49%). If the patients were going to exercise, they wanted to exercise at home (73%) using a combination of aerobic and resistance training (41%), regardless of modality or age category [91]. While most trials have reported beneficial effects on biochemical parameters and possible benefits in terms of reduced mortality, these PRO studies suggest that these promising results are less important for dialysis patients and may not motivate them to stick to an exercise regimen. Rather, they are more interested in how to relieve fatigue and how to recover energy for their daily lives. Therefore, it is essential for us to understand these barriers and to provide continuous support programs to achieve patient satisfaction. In order to keep exercising regularly and actively for a long time, it may be necessary to prescribe a customized "My pace" program, an easy "Accessible" program, and an enjoyable "Together" program: A combined concept of "MAT: My pace, Accessible, and Together".

10. Conclusions

Dialysis-associated health professionals often act as first-line healthcare providers, not unlike home doctors, for dialysis patients. Therefore, they may be considered the best gatekeepers of renal rehabilitation who need to contact other healthcare professionals, such as rehabilitation therapists, diet nutritionists, nursing specialists, social workers, pharmacists, and therapists, to coordinate the patient's renal rehabilitation. Renal rehabilitation is a relatively new concept. Based on the urgent needs of an elderly society, especially in advanced countries, it is necessary to combine our multidisciplinary knowledge, gather new evidence, and create a sustainable environment for renal rehabilitation.

Funding: This research received no external funding. The author received competitive research funds from Otsuka Pharmaceutical Co. Ltd., as well as a lecture fee from Ono Pharmaceutical Co. Ltd.

Institutional Review Board Statement: Not applicable.

Informed Consent Statement: Not applicable.

Data Availability Statement: The data that support the findings of this study are available from the corresponding author, J.H., upon reasonable request. Restrictions apply to the availability of these data. The Figures 3–6 was obtained from the references [21,79] and are available from the authors or publishers with the permission.

Acknowledgments: The author is grateful to Professors Masaaki Inaba, Yoshihiko Kanno, Masanori Abe, and Katsuhito Mori for the opportunity to work in the Japanese Society for Dialysis Therapy; to Professors Kunihiro Yamagata and Masahiro Kohzuki, the President and Former President, respectively, of the JSRR, for the opportunity to work in renal rehabilitation; and to all members of the Nephrology Center and Department of Rehabilitation of Toranomon Hospital.

Conflicts of Interest: The author declares no conflict of interest.

References

1. Ministry_of_Health_Labor_and_Welfare. Trends of Life Expectancy and Healthy Life Expectancy in Japan. Available online: https://www.mhlw.go.jp/stf/wp/hakusyo/kousei/19/backdata/01-01-02-06.html (accessed on 16 February 2021). (In Japanese)
2. Chapter 11: International Comparisons. *Am. J. Kidney Dis.* **2019**, *73*, S549–S594. [CrossRef]
3. Nitta, K.; Goto, S.; Masakane, I.; Hanafusa, N.; Taniguchi, M.; Hasegawa, T.; Nakai, S.; Wada, A.; Hamano, T.; Hoshino, J.; et al. Annual dialysis data report for 2018, JSDT Renal Data Registry: Survey methods, facility data, incidence, prevalence, and mortality. *Ren. Replace. Ther.* **2020**, *6*, 41. [CrossRef]
4. Nitta, K.; Goto, S.; Masakane, I.; Hanafusa, N.; Taniguchi, M.; Hasegawa, T.; Nakai, S.; Wada, A.; Hamano, T.; Hoshino, J.; et al. Annual dialysis data report for 2019, JSDT Renal Data Registry. *J. Jpn. Soc. Dial. Ther.* **2020**, *53*, 579–632. [CrossRef]
5. Hoshino, J.; Yamagata, K.; Nishi, S.; Nakai, S.; Masakane, I.; Iseki, K.; Tsubakihara, Y. Significance of the decreased risk of dialysis-related amyloidosis now proven by results from Japanese nationwide surveys in 1998 and 2010. *Nephrol. Dial. Transpl.* **2016**, *31*, 595–602. [CrossRef]
6. Brahee, D.D.; Guebert, G.M.; Virgin, B. Dialysis-related spondyloarthropathy. *J. Manip. Physiol. Ther.* **2001**, *24*, 127–130. [CrossRef]
7. Charra, B.; Calemard, E.; Uzan, M.; Terrat, J.C.; Vanel, T.; Laurent, G. Carpal tunnel syndrome, shoulder pain and amyloid deposits in long-term haemodialysis patients. In *Proceedings of the European Dialysis and Transplant Association-European Renal Association. European Dialysis and Transplant Association-European Renal Association*; Congress: Washington, DC, USA, 1985; Volume 21, pp. 291–295.

8. Hoshino, J.; Yamagata, K.; Nishi, S.; Nakai, S.; Masakane, I.; Iseki, K.; Tsubakihara, Y. Carpal tunnel surgery as proxy for dialysis-related amyloidosis: Results from the Japanese society for dialysis therapy. *Am. J. Nephrol.* **2014**, *39*, 449–458. [CrossRef]
9. Kazama, J.J.; Yamamoto, S.; Takahashi, N.; Ito, Y.; Maruyama, H.; Narita, I.; Gejyo, F. Abeta-2M-amyloidosis and related bone diseases. *J. Bone Miner. Metab.* **2006**, *24*, 182–184. [CrossRef]
10. Labriola, L.; Jadoul, M. Dialysis-related Amyloidosis: Is It Gone or Should It Be? *Semin Dial.* **2017**, *30*, 193–196. [CrossRef]
11. K/DOQI clinical practice guidelines for bone metabolism and disease in chronic kidney disease. *Am. J. Kidney Dis.* **2003**, *42*, S1–S201. [CrossRef]
12. Jassal, S.V.; Karaboyas, A.; Comment, L.A.; Bieber, B.A.; Morgenstern, H.; Sen, A.; Gillespie, B.W.; De Sequera, P.; Marshall, M.R.; Fukuhara, S.; et al. Functional Dependence and Mortality in the International Dialysis Outcomes and Practice Patterns Study (DOPPS). *Am. J. Kidney Dis.* **2016**, *67*, 283–292. [CrossRef]
13. Johansen, K.L.; Delgado, C.; Bao, Y.; Kurella Tamura, M. Frailty and dialysis initiation. *Semin. Dial.* **2013**, *26*, 690–696. [CrossRef]
14. Lacquaniti, A.; Bolignano, D.; Campo, S.; Perrone, C.; Donato, V.; Fazio, M.R.; Buemi, A.; Sturiale, A.; Buemi, M. Malnutrition in the elderly patient on dialysis. *Ren. Fail.* **2009**, *31*, 239–245. [CrossRef]
15. Moorthi, R.N.; Avin, K.G. Clinical relevance of sarcopenia in chronic kidney disease. *Curr. Opin. Nephrol. Hypertens.* **2017**, *26*, 219–228. [CrossRef]
16. Abdel-Rahman, E.M.; Turgut, F.; Turkmen, K.; Balogun, R.A. Falls in elderly hemodialysis patients. *QJM Mon. J. Assoc. Physicians* **2011**, *104*, 829–838. [CrossRef]
17. Hoshino, J. Renal rehabilitation in CKD patients. *Jpn. J. Nephrol.* **2020**, *62*, 730–735.
18. Eknoyan, G.; Lameire, N.; Eckardt, K.U. KDIGO 2012 Clinical Practice Guideline for the Evaluation and Management of Chronic kidney disease. *Kidney Int. Suppl.* **2013**, *3*, 136–150.
19. Smart, N.A.; Williams, A.D.; Levinger, I.; Selig, S.; Howden, E.; Coombes, J.S.; Fassett, R.G. Exercise & Sports Science Australia (ESSA) position statement on exercise and chronic kidney disease. *J. Sci. Med. Sport* **2013**, *16*, 406–411. [CrossRef] [PubMed]
20. Ferguson, B. ACSM's Guidelines for Exercise Testing and Prescription 9th Ed. 2014. *J. Can. Chiropr. Assoc.* **2014**, *58*, 328.
21. Yamagata, K.; Hoshino, J.; Sugiyama, H.; Hanafusa, N.; Shibagaki, Y.; Komatsu, Y.; Konta, T.; Fujii, N.; Kanda, E.; Sofue, T.; et al. Clinical practice guideline for renal rehabilitation: Systematic reviews and recommendations of exercise therapies in patients with kidney diseases. *Ren. Replace. Ther.* **2019**, *5*, 28. [CrossRef]
22. Afsar, B.; Siriopol, D.; Aslan, G.; Eren, O.C.; Dagel, T.; Kilic, U.; Kanbay, A.; Burlacu, A.; Covic, A.; Kanbay, M. The impact of exercise on physical function, cardiovascular outcomes and quality of life in chronic kidney disease patients: A systematic review. *Int. Urol. Nephrol.* **2018**, *50*, 885–904. [CrossRef] [PubMed]
23. Matsuzawa, R.; Hoshi, K.; Yoneki, K.; Harada, M.; Watanabe, T.; Shimoda, T.; Yamamoto, S.; Matsunaga, A. Exercise Training in Elderly People Undergoing Hemodialysis: A Systematic Review and Meta-analysis. *Kidney Int. Rep.* **2017**, *2*, 1096–1110. [CrossRef] [PubMed]
24. Vanden Wyngaert, K.; Van Craenenbroeck, A.H.; Van Biesen, W.; Dhondt, A.; Tanghe, A.; Van Ginckel, A.; Celie, B.; Calders, P. The effects of aerobic exercise on eGFR, blood pressure and VO2peak in patients with chronic kidney disease stages 3–4: A systematic review and meta-analysis. *PLoS ONE* **2018**, *13*, e0203662. [CrossRef]
25. Bennett, P.N.; Thompson, S.; Wilund, K.R. An introduction to Exercise and Physical Activity in Dialysis Patients: Preventing the unacceptable journey to physical dysfunction. *Semin. Dial.* **2019**, *32*, 281–282. [CrossRef] [PubMed]
26. Evangelidis, N.; Craig, J.; Bauman, A.; Manera, K.; Saglimbene, V.; Tong, A. Lifestyle behaviour change for preventing the progression of chronic kidney disease: A systematic review. *BMJ Open* **2019**, *9*, e031625. [CrossRef]
27. Pei, G.; Tang, Y.; Tan, L.; Tan, J.; Ge, L.; Qin, W. Aerobic exercise in adults with chronic kidney disease (CKD): A meta-analysis. *Int. Urol. Nephrol.* **2019**, *51*, 1787–1795. [CrossRef] [PubMed]
28. Thompson, S.; Wiebe, N.; Padwal, R.S.; Gyenes, G.; Headley, S.A.E.; Radhakrishnan, J.; Graham, M. The effect of exercise on blood pressure in chronic kidney disease: A systematic review and meta-analysis of randomized controlled trials. *PLoS ONE* **2019**, *14*, e0211032. [CrossRef]
29. Viana, J.L.; Martins, P.; Parker, K.; Madero, M.; Perez Grovas, H.; Anding, K.; Degenhardt, S.; Gabrys, I.; Raugust, S.; West, C.; et al. Sustained exercise programs for hemodialysis patients: The characteristics of successful approaches in Portugal, Canada, Mexico, and Germany. *Semin. Dial.* **2019**, *32*, 320–330. [CrossRef]
30. Zhang, L.; Wang, Y.; Xiong, L.; Luo, Y.; Huang, Z.; Yi, B. Exercise therapy improves eGFR, and reduces blood pressure and BMI in non-dialysis CKD patients: Evidence from a meta-analysis. *BMC Nephrol.* **2019**, *20*, 398. [CrossRef]
31. Ferrari, F.; Helal, L.; Dipp, T.; Soares, D.; Soldatelli, Â.; Mills, A.L.; Paz, C.; Tenório, M.C.C.; Motta, M.T.; Barcellos, F.C.; et al. Intradialytic training in patients with end-stage renal disease: A systematic review and meta-analysis of randomized clinical trials assessing the effects of five different training interventions. *J. Nephrol.* **2020**, *33*, 251–266. [CrossRef]
32. Labib, M.; Bohm, C.; MacRae, J.M.; Bennett, P.N.; Wilund, K.R.; McAdams-DeMarco, M.; Jhamb, M.; Mustata, S.; Thompson, S. An International Delphi Survey on Exercise Priorities in CKD. *Kidney Int. Rep.* **2020**. [CrossRef]
33. Heiwe, S.; Tollback, A.; Clyne, N. Twelve weeks of exercise training increases muscle function and walking capacity in elderly predialysis patients and healthy subjects. *Nephron* **2001**, *88*, 48–56. [CrossRef] [PubMed]
34. Clyne, N.; Ekholm, J.; Jogestrand, T.; Lins, L.E.; Pehrsson, S.K. Effects of exercise training in predialytic uremic patients. *Nephron* **1991**, *59*, 84–89. [CrossRef] [PubMed]

35. Painter, P.L.; Nelson-Worel, J.N.; Hill, M.M.; Thornbery, D.R.; Shelp, W.R.; Harrington, A.R.; Weinstein, A.B. Effects of exercise training during hemodialysis. *Nephron* **1986**, *43*, 87–92. [CrossRef]
36. Avesani, C.M.; Trolonge, S.; Deleaval, P.; Baria, F.; Mafra, D.; Faxen-Irving, G.; Chauveau, P.; Teta, D.; Kamimura, M.A.; Cuppari, L.; et al. Physical activity and energy expenditure in haemodialysis patients: An international survey. *Nephrol. Dial. Transplant.* **2012**, *27*, 2430–2434. [CrossRef]
37. Heiwe, S.; Clyne, N.; Tollback, A.; Borg, K. Effects of regular resistance training on muscle histopathology and morphometry in elderly patients with chronic kidney disease. *Am. J. Phys. Med. Rehabil.* **2005**, *84*, 865–874. [CrossRef]
38. Tamaki, M.; Miyashita, K.; Wakino, S.; Mitsuishi, M.; Hayashi, K.; Itoh, H. Chronic kidney disease reduces muscle mitochondria and exercise endurance and its exacerbation by dietary protein through inactivation of pyruvate dehydrogenase. *Kidney Int.* **2014**, *85*, 1330–1339. [CrossRef] [PubMed]
39. Tamaki, M.; Hagiwara, A.; Miyashita, K.; Wakino, S.; Inoue, H.; Fujii, K.; Fujii, C.; Sato, M.; Mitsuishi, M.; Muraki, A.; et al. Improvement of Physical Decline Through Combined Effects of Muscle Enhancement and Mitochondrial Activation by a Gastric Hormone Ghrelin in Male 5/6Nx CKD Model Mice. *Endocrinology* **2015**, *156*, 3638–3648. [CrossRef]
40. Tsubakihara, Y.; Nishi, S.; Akiba, T.; Hirakata, H.; Iseki, K.; Kubota, M.; Kuriyama, S.; Komatsu, Y.; Suzuki, M.; Nakai, S.; et al. 2008 Japanese Society for Dialysis Therapy: Guidelines for renal anemia in chronic kidney disease. *Ther. Apher. Dial.* **2010**, *14*, 240–275. [CrossRef]
41. Ott, S.M. Therapy for patients with CKD and low bone mineral density. *Nat. Rev. Nephrol.* **2013**, *9*, 681–692. [CrossRef]
42. Fahal, I.H. Uraemic sarcopenia: Aetiology and implications. *Nephrol. Dial. Transplant.* **2014**, *29*, 1655–1665. [CrossRef]
43. Levey, A.S.; de Jong, P.E.; Coresh, J.; El Nahas, M.; Astor, B.C.; Matsushita, K.; Gansevoort, R.T.; Kasiske, B.L.; Eckardt, K.U. The definition, classification, and prognosis of chronic kidney disease: A KDIGO Controversies Conference report. *Kidney Int.* **2011**, *80*, 17–28. [CrossRef]
44. Kurella Tamura, M.; Covinsky, K.E.; Chertow, G.M.; Yaffe, K.; Landefeld, C.S.; McCulloch, C.E. Functional status of elderly adults before and after initiation of dialysis. *N. Engl. J. Med.* **2009**, *361*, 1539–1547. [CrossRef] [PubMed]
45. Sterky, E.; Stegmayr, B.G. Elderly patients on haemodialysis have 50% less functional capacity than gender- and age-matched healthy subjects. *Scand. J. Urol. Nephrol.* **2005**, *39*, 423–430. [CrossRef]
46. Johansen, K.L.; Chertow, G.M.; Jin, C.; Kutner, N.G. Significance of frailty among dialysis patients. *J. Am. Soc. Nephrol.* **2007**, *18*, 2960–2967. [CrossRef]
47. Fried, L.P.; Tangen, C.M.; Walston, J.; Newman, A.B.; Hirsch, C.; Gottdiener, J.; Seeman, T.; Tracy, R.; Kop, W.J.; Burke, G.; et al. Frailty in older adults: Evidence for a phenotype. *J. Gerontol. Ser. A Biol. Sci. Med. Sci.* **2001**, *56*, M146–M156. [CrossRef]
48. Morley, J.E.; Vellas, B.; van Kan, G.A.; Anker, S.D.; Bauer, J.M.; Bernabei, R.; Cesari, M.; Chumlea, W.C.; Doehner, W.; Evans, J.; et al. Frailty consensus: A call to action. *J. Am. Med. Dir. Assoc.* **2013**, *14*, 392–397. [CrossRef] [PubMed]
49. Satake, S.; Shimada, H.; Yamada, M.; Kim, H.; Yoshida, H.; Gondo, Y.; Matsubayashi, K.; Matsushita, E.; Kuzuya, M.; Kozaki, K.; et al. Prevalence of frailty among community-dwellers and outpatients in Japan as defined by the Japanese version of the Cardiovascular Health Study criteria. *Geriatr. Gerontol. Int.* **2017**, *17*, 2629–2634. [CrossRef] [PubMed]
50. Ma, L.; Sun, F.; Tang, Z. Social Frailty Is Associated with Physical Functioning, Cognition, and Depression, and Predicts Mortality. *J. Nutr. Health Aging* **2018**, *22*, 989–995. [CrossRef] [PubMed]
51. Panza, F.; Solfrizzi, V.; Barulli, M.R.; Santamato, A.; Seripa, D.; Pilotto, A.; Logroscino, G. Cognitive Frailty: A Systematic Review of Epidemiological and Neurobiological Evidence of an Age-Related Clinical Condition. *Rejuvenation Res.* **2015**, *18*, 389–412. [CrossRef]
52. Tentori, F.; Elder, S.J.; Thumma, J.; Pisoni, R.L.; Bommer, J.; Fissell, R.B.; Fukuhara, S.; Jadoul, M.; Keen, M.L.; Saran, R.; et al. Physical exercise among participants in the Dialysis Outcomes and Practice Patterns Study (DOPPS): Correlates and associated outcomes. *Nephrol. Dial. Transplant.* **2010**, *25*, 3050–3062. [CrossRef]
53. Hoshino, J.; Muenz, D.; Zee, J.; Sukul, N.; Speyer, E.; Guedes, M.; Lopes, A.A.; Asahi, K.; van Haalen, H.; James, G.; et al. Associations of Hemoglobin Levels With Health-Related Quality of Life, Physical Activity, and Clinical Outcomes in Persons With Stage 3-5 Nondialysis CKD. *J. Ren. Nutr.* **2020**. [CrossRef] [PubMed]
54. Chen, I.R.; Wang, S.M.; Liang, C.C.; Kuo, H.L.; Chang, C.T.; Liu, J.H.; Lin, H.H.; Wang, I.K.; Yang, Y.F.; Chou, C.Y.; et al. Association of Walking with Survival and RRT Among Patients with CKD Stages 3–5. *Clin. J. Am. Soc. Nephrol.* **2014**. [CrossRef]
55. Matsuzawa, R.; Matsunaga, A.; Wang, G.; Kutsuna, T.; Ishii, A.; Abe, Y.; Takagi, Y.; Yoshida, A.; Takahira, N. Habitual physical activity measured by accelerometer and survival in maintenance hemodialysis patients. *Clin. J. Am. Soc. Nephrol.* **2012**, *7*, 2010–2016. [CrossRef] [PubMed]
56. Beddhu, S.; Wei, G.; Marcus, R.L.; Chonchol, M.; Greene, T. Light-intensity physical activities and mortality in the United States general population and CKD subpopulation. *Clin. J. Am. Soc. Nephrol.* **2015**, *10*, 1145–1153. [CrossRef] [PubMed]
57. Robinson-Cohen, C.; Littman, A.J.; Duncan, G.E.; Roshanravan, B.; Ikizler, T.A.; Himmelfarb, J.; Kestenbaum, B.R. Assessment of physical activity in chronic kidney disease. *J. Ren. Nutr. Off. J. Counc. Ren. Nutr. Natl. Kidney Found.* **2013**, *23*, 123–131. [CrossRef]
58. Wasserman, K.; Kessel, A.; Burton, G. Interaction of Physiological Mechanisms During Exercise. *J. Appl. Physiol.* **1967**, *22*, 71–85. [CrossRef]

59. Mezzani, A.; Hamm, L.F.; Jones, A.M.; McBride, P.E.; Moholdt, T.; Stone, J.A.; Urhausen, A.; Williams, M.A. Aerobic exercise intensity assessment and prescription in cardiac rehabilitation: A joint position statement of the European Association for Cardiovascular Prevention and Rehabilitation, the American Association of Cardiovascular and Pulmonary Rehabilitation, and the Canadian Association of Cardiac Rehabilitation. *J. Cardiopulm. Rehabil. Prev.* **2012**, *32*, 327–350. [CrossRef]
60. Balady Gary, J.; Arena, R.; Sietsema, K.; Myers, J.; Coke, L.; Fletcher Gerald, F.; Forman, D.; Franklin, B.; Guazzi, M.; Gulati, M.; et al. Clinician's Guide to Cardiopulmonary Exercise Testing in Adults. *Circulation* **2010**, *122*, 191–225. [CrossRef]
61. Gulati, M.; Black, H.R.; Arnsdorf, M.F.; Shaw, L.J.; Bakris, G.L. Kidney dysfunction, cardiorespiratory fitness, and the risk of death in women. *J. Womens Health* **2012**, *21*, 917–924. [CrossRef]
62. Berg, J.M.; Tymoczko, J.A.; Stryer, L. *Biochemistry*, 6th ed.; W. H. Freeman and Company: New York, NY, USA, 2008.
63. Wilkinson, D.J.; Hossain, T.; Hill, D.S.; Phillips, B.E.; Crossland, H.; Williams, J.; Loughna, P.; Churchward-Venne, T.A.; Breen, L.; Phillips, S.M.; et al. Effects of leucine and its metabolite β-hydroxy-β-methylbutyrate on human skeletal muscle protein metabolism. *J. Physiol.* **2013**, *591*, 2911–2923. [CrossRef]
64. Margolis, L.M.; Allen, J.T.; Hatch-McChesney, A.; Pasiakos, S.M. Coingestion of Carbohydrate and Protein on Muscle Glycogen Synthesis after Exercise: A Meta-analysis. *Med. Sci. Sports Exerc.* **2021**, *53*, 384–393. [CrossRef]
65. Thomas, D.T.; Erdman, K.A.; Burke, L.M. American College of Sports Medicine Joint Position Statement. Nutrition and Athletic Performance. *Med. Sci. Sports Exerc.* **2016**, *48*, 543–568. [CrossRef] [PubMed]
66. Johansen, K.L.; Shubert, T.; Doyle, J.; Soher, B.; Sakkas, G.K.; Kent-Braun, J.A. Muscle atrophy in patients receiving hemodialysis: Effects on muscle strength, muscle quality, and physical function. *Kidney Int.* **2003**, *63*, 291–297. [CrossRef] [PubMed]
67. Molina, P.; Carrero, J.J.; Bover, J.; Chauveau, P.; Mazzaferro, S.; Torres, P.U. Vitamin D, a modulator of musculoskeletal health in chronic kidney disease. *J. Cachexia Sarcopenia Muscle* **2017**, *8*, 686–701. [CrossRef]
68. Rhee, C.M.; Kalantar-Zadeh, K. Resistance exercise: An effective strategy to reverse muscle wasting in hemodialysis patients? *J. Cachexia Sarcopenia Muscle* **2014**, *5*, 177–180. [CrossRef]
69. Wang, X.H.; Mitch, W.E. Mechanisms of muscle wasting in chronic kidney disease. *Nat. Rev. Nephrol.* **2014**, *10*, 504–516. [CrossRef]
70. Nakamura, S.; Sato, Y.; Kobayashi, T.; Kaneko, Y.; Ito, E.; Soma, H.; Okada, H.; Miyamoto, K.; Oya, A.; Matsumoto, M.; et al. Vitamin D protects against immobilization-induced muscle atrophy via neural crest-derived cells in mice. *Sci. Rep.* **2020**, *10*, 12242. [CrossRef] [PubMed]
71. Haas, J.D.; Brownlie, T.t. Iron deficiency and reduced work capacity: A critical review of the research to determine a causal relationship. *J. Nutr.* **2001**, *131*, 676S–688S, discussion 688S–690S. [CrossRef] [PubMed]
72. Sato, E.; Mori, T.; Mishima, E.; Suzuki, A.; Sugawara, N.; Kurasawa, N.; Saigusa, D.; Miura, D.; Morikawa-Ichinose, T.; Saito, R.; et al. Metabolic alterations by indoxyl sulfate in skeletal muscle induce uremic sarcopenia in chronic kidney disease. *Sci. Rep.* **2016**, *6*, 36618. [CrossRef]
73. Nishikawa, M.; Ishimori, N.; Takada, S.; Saito, A.; Kadoguchi, T.; Furihata, T.; Fukushima, A.; Matsushima, S.; Yokota, T.; Kinugawa, S.; et al. AST-120 ameliorates lowered exercise capacity and mitochondrial biogenesis in the skeletal muscle from mice with chronic kidney disease via reducing oxidative stress. *Nephrol. Dial. Transplant.* **2015**, *30*, 934–942. [CrossRef]
74. Deger, S.M.; Hung, A.M.; Ellis, C.D.; Booker, C.; Bian, A.; Chen, G.; Abumrad, N.N.; Ikizler, T.A. High Dose Omega-3 Fatty Acid Administration and Skeletal Muscle Protein Turnover in Maintenance Hemodialysis Patients. *Clin. J. Am. Soc. Nephrol.* **2016**, *11*, 1227–1235. [CrossRef]
75. Shinaberger, C.S.; Greenland, S.; Kopple, J.D.; Van Wyck, D.; Mehrotra, R.; Kovesdy, C.P.; Kalantar-Zadeh, K. Is controlling phosphorus by decreasing dietary protein intake beneficial or harmful in persons with chronic kidney disease. *Am. J. Clin. Nutr.* **2008**, *88*, 1511–1518. [CrossRef]
76. O'Hare, A.M.; Tawney, K.; Bacchetti, P.; Johansen, K.L. Decreased survival among sedentary patients undergoing dialysis: Results from the dialysis morbidity and mortality study wave 2. *Am. J. Kidney Dis.* **2003**, *41*, 447–454. [CrossRef]
77. Yurtkuran, M.; Alp, A.; Yurtkuran, M.; Dilek, K. A modified yoga-based exercise program in hemodialysis patients: A randomized controlled study. *Complementary Ther. Med.* **2007**, *15*, 164–171. [CrossRef] [PubMed]
78. Johansen, K.L.; Painter, P. Exercise in individuals with CKD. *Am. J. Kidney Dis.* **2012**, *59*, 126–134. [CrossRef]
79. The_Japanese_Society_of_Renal_Rehabilitation. *Guideline for Renal Rehabilitation*; Nankodo: Tokyo, Japan, 2018.
80. Sheng, K.; Zhang, P.; Chen, L.; Cheng, J.; Wu, C.; Chen, J. Intradialytic exercise in hemodialysis patients: A systematic review and meta-analysis. *Am. J. Nephrol.* **2014**, *40*, 478–490. [CrossRef]
81. Kornhauser, C.; Malacara, J.-M.; Macías-Cervantes, M.-H.; Rivera-Cisneros, A.-E. Effect of exercise intensity on albuminuria in adolescents with Type 1 diabetes mellitus. *Diabet. Med. A J. Br. Diabet. Assoc.* **2012**, *29*, 70–73. [CrossRef] [PubMed]
82. Peng, H.; Wang, Q.; Lou, T.; Qin, J.; Jung, S.; Shetty, V.; Li, F.; Wang, Y.; Feng, X.H.; Mitch, W.E.; et al. Myokine mediated muscle-kidney crosstalk suppresses metabolic reprogramming and fibrosis in damaged kidneys. *Nat. Commun.* **2017**, *8*, 1493. [CrossRef] [PubMed]
83. Ito, D.; Cao, P.; Kakihana, T.; Sato, E.; Suda, C.; Muroya, Y.; Ogawa, Y.; Hu, G.; Ishii, T.; Ito, O.; et al. Chronic Running Exercise Alleviates Early Progression of Nephropathy with Upregulation of Nitric Oxide Synthases and Suppression of Glycation in Zucker Diabetic Rats. *PLoS ONE* **2015**, *10*, e0138037. [CrossRef]
84. Group, J.C.S.J.W. Guidelines for Rehabilitation in Patients With Cardiovascular Disease (JCS 2012)—Digest Version—. *Circ. J.* **2014**, *78*, 2022–2093. [CrossRef]

85. Aging, N. Four Types of Exercise Can Improve Your Health and Physical Ability. Available online: https://www.nia.nih.gov/health/four-types-exercise-can-improve-your-health-and-physical-ability#:~{}:text=Research%20has%20shown%20that%20it%E2%80%99s%20important%20to%20get,variety%20helps%20reduce%20boredom%20and%20risk%20of%20injury (accessed on 19 April 2021).
86. Hellberg, M.; Hoglund, P.; Svensson, P.; Clyne, N. Randomized Controlled Trial of Exercise in CKD-The RENEXC Study. *Kidney Int. Rep.* **2019**, *4*, 963–976. [CrossRef] [PubMed]
87. Zhou, Y.; Hellberg, M.; Hellmark, T.; Hoglund, P.; Clyne, N. Muscle mass and plasma myostatin after exercise training: A substudy of Renal Exercise (RENEXC)-a randomized controlled trial. *Nephrol. Dial. Transplant.* **2019**. [CrossRef]
88. Clarke, A.L.; Young, H.M.; Hull, K.L.; Hudson, N.; Burton, J.O.; Smith, A.C. Motivations and barriers to exercise in chronic kidney disease: A qualitative study. *Nephrol. Dial. Transplant.* **2015**, *30*, 1885–1892. [CrossRef]
89. Abdel-Kader, K.; Unruh, M.L.; Weisbord, S.D. Symptom burden, depression, and quality of life in chronic and end-stage kidney disease. *Clin. J. Am. Soc. Nephrol.* **2009**, *4*, 1057–1064. [CrossRef]
90. Tong, A.; Manns, B.; Wang, A.Y.M.; Hemmelgarn, B.; Wheeler, D.C.; Gill, J.; Tugwell, P.; Pecoits-Filho, R.; Crowe, S.; Harris, T.; et al. Implementing core outcomes in kidney disease: Report of the Standardized Outcomes in Nephrology (SONG) implementation workshop. *Kidney Int.* **2018**, *94*, 1053–1068. [CrossRef] [PubMed]
91. Moorman, D.; Suri, R.; Hiremath, S.; Jegatheswaran, J.; Kumar, T.; Bugeja, A.; Zimmerman, D. Benefits and Barriers to and Desired Outcomes with Exercise in Patients with ESKD. *Clin. J. Am. Soc. Nephrol.* **2019**, *14*, 268–276. [CrossRef] [PubMed]

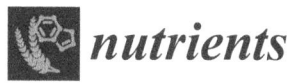

Review

Significance of Adipose Tissue Maintenance in Patients Undergoing Hemodialysis

Senji Okuno

Kidney Center, Shirasagi Hospital, 7-11-23, Kumata, Higashisumiyoshi-ku, Osaka 546-0002, Japan; okuno@shirasagi-hp.or.jp; Tel.: +81-6-6714-1661

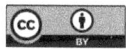

Citation: Okuno, S. Significance of Adipose Tissue Maintenance in Patients Undergoing Hemodialysis. *Nutrients* 2021, 13, 1895. https://doi.org/10.3390/nu13061895

Academic Editor: Antonio Brunetti

Received: 6 April 2021
Accepted: 27 May 2021
Published: 31 May 2021

Publisher's Note: MDPI stays neutral with regard to jurisdictional claims in published maps and institutional affiliations.

Copyright: © 2021 by the author. Licensee MDPI, Basel, Switzerland. This article is an open access article distributed under the terms and conditions of the Creative Commons Attribution (CC BY) license (https://creativecommons.org/licenses/by/4.0/).

Abstract: In the general population, obesity is known to be associated with adverse outcomes, including mortality. In contrast, high body mass index (BMI) may provide a survival advantage for hemodialysis patients, which is known as the obesity paradox. Although BMI is the most commonly used measure for the assessment of obesity, it does not distinguish between fat and lean mass. Fat mass is considered to serve as an energy reserve against a catabolic condition, while the capacity to survive starvation is also thought to be dependent on its amount. Thus, fat mass is used as a nutritional marker. For example, improvement of nutritional status by nutritional intervention or initiation of hemodialysis is associated with an increase in fat mass. Several studies have shown that higher levels of fat mass were associated with better survival in hemodialysis patients. Based on body distribution, fat mass is classified into subcutaneous and visceral fat. Visceral fat is metabolically more active and associated with metabolic abnormalities and inflammation, and it is thus considered to be a risk factor for cardiovascular disease and mortality. On the other hand, subcutaneous fat has not been consistently linked to adverse phenomena and may reflect nutritional status as a type of energy storage. Visceral and subcutaneous adipose tissues have different metabolic and inflammatory characteristics and may have opposing influences on various outcomes, including mortality. Results showing an association between increased subcutaneous fat and better survival, along with other conditions, such as cancer or cirrhosis, in hemodialysis patients have been reported. This evidence suggests that fat mass distribution (i.e., visceral fat and subcutaneous fat) plays a more important role for these beneficial effects in hemodialysis patients.

Keywords: fat mass; visceral fat; subcutaneous fat; nutrition; mortality; body mass index; obesity paradox

1. Introduction

In patients with chronic kidney disease (CKD), especially those undergoing maintenance hemodialysis therapy, poor nutritional status is a common and important complication. Various terms and definitions have been applied for conditions associated with malnutrition, such as loss of muscle and fat tissue, and inflammation, including uremic malnutrition [1], protein–energy malnutrition [2], malnutrition–inflammation atherosclerosis syndrome [3], and malnutrition–inflammation complex syndrome [4]. To avoid confusion, the International Society of Renal Nutrition and Metabolism (ISRNM) has recommended the term protein–energy wasting (PEW) [5]. The four main established categories now recognized for diagnosis of PEW are biochemical criteria and include low body weight and reduced total body fat, weight loss, decrease in muscle mass, and low protein or energy intake.

Several studies have shown that PEW is a significant risk factor for low quality of life, muscle weakness, hospitalization, and mortality; thus, nutritional assessment of hemodialysis patients is important to avoid development and progression of PEW. Body fat mass is considered to be a nutritional parameter, since low fat mass is one of the factors examined for diagnosis of PEW. In the general population, an increase in fat mass, particularly visceral fat mass, is considered to be a risk factor for cardiovascular disease (CVD) and mortality, whereas in hemodialysis patients, such an increase may represent improved nutritional status and better survival. This review focuses on the associations of fat mass and its distribution (i.e., visceral fat and subcutaneous fat) with outcomes, particularly mortality, in patients undergoing hemodialysis. The purpose of this article is to clarify an ambiguous role of fat mass, so-called reverse epidemiology, with the difference among the general population and hemodialysis patients. The search terms I used to collect the bibliography were fat mass, adipose tissue, obesity, dialysis, kidney, mortality, and nutrition. A comprehensive literature search was preformed using PubMed from January 1980 to January 2021.

2. Higher Body Mass Index Is Related to Better Survival in Hemodialysis Patients

Obesity, primarily defined by excess body fat mass, is highly prevalent and increasing worldwide and has been found to be associated with serious outcomes, including diabetes, hypertension, CVD, and mortality [6,7]. Body mass index (BMI) is considered to be a reasonably good measure of general adiposity, and thus, the most common method for defining obesity is based on that. Despite the high risk of adverse outcomes in the general population, high BMI may be associated with a survival advantage in CKD patients, which is known as the obesity paradox or reverse epidemiology of obesity [8,9]. Other than CKD, the obesity paradox has also been observed in various clinical settings, including cases of chronic heart failure [10], chronic obstructive pulmonary disease [11], and cancer [12], as well as elderly patients [13].

In 1982, Degoulet et al. reported that high BMI in 1453 French hemodialysis patients was not associated with cardiovascular mortality or all-cause mortality [14]. Using data from the United States Renal Data System (USRDS), Leavey et al. also found no evidence of increased mortality risk related to higher values of BMI in 3607 hemodialysis patients (BMI 24.4 ± 5.3 kg/m^2 (mean $\pm$ SE)) in follow-up examinations conducted over a five-year period [15]. In another study, Fleischmann et al. noted that compared with normal-weight (BMI 20–27.5 kg/m^2), the one-year survival rate was significantly greater in overweight hemodialysis patients (BMI $\geq$ 27.5 kg/m^2, 38% of 1346 patients), a paradoxical finding when compared to the general population [16]. Additionally, that study showed that with a one-unit increase in BMI over 27.5 kg/m^2, the relative risk for mortality was reduced by 30% ($p < 0.04$).

Johansen et al. investigated the relationship between BMI and survival in USRDS data obtained for 418,055 patients who had started hemodialysis [17]. They found that high BMI was associated with increased survival over a two-year averaged follow-up period after adjustments for demographic, laboratory, and comorbidity data, even in subjects with extremely high BMI. Furthermore, high BMI was also associated with reduced risk of hospitalization. These results were observed for Caucasian, African American, and Hispanic subjects, but not for Asians. Additionally, alternative estimates of adiposity, including the Benn index and estimated fat mass, yielded similar results, and adjustments for lean body mass did not substantially alter the findings. A meta-analysis was also conducted, which showed that for every 1 kg/m^2 increase in BMI, the reduction in risk of all-cause mortality was 3% (hazard ratio (HR) 0.97; 95% CI 0.96–0.98, n = 89,332), and the risk of cardiovascular mortality was reduced by 4% (HR 0.96; 95% CI 0.92–1.00, n = 8918) in the study cohort [18].

Hemodialysis patients can often experience fluctuations in body weight resulting from changes in dietary intake and comorbidity status, and several studies have shown that body weight changes are strongly associated with mortality [19]. Chazot et al. conducted a prospective observational study of 5592 incident hemodialysis patients (age 64.4 ± 16.5 years, 40.9% females, 27.7% diabetics) in Southern Europe who were followed for 2.0 ± 1.6 years [20]. The four categories used for baseline BMI—underweight, normal range, overweight, and obese—were found to significantly influence survival. With the normal BMI range used as a reference, HR (95% CI) was 0.74 (0.67–0.90) for overweight and 0.78 (0.56–0.87) for obese patients, suggesting an association of higher BMI, even in obese subjects, with better survival. Moreover, when compared to patients in whom body weight remained stable during the first year after initiation of hemodialysis, survival was significantly lower in those with a decrease in body weight (less than −5.8% in one year) with an HR of 1.60 (95% CI 1.20–2.14).

Kalantar-Zadeh et al. explored the effects of both baseline and changes in BMI on all-cause and cardiovascular mortality in a two-year study of 54,535 patients receiving maintenance hemodialysis in the United States (age 61.7 ± 15.5 years, 54% males, 45% diabetics) [21]. They found that obesity, including morbid obesity, was associated with better survival and reduced cardiovascular death even after accounting for changes in BMI and laboratory values over time. In examinations of the regression slope of change in weight over time, progressively worsening loss was associated with poor survival, whereas weight gain showed a tendency for decreased cardiovascular death.

Chang et al. examined the association of changes in body weight after initiation of hemodialysis treatment with all-cause mortality in a study conducted in the United States that included 58,106 patients [22]. Compared with the reference group (−2% to 2% weight change occurring between first and fifth months), the mortality HR (95% CI) value during the first five months for patients with −6% to −2% weight loss was 1.08 (1.02–1.14), while that in those with greater than or equal to −6% weight loss was 1.14 (1.07–1.22). When weight changes from 5 to 12 months were considered, the association between such change and mortality was even stronger. Each 4% increase in weight between the 5th and 12th months was associated with an HR value of 0.92 (95% CI 0.90–0.93; $p < 0.001$), whereas the same degree of weight change was associated with an HR value of 0.96 (95% CI 0.95–0.98; $p < 0.001$) over the first 5 months.

Doshi et al. examined the association between BMI and all-cause mortality in a study of 123,624 adult maintenance hemodialysis patients in the United States (age 61 ± 15 years, 45% females, 32% African Americans) using marginal structural model analysis, a technique that accounts for time-varying confounders [23]. They confirmed that BMI had a linear incremental inverse association with mortality. In marginal structural model analysis results, as compared with the reference (BMI 25 to <27.5 kg/m^2), BMI < 18 kg/m^2 was associated with 3.2-fold higher death risk (HR 3.17; 95% CI 3.05–3.29), while mortality risk declined with increasing BMI, with the greatest survival advantage, 31% lower risk (HR 0.69; 95% CI 0.64–0.75), observed in patients with a BMI value ranging from 40 to <45 kg/m^2.

Stenvinkel et al. examined the relationship between BMI and all-cause mortality in 5904 European incident hemodialysis patients, accounting for inflammation [24]. Patients were classified based on the presence ($n = 3231$) or absence ($n = 2673$) of inflammation (defined as C-reactive protein ≥ 10 mg/L and/or albumin ≤ 35 g/L) and then further divided into quintiles by BMI. Higher BMI was associated with lower mortality risk in patients with inflammation, whereas no protective effect was associated with the higher BMI quintile in patients without inflammation. In the Dialysis Outcomes and Practice Patterns Study (DOPPS), Leavey et al. evaluated relationships between BMI and mortality in hemodialysis subpopulations defined by continent, ethnicity, gender, tertile of illness severity (based on a score derived from comorbid conditions and serum albumin concentration), age, smoking, and diabetic status [25]. The relative mortality risk was found to decrease with increasing BMI. That result was statistically significant in all subjects, except for the smallest subgroup of patients who were <45 years old and also in the healthiest tertile of comorbidity.

It has also been reported that the association between weight change and mortality is less apparent in obese hemodialysis patients. In 6296 European patients with prospective data collected every 6 months for 3 years (age 64 ± 14 years, 61% males, 31% diabetics, BMI: 25.3 ± 4.9 kg/m^2), Cabezas-Rodriguez et al. examined the influence of BMI on the association of short-term weight change with mortality [26]. Compared with stable weight (±1%), weight loss (>1% weight decline) in the whole cohort was strongly associated with higher mortality, while weight gain (>1% weight increase) had an association with lower mortality. After stratification by BMI categories, this remained true when nonobese categories were used, especially in underweight patients. As for obese patients, the association of weight loss with mortality was attenuated and no longer statistically significant (HR 1.28; 95% CI 0.74–2.14), and no survival benefit was seen in association with gaining weight (HR 0.98; 95% CI 0.59–1.62), indicating potential resistance to the development of wasting in obese hemodialysis patients. These results suggested that the association between body size and mortality in hemodialysis patients might be affected by baseline health and nutritional status.

Previous studies of the association between BMI and mortality have shown conflicting results obtained with nondialysis-dependent CKD patients [27]. Madero et al. reported that high BMI had no protective effect on 1759 CKD patients with a mean estimated glomerular filtration rate (eGFR) of 39 ± 21 mL/min/1.73 m^2 [28]. In 920 Swedish patients with advanced kidney dysfunction (serum creatinine level >3.4 mg/dL in males, >2.8 mg/dL in females), Evans et al. reported that high BMI was associated with lower mortality [29]. Similarly, in a study of 521 male veterans in the United States with CKD (age 68.8 ± 10.4 years, eGFR 37.5 ± 16.8 mL/min/1.73 m^2), Kovesdy et al. reported that higher BMI was associated with lower mortality in groups with BMI in the 10th to 50th, 50th to 90th, and >90th percentiles versus the <10th percentile, noting values of 0.75 (95% CI 0.46–1.22), 0.56 (95% CI 0.33–0.94), and 0.39 (95% CI 0.17–0.87), respectively [30]. Lu et al. examined the associations of BMI with all-course mortality and disease progression in a cohort of 453,946 United States veterans with nondialysis-dependent CKD (eGFR < 60 mL/min/1.73 m^2) [31]. Their results showed a relatively consistent U-shaped association of BMI with clinical outcomes. For example, BMI $\geq$ 35 mg/m^2 was associated with worse outcome in patients with an earlier stage of CKD, while that association was attenuated in those with eGFR < 30 mL/min/1.73 m^2.

3. Determination of Visceral and Subcutaneous Fat and Muscle Mass

BMI is the most commonly used measure for the assessment of obesity in both research and clinical practice, though it does not distinguish between fat and lean mass [32,33]. Thus, even though greater BMI has beneficial effects for survival, fat and lean mass should be separately evaluated to elucidate the association of body composition with mortality.

Anthropometry is widely used for determining body composition because of its ease to use, wide availability, low cost, and favorable safety profile, though fluid status has been shown to influence calculations in hemodialysis patients [34,35]. Mid-arm circumference (MAC) and mid-arm muscle circumference (MAMC) are anthropometric methods developed to assess lean body mass, while skinfold thickness (SFT) at four sites (triceps, biceps, subscapular, ileac crest) is used to assess total body fat mass. For assessing abdominal obesity, waist circumference, waist-to-hip ratio, and waist-to-height ratio are applied. Kamimura et al. evaluated body fat mass using skinfold thickness and a bioelectrical impedance analysis (BIA) technique in 90 clinically stable hemodialysis patients. Body fat mass measurements based on skinfold thickness (13.5 ± 6.2 kg) and BIA (13.7 ± 6.7 kg) were similar, and strong correlations were found between results obtained with these two methods (r = 0.87) [36]. Oe et al. also noted that values for lean mass and fat mass obtained via skinfold anthropometry and BIA were significantly correlated [37].

BIA, a noninvasive rapid and reliable method with low cost, is also commonly used to evaluate body composition for both epidemiological and clinical purposes [38]. A principle of BIA techniques is that the transit time of a low-voltage electric current through the body is dependent on body composition characteristics [39].

Dual energy X-ray absorptiometry (DXA) is considered to be a more accurate and reliable reference method for measurements of fat and lean mass. With this method, the differential of two X-ray beams as they pass through the body is determined so as to distinguish bone from soft tissue, then the findings are subsequently used to divide soft tissue mass into fat and fat-free soft-tissue mass (lean mass). However, measurements of lean mass by DXA are influenced by hydration, whereas that has scarce effects on fat mass measurements [40,41]. Reproducibility of fat mass measurements by DXA has also been shown to be excellent, with variations <2% among patients undergoing hemodialysis [42]. Nishizawa et al. showed that DXA-determined fat mass index (kg/m^2) in 104 patients undergoing hemodialysis (age 53.9 ± 9.1 years, hemodialysis duration 7.5 ± 5.1 years, 39 males and 64 females) was 5.2 ± 0.2 kg/m^2, significantly lower than the value obtained with 167 age- and gender-matched healthy control subjects of 5.8 ± 0.2 kg/m^2 (age 52.9 ± 9.0 years, 53 males and 114 females) ($p < 0.05$) [42].

The most reliable methods for determining body composition in clinical practice might be computed tomography (CT) and magnetic resonance imaging (MRI) [35], as both can be utilized to assess fat mass distribution and also distinguish between subcutaneous and visceral fat with direct measurements. The results obtained are accurate and reproducible as compared with simulated phantom studies. However, CT and MRI are impractical for general population screening due to their high cost, and CT exposes the subject to radiation. Although DXA cannot directly discriminate between visceral and subcutaneous fat, visceral fat mass estimated by DXA has been shown to be strongly correlated with the visceral fat area determined by CT and visceral fat mass by MRI [43].

4. Fat Mass—A Useful Nutritional Marker and Its Significance for Survival

It is considered that fat mass may serve as an energy reserve against a catabolic condition, and the capacity to survive starvation has also been shown to be dependent on its amount [44]. In obese model rats developed by a high-fat diet, increased fat mass provided fuel availability and conservation of lean mass with starvation compared to control rats [45]. Therefore, fat mass is regarded as an important indicator of nutritional status in hemodialysis patients. Additionally, low fat mass, one of the characteristics examined for PEW diagnosis [5], is often complicated in hemodialysis patients and thought to contribute to the high rates of morbidity and mortality observed in those cases. Consequently, it is assumed that fat mass is decreased in hemodialysis patients with PEW. In a study of 468 prevalent hemodialysis patients (median age 66 years, median hemodialysis duration 37 months, 34% females, 50% diabetics), Anton-Perez et al. reported the results of a multivariate regression analysis showing a linear inverse relationship between lower fat mass determined by BIA with a greater number of PEW syndrome categories [46]. Similarly, in 186 advanced CKD patients (age 66.1 ± 16 years, 101 males and 85 females), Perez-Torres et al. found that the prevalence of PEW was 30.1% and evidence of lower fat mass in PEW patients [47].

Various clinical and biochemical parameters can be used to evaluate nutritional status in individuals with CKD. Among nutritional scoring systems, subjective global assessment (SGA) and malnutrition–inflammation score (MIS) are often utilized. SGA is based on a combination of subjective and objective features obtained from patient medical history and physical examination findings. In a comparison of SGA with nutritional status determined by total-body nitrogen, which directly quantifies body protein content, SGA was shown to be able to differentiate severely malnourished dialysis patients from those with normal nutrition [48]. A modified version of SGA was used in the DOPPS, which found that lower values obtained with that modified version were associated with higher risk of mortality in hemodialysis patients [49]. Kalantar-Zadeh et al. examined 41 hemodialysis patients (age 57 ± 12 years, hemodialysis duration 3.0 ± 2.1 years, males 49%) using the modified SGA system and showed that subcutaneous fat mass assessed by biceps skinfold thickness was significantly negatively correlated with malnutrition score [50]. In another study, Paudel et al. found that 96 (21%) of 455 peritoneal dialysis patients were malnourished, based on an SGA score between 1 and 5, and those malnourished patients exhibited a significantly lower fat tissue index determined by BIA [51]. In a study of 1334 older adults (age ≥ 65 years) not receiving dialysis with advanced CKD and an eGFR <20 mL/min/1.73 m^2, Windahl et al. reported that fat mass was decreased according to the SGA subscale [52].

MIS is an adaptation of SGA for hemodialysis patients and has 10 components derived from medical history, physical examination findings, BMI, and laboratory parameters such as serum albumin and transferrin level [53]. Studies have shown that MIS results can be used to predict poor outcome in hemodialysis, peritoneal dialysis, and nondialyzed CKD patients [54,55]. Wang et al. investigated 144 CKD stage 1–4 patients (median age 53 years; IQR 38–63 years, 94 males and 50 females) and reported that MIS was negatively correlated with BIA-measured fat tissue index ($r = -0.179$, $p = 0.032$) [56]. In another study that included 91 patients (age 60 ± 14 years, 70.3% males, BMI 24 ± 4.1 kg/m^2) being treated with hemodialysis, Arias-Guillen et al. compared body composition evaluated by BIA between groups with or without PEW with that defined as MIS above 5 and reported that subjects with PEW showed a significantly lower fat tissue index [57].

5. Factors Affecting Fat Mass Changes

5.1. Nutritional Support

Several studies have shown that nutritional interventions, such as oral nutritional supplementation and intradialytic parenteral nutrition, can improve the nutritional status of hemodialysis patients [58]. Pupim et al. reported that protein turnover study results showed a highly positive whole body net balance during hemodialysis for both intradialytic parenteral nutrition and oral supplementation as compared with a control group [59]. In addition, skeletal muscle protein homeostasis examined during the hemodialysis session was also found to be improved with both intradialytic parenteral nutrition and oral supplementation. Furthermore, Fouque et al. found that use of energy-dense phosphate-restricted renal-specific oral supplementation in hemodialysis patients with low protein intake resulted in improved SGA and quality of life [60].

Improvement of nutritional status with oral supplementation is also indicated by an increase in fat mass, with fat mass change considered to function as a parameter indicating nutritional changes. Caetano et al. investigated the effects of intradialytic oral supplementation along with a protein-rich meal on body composition in 99 hemodialysis patients with a serum albumin level <38 g/L (age 69.9 ± 12.9 years, hemodialysis duration 60.0 ± 50.0 months) [61]. In the intervention group, patients ate a protein-rich meal during each treatment session for six months, while the control group ingested their usual snack brought from home. Although lean mass was decreased in both the intervention and control groups, fat mass at the end of the study was significantly increased in the intervention group in contrast to a decline in the control. Similarly, in 36 patients undergoing hemodialysis, Martin-Alemany et al. found that fat mass assessed by triceps skinfold thickness was significantly increased in association with oral nutritional supplementation or that and resistance exercise for a period of 12 weeks [62].

Nutritional supplementation may also improve survival of hemodialysis patients. Weiner et al. reported that oral protein supplementation given during the dialysis procedure was associated with a 29% reduction in risk of all-cause mortality (HR 0.71; 95% CI 0.58–0.86) in hemodialysis patients with a serum albumin level ≤ 3.5 g/dL [63]. Similarly, Lacson et al. found mortality risk decreased to 0.91 (95% CI 0.85–0.98) in intention-to-treat analysis and 0.66 (95% CI 0.61–0.71) in as-treated analysis, after adjustment for confounding factors, in hemodialysis patients with serum albumin ≤ 3.5 g/dL [64]. These results suggest that fat mass increased by nutritional supplementation in hemodialysis patients might be associated with survival improvement.

5.2. Initiation of Hemodialysis

Following initiation of hemodialysis, most patients generally gain a sense of improved wellbeing and better appetite, as most symptoms associated with uremia, such as loss of appetite, nausea, and general fatigue, are diminished or disappear. Thus, it is considered that nutritional status is improved by initiation of hemodialysis, and in an investigation of a stable cohort, Goldwasser et al. reported that serum albumin and creatinine levels rose by 12% to 13% during the first half-year of hemodialysis [65]. Fat mass as a nutritional marker may also increase following initiation of hemodialysis because of improved nutritional status. We conducted a study of changes in fat mass in hemodialysis patients and found that it was increased in the first year after initiation of treatment [66]. In 72 patients with

CKD (age 62 ± 12 years, 42 males and 30 females), body fat mass was determined by DXA at one month after initiation of maintenance hemodialysis and again approximately one year later. The second measurement showed significantly greater fat (11.38 ± 3.84 vs. 10.09 ± 4.12 kg, $p < 0.0001$). Additionally, change in fat mass per month was negatively correlated with baseline serum albumin concentration ($r = -0.449$; $p < 0.0001$) and basal fat mass ($r = -0.423$; $p < 0.001$). Our results suggested that fat mass increase after initiation of hemodialysis may be greater in patients with worse initial nutritional status. In a study of 8227 incident hemodialysis patients, Marcelli et al. also found that fat mass index evaluated by BIA was increased by approximately 0.95 kg/m^2 in the first 2 years after the start of hemodialysis [67]. Similar to our results, in addition to female gender and diabetes status, basal fat mass index was found to be associated with a significantly greater increase in fat mass index. Similarly, Keane et al. observed a mean increase in fat mass of 0.65 kg determined by BIA over a 2-year follow-up period after initiation of hemodialysis in 299 patients [68].

In a cross-sectional study, we examined the association between fat mass and hemodialysis duration to clarify the period of increasing fat mass [69]. In 561 patients with a hemodialysis duration less than 180 months (age 62.3 ± 11.5 years, 336 males and 225 females), fat mass index for each year of hemodialysis tended to increase during the first three years of treatment and then showed a decreasing trend thereafter. The fat mass index value for the third year (5.85 ± 2.92 kg/m^2) was significantly higher compared to the other years. Furthermore, that index was positively correlated with hemodialysis duration in the first three years ($r = 0.124$; $p < 0.05$), and then a negative correlation was seen with duration greater than three years ($r = -0.192$; $p < 0.001$). These results indicated increases in fat mass during the first three years after hemodialysis initiation.

5.3. Inflammation

Inflammation is well known to be strongly associated with malnutrition in CKD patients, and a decrease in fat mass can be predicted in those in a state of high inflammation. We conducted a study to examine the association of inflammation, represented by C-reactive protein (CRP) level, with changes in fat mass in 389 hemodialysis patients who had a treatment duration of more than one year [70]. Body fat mass was determined twice using DXA, with a one-year interval between measurements. The results showed that change in fat mass was significantly negatively correlated with CRP ($r = -0.165$; $p < 0.005$). Additionally, multiple regression analysis indicated that CRP significantly ($\beta = -0.163$; $p < 0.005$) affected fat mass change, independent of hemodialysis duration, serum albumin level, baseline fat mass, and other confounding clinical factors ($R^2 = 0.127$; $p < 0.001$).

5.4. Diabetes

Several studies have shown that the presence of diabetes is associated with poor nutritional status in CKD patients [71]. We compared changes in fat mass in hemodialysis patients with and without diabetes by determining body fat mass twice by DXA with a 1-year interval in 217 male hemodialysis patients (age 60 ± 13 years, 32% diabetics) who had a duration of hemodialysis from 1 to 10 years (4.9 ± 2.5 years) [72]. Body fat mass was significantly decreased from 12.1 ± 4.4 to 11.0 ± 4.7 kg ($p < 0.01$) during the 1-year study period in the diabetes patients, whereas that was not seen in the nondiabetes patients (12.2 ± 5.0 vs. 11.9 ± 4.9 kg; $p = 0.15$). Further, percentage change in fat mass in one year in the diabetes patients was significantly greater than that in those without diabetes (−7.9 ± 3.4% vs. 0.1 ± 1.9%; $p < 0.05$). Of several clinical parameters examined, protein catabolic rate had a significantly positive correlation with change in fat mass, suggesting that poor protein intake may be a risk factor for fat mass decrease.

6. Fat Mass and Mortality

In the general population, it is considered that the relationships of body fat mass and BMI with mortality are similar. The association between body fat mass (assessed by BIA) and all-cause mortality was investigated by Bigaaed et al. in 27,178 males and 29,875 females in the general population (age 50–64 years) [73]. The median follow-up period was 5.8 years, and 1851 died during the study. They found a J-shape association of body fat mass index with mortality in both the male and female subjects.

Although excess body fat mass is a risk factor for mortality in the general population, high fat mass in hemodialysis patients appears to be protective. In a study of 808 Japanese hemodialysis patients (age 55.1 ± 11.4 years, hemodialysis duration 70.1 ± 66.2 months, 61.3% males, 19.9% diabetics), Kakiya et al. reported that increased fat mass index determined by DXA was associated with decreased all-cause mortality (HR 0.926; 95% CI 0.891–0.962; 1 kg/m^2 increase) and noncardiovascular mortality (HR 0.850; 95% CI 0.806–0.896; 1 kg/m^2 increase) during the mean follow-up period of 53 months, after adjustment for confounding variables such as diabetes, serum albumin, and creatinine level [74]. In addition, higher lean mass index was associated with lower cardiovascular mortality (HR 0.874; 95% CI 0.814–0.938; 1 kg/m^2 increase). Similarly, Honda et al., in an investigation of 328 CKD patients starting dialysis (age 53 ± 12 years, 201 males), found that low fat mass index (evaluated by DXA) was an independent predictor of higher mortality during a six-year follow-up period, after adjustments for age, diabetes, CVD status, inflammation, and other confounders (HR 2.179; 95% CI 1.058–4.488; p = 0.0345; low tertile as compared with others) [75].

Yajima et al. analyzed the association of fat mass (determined by BIA) and mortality in 162 hemodialysis patients. During the follow-up period (median 2.5 years, range 1.0–4.5 years), 29 of the subjects died. Univariate Cox proportional hazards analysis showed that both higher BMI (HR 0.87; 95% CI 0.76–0.98; p = 0.022) and fat tissue index (HR 0.86; 95% CI 0.74–0.98; p = 0.021) were significant predictors of lower all-cause mortality. In findings obtained with multivariate Cox proportional hazards analysis after adjusting for age, gender, albumin, diabetes, hypertension, and history of CVD, the adjusted HR value was 0.40 (95% CI 0.17–0.90; p = 0.027), above the median value for the higher fat tissue index group [76].

In another study, Noori et al. analyzed 742 maintenance hemodialysis patients (age 54 ± 15 years, dialysis duration 28 ± 26 months, 53% diabetics, BMI 26.5 ± 5.8 kg/m^2, 31% African Americans), with males (n = 391) and females (n = 351) categorized separately into four quartiles based on near-infrared interactance-determined fat and lean mass. After adjustments for case-mix and inflammatory markers, the highest quartiles for fat mass and lean mass in females were both associated with greater survival compared to the lowest quartile, with estimated HR values of 0.38 (95% CI 0.20–0.71) and 0.34 (95% CI 0.17–0.67), respectively. In males, the highest quartile for fat mass but not lean mass was associated with greater survival, and those had estimated HR values of 0.51 (95% CI 0.27–0.96) and 1.17 (95% CI 0.60–2.27), respectively [77]. Marcelli et al. investigated an international European cohort of 37,345 hemodialysis patients (age 62.7 ± 15.2 years) and found that low fat tissue index (<10th percentile), determined with BIA, was associated with significantly increased mortality compared to the reference fat tissue index between the 10th and 90th percentile (HR 1.19; 95% CI 1.08–1.31; p < 0.001) [78]. Moreover, Caetano et al. [79] and Duong et al. [80] reported that low fat mass determined using BIA was significantly associated with higher risk of mortality in hemodialysis patients. Based on these results, it is suggested that greater fat mass is associated with better survival in hemodialysis patients in contrast to the general population.

We performed a study to examine the influence of fat mass change on mortality during a 1-year interval in 190 female patients (age 61.9 ± 11.3 years, hemodialysis duration 7.2 ± 6.4 years, 26.3% diabetics, BMI 20.3 ± 3.2 kg/m^2, fat mass 15.0 ± 6.0 kg) undergoing maintenance hemodialysis with DXA [81]. Among this cohort, 110 showed a decrease in annual fat mass, while 80 showed an increase. During the follow-up period of 5 years, 65

(34.3%) of the patients died, and Kaplan–Meier analysis demonstrated that those who lost fat mass had a significantly lower survival rate during the follow-up period compared with those who gained fat mass ($p = 0.021$), with the 5-year survival rates shown to be 58.2% and 76.3%, respectively. Furthermore, multivariate Cox regression analysis indicated that a decrease in annual fat mass (HR 0.504; 95% CI 0.264–0.961; $p = 0.0375$; loser vs. gainer) as well as the value for annual fat mass change (HR 0.855; 95% CI 0.763–0.958; $p = 0.0072$; for 1 kg increase) were significant predictors of all-cause mortality, after adjustments for age, hemodialysis duration, presence of diabetes, body mass index, serum albumin level, and other variables. An increase in annual fat mass of 1 kg was found to reduce mortality by 14.5%. These results demonstrated that a decrease in fat mass is an independent predictor for increased all-cause mortality in hemodialysis patients. Similarly, in a study of 535 adult hemodialysis patients whose body fat mass was directly measured with near-infrared interactance, 46 with body fat mass <12% showed mortality at a rate 4 times greater compared to 199 patients with body fat mass content between 24% and 36% (HR 4.01; 95% CI 1.61–9.99; $p = 0.003$), following multivariate adjustments for demographics, and surrogates of muscle mass and inflammation [82]. That study also found that in hemodialysis patients whose body fat mass was re-measured after 6 months ($n = 411$), fat loss ($\leq -1\%$) was associated with a two-times greater death risk than that of patients who gained fat ($\geq 1\%$), after a multivariate adjustment (HR 2.04; 95% CI 1.05–4.05; $p = 0.04$).

7. Important Role of Visceral Fat in Development of Various Clinical Outcomes as Compared to Subcutaneous Fat

7.1. Visceral Fat and Inflammation

Fat mass can be classified into visceral and subcutaneous based on distribution, and those are metabolically different. The metabolically more active visceral fat is a key factor in the development of insulin resistance, type 2 diabetes, hypertension, dyslipidemia, and atherosclerosis [83]. Moreover, visceral fat, which produces more inflammatory cytokines, such as interleukin 6 (IL-6) and tumor necrosis factor α (TNF-α), is characterized by inflammation and considered to be a risk factor for CVD and increased mortality [84]. In contrast, subcutaneous fat has not been consistently linked to these adverse phenomena and may reflect overall nutritional status as energy storage in both the general population and CKD patients [85].

Waist circumference, an indicator of visceral fat, has been shown to be associated with inflammatory markers in general population cohorts. Schrager et al. reported that waist circumference was associated with higher levels of inflammation markers than overall obesity in community-dwelling older people (age ≥ 65 years, 378 males and 493 females) [86]. In an evaluation of the association between adiposity and inflammation markers in 179 older adults (age 77 ± 4 years, 70% females), Brinkley et al. found that large waist circumference (≥ 102 cm for males, ≥ 88 cm for females) was more strongly correlated with inflammation markers than total fat mass determined by DXA [87].

Previous studies have shown that greater waist circumference is associated with higher levels of inflammation in hemodialysis patients [88], similar to the general population, and thus, visceral fat may also play an inflammatory role in these patients. Delgado et al. enrolled 609 patients undergoing hemodialysis (age 56.1 ± 14.3 years, 57% males, 43% diabetics) and found that waist circumference was positively correlated with CRP and IL-6 concentrations, and inversely with serum albumin and prealbumin concentration. In contrast, the total percentage of fat adjusted for waist circumference, used as a proxy for subcutaneous fat, was inversely correlated with CRP and IL-6 concentration and positively with prealbumin and albumin concentration [89]. In a study of 15,314 CKD patients who participated in the Third National Health and Nutrition Examination Survey (NHANES III), Beddhu et al. noted that abdominal obesity was associated with inflammation (CRP >3 mg/L) [90].

To examine the relationship between fat mass distribution and inflammation, we investigated the association of body composition, determined by DXA, and CRP in 452 hemodialysis patients (age 64 ± 11 years, hemodialysis duration 89 ± 77 months, 63% males, 37% diabetics) [91]. The patients were divided into two groups according to serum high-sensitivity CRP (hsCRP) level—normal CRP (n = 346; hsCRP < 0.3 mg/dL, i.e., normal level) and high CRP (n = 106; hsCRP $\geq$ 0.3 mg/dL). Fat mass in the high CRP group was significantly greater, while there was no significant difference for lean mass between the groups. Additionally, truncal fat mass (surrogate for visceral fat mass) was significantly greater in the high compared to the normal CRP group, with no significant difference in nontruncal fat mass (surrogate for subcutaneous fat mass) between them. In multiple regression analysis, truncal fat mass (β = 0.227; p < 0.01) was significantly and independently associated with serum hsCRP level, after adjustments for age, gender, diabetes, and other confounders (R^2 = 0.137; p < 0.01), whereas nontruncal fat mass was not.

In a study of 197 CKD patients (age 52 $\pm$ 1 years, 123 males) examined shortly before starting dialysis, Axelsson et al. reported that truncal fat mass, estimated by DXA, was significantly positively correlated with both CRP (ρ = 0.23; p < 0.01) and IL-6 (ρ = 0.21; p < 0.01) levels [92]. Kaysen et al. examined visceral adipose tissue using MRI in 48 patients with prevalent hemodialysis and showed that ceruloplasmin, an acute phase inflammatory protein, was strongly associated with visceral adipose tissue [93]. Further, Gohda et al. examined the visceral fat area shown in CT results in 80 patients with prevalent hemodialysis and found that the visceral fat area was a predominant determinant of CRP [94]. These results suggest that visceral or truncal fat mass is an important contributor to increased inflammation in hemodialysis patients, similar to the general population.

7.2. Visceral Fat and CVD Risk

Visceral fat was found to be associated with CVD risk in a general population study. Canoy et al. examined the prospective relationship between fat distribution indices and coronary heart disease among 11,117 males and 13,391 females ranging from 45 to 79 years old [95]. During a mean follow-up period of 9.1 years, 1708 males and 892 females developed coronary heart disease. The risk for developing subsequent coronary heart disease was increased with elevation of waist-to-hip ratio and waist circumference. The HR value (95% CI) of the top compared to the bottom fifth of waist-to-hip ratio was 1.55 (1.28–1.73) in males and 1.91 (1.44–2.54) in females, after adjustments for BMI and other coronary heart disease risk factors. Additionally, risk estimates for waist circumference without hip circumference adjustment were 10% to 18% lower.

Visceral fat might also be associated with outcomes including cardiovascular events in hemodialysis patients [96]. In an Asian hemodialysis cohort (n = 91, age 58.7 $\pm$ 12.5 years, 56.0% males) analyzed over a three-year period, Wu et al. reported that central obesity, determined based on a waist circumference $\geq$90 cm in males and $\geq$80 cm in females, was a significant predictor of cardiovascular events (HR 4.91; 95% CI 1.3–18.9; p = 0.02) and all-cause hospitalization (HR 1.83; 95% CI 1.1–3.1; p = 0.03), shown in multivariate Cox regression analysis results [97].

The negative metabolic consequences of excess visceral fat are preserved in CKD patients [98]. In the study conducted by Sanches et al. of 122 patients with CKD and not yet receiving dialysis therapy (age 55.3 $\pm$ 11.3 years, 75 males and 47 females, 30% diabetics, BMI 27.1 $\pm$ 5.2 kg/m^2, eGFR 35.4 $\pm$ 15.2 mL/min/1.73 m^2), waist circumference was strongly correlated with visceral fat determined by CT (r = 0.75 for males, r = 0.81 for males, p < 0.01), and visceral fat was associated with risk factors for cardiovascular disease, such as triacylglycerol levels [99]. In another investigation of 1669 subjects with CKD (age 70.3 years, 56% females), defined as a baseline eGFR of 15–60 mL/min/1.73 m^2, Elsayed et al. examined the association between waist-to-hip ratio and risk for cardiac events (myocardial infarction, fatal coronary disease) [100]. During a mean follow-up period of 9.3 years, there were 334 cardiac events. Using multivariable-adjusted Cox models, the highest waist-to-hip ratio group (n = 386) was found to be associated with increased risk of cardiac events as compared with the lowest waist-to-hip ratio group (n = 590, HR 1.36; 95% CI 1.01–1.83).

7.3. Subcutaneous Fat and Metabolic Risk

In contrast to visceral fat, subcutaneous fat may have beneficial metabolic effects and possibly reflects overall nutritional status as energy storage in the general population [101]. In 115 healthy, overweight/moderately obese adults with BMI ranging from 25 to 36.9 kg/m^2, McLaughlin et al. found that despite nearly identical mean BMI values in the insulin-resistant and insulin-sensitive groups, visceral adipose tissue, quantified by CT results, was significantly higher in the insulin resistance group, whereas subcutaneous adipose tissue was significantly lower [102]. Inclusion of both visceral adipose tissue and subcutaneous adipose tissue in the same multiple logistic regression analysis demonstrated independent associations, in opposite directions, for both visceral (OR: 1.77; 95% CI 1.04–3.02) and subcutaneous (OR: 0.56; 95% CI 0.34–0.94) adipose tissue with insulin resistance as compared to insulin sensitivity, after adjusting for BMI and gender.

Tanko et al. enrolled 1356 elderly females from 60 to 85 years old and reported that subcutaneous fat, determined by DXA, had an independent negative correlation with both atherogenic metabolic risk factors, such as glucose and lipid metabolites, and aortic calcification, assessed by lateral radiograph findings, in contrast to visceral fat, used as a central adiposity surrogate [103]. The most severe instances of insulin resistance—dyslipidemic syndrome and aortic calcification—were found in subjects with high central and low subcutaneous fat percentages. In a study of 3001 participants in the Framingham Heart Study who were free from clinical cardiovascular disease (mean age 50 years, 48% females), Fox et al. found that visceral adipose tissue but not subcutaneous abdominal adipose tissue, both determined by CT results, contributed significantly to metabolic risk factors, after adjustments for covariant factors, including BMI [85].

The effects of subcutaneous and visceral fat on metabolic risk and inflammation have also been observed in animal models. In mice given a high-fat diet, glucose tolerance was improved in those implanted intra-abdominally with subcutaneous adipose tissue as compared to mice with epididymal visceral adipose tissue implanted intra-abdominally [104]. Mice that received subcutaneous adipose tissue also displayed a marked reduction in the plasma concentration of several proinflammatory cytokines, such as TNF-α and IL-17.

7.4. Visceral Fat and Mortality

Several studies that included general population subjects and CKD patients [105] have shown that increased visceral fat is associated with a higher risk of mortality. Leitzmann et al. prospectively examined waist circumference in relation to cause-specific death in a large cohort of males and females in the United States (n = 225,712). Increased waist circumference was consistently associated with increased risk of death due to any cause as well as major causes of death, including CVD, independent of BMI, age, gender, ethnicity, smoking status, and alcohol intake [106]. Similarly, Lahmann et al. reported that a higher waist-to-hip ratio was a strong predictor of all-cause mortality independent of percentage of body fat mass in 16,814 middle-aged and older females examined in Sweden [107].

Postorino et al. performed a prospective cohort study of 537 hemodialysis patients (age 63 ± 15 years) [32]. Using BMI-adjusted Cox models, waist circumference was found to be a direct predictor of all-cause and cardiovascular mortality ($p < 0.001$), whereas BMI showed an inverse relationship ($p < 0.001$) with those outcomes. The rates of overall and cardiovascular death were maximum in patients with a relatively lower BMI score (below median) and higher waist circumferences (at least median), but minimal in patients with a higher BMI score (at least median) and small waist circumferences (below median). The prognostic power of waist circumference per 10 cm increase for all-cause (HR 1.23; 95% CI 1.02–1.47; $p = 0.03$) and cardiovascular (HR 1.37; 95% CI 1.09–1.73; $p = 0.006$) mortality remained significant after adjustments for cardiovascular comorbidities, as well as traditional and emerging risk factors. Waist-to-hip ratio was also demonstrated to be related to all-cause ($p = 0.009$) and cardiovascular ($p = 0.07$) mortality. Similarly, higher BMI has been found to be protective against and greater waist circumference predictive of mortality in an elderly population [108], as well as kidney transplant patients [109].

In a study of 97 hemodialysis patients, Xiong et al. found that visceral fat determined by BIA was associated with cardiovascular events (HR 9.21; 95% CI 1.49–56.76; visceral fat area ≥ 71.3 cm^2 vs. <71.3 cm^2; $p = 0.017$), cardiovascular mortality (HR 1.11; 95% CI 1.01–1.22; 1-cm^2 increase in fat mass area; $p = 0.035$), and all-cause mortality (HR 1.08; 95% CI 1.02–1.14; 1-cm^2 increase in fat mass area; $p = 0.011$) [110]. Okamoto et al. followed 126 patients on maintenance hemodialysis for 60 months and reported multivariate Cox proportional hazards analysis results showing that a visceral fat area of >71.5 cm^2, determined by CT, was an independent predictor of cardiovascular death (HR 4.46; 95% CI 1.24–16.05; $p = 0.022$) [111].

In a study of 5805 CKD Stage 1–4 patients with BMI ≥ 18.5 kg/m^2, Kramer et al. showed that the association between waist circumference and all-cause mortality was fairly linear, and HR values for mortality were significantly higher for waist circumference ≥ 98 cm in females and ≥ 112 cm in males, as compared to the reference waist circumference values (<80 and <94 cm, respectively) [112]. After adjustments for all covariates, including BMI, HR for all-cause mortality for waist circumference ≥ 108 cm in females and ≥ 122 cm in males was 2.09 (95% CI 1.26–3.46) as compared to the reference values. After fully adjusting for continuous variables, each 1 cm increase in waist circumference was associated with a 2% increase in risk of mortality (95% CI 1.01–1.04).

7.5. Subcutaneous Fat and Mortality

Visceral and subcutaneous adipose tissues have different metabolic and inflammatory characteristics, and they thus may have an opposing influence on several outcomes, including mortality. In a general population study, preferential fat deposition in subcutaneous and visceral locations was suggested to be more important than the total amount of body fat in regard to mortality. Lee et al. investigated the relationship between body fat distribution and all-cause mortality in 32,593 subjects who underwent an abdominal CT examination as part of a health check-up [113]. There were 253 deaths during the mean follow-up period of 5.7 years. Their findings showed that an increased visceral fat area was related to increased all-cause mortality, while an increased subcutaneous fat area was associated with a decrease in all-cause mortality. However, in multivariate Cox proportional hazard regression analysis, only the visceral fat area was found to be independently associated with all-cause mortality.

The association between subcutaneous fat and mortality has also been observed in regard to other conditions, such as cancer [114] and cirrhosis [115]. In a study conducted by Ebadi et al., the association between subcutaneous fat and mortality in 1473 gastrointestinal and respiratory cancer and 273 metastatic renal cell carcinoma patients was investigated using CT results. A low subcutaneous adipose tissue index (<50.0 cm^2/m^2 in males, <42.0 cm^2/m^2 in females) was shown to be independently associated with increased mortality (HR 1.26; 95% CI 1.11–1.43; $p < 0.001$) and shorter survival (13.1 months; 95% CI 11.4–14.7) compared to patients with a high subcutaneous adipose tissue index (19.3 months; 95% CI 17.6–21.0; $p < 0.001$) [116]. Antoun et al. also reported findings of 120 patients with metastatic castration-resistant prostate cancer, which showed that those with a higher subcutaneous adipose tissue index had significantly longer overall survival [117]. The median survival was 15 months (95% CI 9–18) for patients with a subcutaneous adipose tissue index lower than the median value and 18 months (95% CI 13–30) for those with a subcutaneous adipose tissue index above that ($p = 0.008$).

The relationships of fat and muscle mass with mortality were examined by Huang et al. in 1709 hemodialysis patients (age 57.7 $\pm$ 14.0 years, hemodialysis duration 3.7 $\pm$ 4.4 years, 56% females, 44% diabetics) who participated in the hemodialysis study (HEMO) [118]. During a median follow-up period of 2.5 years, there were 802 deaths. In adjusted models with continuous covariates, higher triceps skinfold thickness was significantly associated with decreased risk of mortality, while higher mid-arm muscle circumference showed a trend toward decreased mortality. The HR values per 1 S.D. increase were 0.84 (95% CI 0.76–0.92) for triceps skinfold thickness and 0.93 (95% CI 0.86–1.00) for mid-arm muscle circumference. The highest quartiles of triceps skinfold thickness and mid-arm muscle circumference were significantly associated with lower all-cause mortality in comparison with the lowest quartile in adjusted models. Furthermore, triceps skinfold thickness and mid-arm muscle circumference were independently associated with lower risk of mortality when both variables were combined in the same multivariable model. Considering that skinfold thickness is a measure of subcutaneous fat, their results indicated that a high level of subcutaneous fat mass may be associated with better survival in hemodialysis patients. Subcutaneous fat mass has a far greater contribution to total fat mass, as visceral fat mass accounts for only 7–15% of total body fat mass, and thus, it may substantially influence the association of total fat mass and outcomes.

8. The Mechanism by Which Maintained Adiposity Improves Survival in Hemodialysis Patients

In addition to its advantage as a source of fuel, adipose tissue can also exert its beneficial effects through multiple mechanisms, both directly and indirectly in hemodialysis patients [44]. In addition to the direct effect of adipocytes in maintaining good health, adipose tissue produces the TNF-α-soluble receptor that attenuates the adverse effects of TNF-α itself [119], and obese individuals have higher lipoprotein concentrations, which counteract the inflammatory effects of circulating endotoxins.

Subcutaneous fat is positively associated with insulin sensitivity [102] and a slower rate of lipolysis and free fatty acid release into the circulation. Several studies have suggested that subcutaneous fat may exert protective effects against inflammation [91,104]. Subcutaneous fat is considered to be the main source of adiponectin, which is involved in a variety of physiological functions, including energy regulation, inflammation, and insulin sensitivity [120].

Furthermore, overweight and obese individuals have a higher absolute amount of muscle mass thanks to an excess load of increased adiposity. This increased amount of lean tissue might confer an additional protective edge during times of catabolism [121].

Conversely, the absence of adipose tissue causes metabolic dysfunction, including insulin resistance, hyperglycemia, hyperlipidemia, and fatty liver, which can be completely reversed with the transplantation of adipose tissue [122]. Similarly, reductions in total body fat are associated with decreased humoral immunity [123].

9. Conclusions

Nutritional status is closely associated with outcomes including mortality in hemodialysis patients and shows continual fluctuations; thus, regular examinations for assessment of nutrition factors are necessary. Although obesity and excessive fat mass are linked to CVD and mortality in the general population, fat mass is considered to be an important nutritional indicator in hemodialysis patients, who are typically malnourished; thus, its measurement is important for a good understanding of nutritional status. It is also important to note that fat mass is classified into visceral and subcutaneous fat based on distribution, and that those have metabolic differences. Visceral fat is closely associated with metabolism abnormalities and inflammation and considered to be a risk factor for adverse outcomes, such as CVD and mortality, in the general population as well as in hemodialysis patients. In contrast, subcutaneous fat may be protective against wasting and catabolism in patients undergoing hemodialysis. However, fat mass may have potentially beneficial effects on important outcomes in hemodialysis patients, as accumulating evidence suggests that fat mass distribution (i.e., visceral fat and subcutaneous fat) plays a more important role in these beneficial effects.

Funding: This research received no external funding.

Conflicts of Interest: The author declares no conflict of interest.

References

1. Pupim, L.B.; Ikizler, T.A. Uremic malnutrition: New insights into an old problem. *Semin. Dial.* **2003**, *16*, 224–232. [CrossRef] [PubMed]
2. Lindholm, B.; Heimburger, O.; Stenvinkel, P. What are the causes of protein-energy malnutrition in chronic renal insufficiency? *Am. J. Kidney Dis.* **2002**, *39*, 422–425. [CrossRef]
3. Stenvinkel, P.; Heimburger, O.; Paultre, F.; Diczfalusy, U.; Wang, T.; Berglund, L.; Jogestrand, T. Strong association between malnutrition, inflammation, and atherosclerosis in chronic renal failure. *Kidney Int.* **1999**, *55*, 1899–1991. [CrossRef] [PubMed]
4. Kalantar-Zadeh, K.; Ikizler, T.A.; Block, G.; Avram, M.M.; Kopple, J.D. Malnutrition-Inflammation complex syndrome in dialysis patients: Causes and consequences. *Am. J. Kidney Dis.* **2003**, *42*, 864–881. [CrossRef]
5. Fouque, D.; Kalantar-Zadeh, K.; Kopple, J.; Cano, N.; Chauveau, P.; Cuppari, L.; Franch, H.; Guamieri, G.; Ikizler, T.A.; Kaysen, G.; et al. A proposed nomenclature and diagnostic criteria for protein-energy wasting in acute and chronic kidney disease. *Kidney Int.* **2008**, *73*, 391–398. [CrossRef] [PubMed]
6. Gaal, L.F.V.; Mertens, I.L.; Block, C.E.D. Mechanisms linking obesity with cardiovascular disease. *Nature* **2006**, *444*, 875–880. [CrossRef]
7. Prospective Studies Collaboration; Whitlock, G.; Lewington, S.; Sherliker, P.; Clarke, R.; Emberson, J.; Halsey, J.; Qizilbash, N.; Collins, R.; Peto, R. Body-Mass index and cause-specific mortality in 900,000 adults: Collaborative analysis of 57 prospective studies. *Lancet* **2009**, *373*, 1083–1096.
8. Naderi, N.; Kleine, C.E.; Park, C.; Hsiung, J.T.; Soohoo, M.; Tantisattamo, E.; Streja, E.; Kalantar-Zadeh, K.; Moradi, H. Obesity paradox in advanced kidney disease: From bedside to the bench. *Prog. Cardiovasc. Dis.* **2018**, *61*, 168–181. [CrossRef]
9. Park, J.; Ahmadi, S.F.; Streja, E.; Molnar, M.Z.; Flegal, K.M.; Gillen, D.; Kovesdy, C.P.; Kalantar-Zadeh, K. Obesity paradox in end-stage kidney disease patients. *Prog. Cardiovasc. Dis.* **2014**, *56*, 415–425. [CrossRef]
10. Horwich, T.B.; Fonarow, G.C.; Hamilton, M.A.; MacLellan, W.R.; Woo, M.A.; Tillisch, J.H. The relationship between obesity and mortality in patients with heart failure. *J. Am. Coll. Cardiol.* **2001**, *38*, 789–795. [CrossRef]
11. Divo, M.J.; Cabrera, C.; Casanova, C.; Marin, J.M.; Pinto-Plata, V.M.; de-Torres, J.P.; Zulueta, J.; Zagaceta, J.; Sanchez-Salcedo, P.; Berto, J.; et al. Comorbidity distribution, clinical expression and survival in COPD patients with different body mass index. *Chronic. Obstr. Pulm. Dis.* **2014**, *1*, 229–238. [CrossRef] [PubMed]
12. Lennon, H.; Sperrin, M.; Badrick, E.; Renehan, A.G. The obesity paradox in cancer: A review. *Curr. Oncol. Rep.* **2016**, *18*, 56. [CrossRef]
13. Ahmadi, S.F.; Streja, E.; Zahmatkesh, G.; Streja, D.; Kashyap, M.; Moradi, H.; Molnar, M.Z.; Reddy, U.; Amin, A.N.; Kovesdy, C.P.; et al. Reverse epidemiology of traditional cardiovascular risk factors in the geriatric population. *J. Am. Med. Dir. Assoc.* **2015**, *16*, 933–999. [CrossRef] [PubMed]
14. Degoulet, P.; Legrain, M.; Reach, I.; Aime, F.; Devries, C.; Rojas, P.; Jacobs, C. Mortality risk factors in patients treated by chronic hemodialysis. Report of the Diaphane collaborative study. *Nephron* **1982**, *31*, 103–110. [CrossRef] [PubMed]
15. Leavey, S.F.; Strawderman, R.L.; Jones, C.A.; Port, F.K.; Held, P. Simple nutritional indicators as independent predictors of mortality in hemodialysis patients. *Am. J. Kidney Dis.* **1998**, *31*, 997–1006. [CrossRef]
16. Fleischmann, E.; Teal, N.; Dudley, J.; May, W.; Bower, J.D.; Salahudeen, A.K. Influence of excess weight on mortality and hospital stay in 1346 hemodialysis patients. *Kidney Int.* **1999**, *55*, 1560–1567. [CrossRef]
17. Johansen, K.L.; Young, B.; Kaysen, G.A.; Chertow, G.M. Association of body size with outcomes among patients beginning dialysis. *Am. J. Clin. Nutr.* **2004**, *80*, 324–332. [CrossRef]
18. Ladhani, M.; Craig, J.C.; Irving, M.; Clayton, P.A.; Wong, G. Obesity and the risk of cardiovascular and all-cause mortality in chronic kidney disease: A systematic review and meta-analysis. *Nephrol. Dial. Tansplant.* **2017**, *32*, 439–449. [CrossRef]
19. Kalantar-Zadeh, K.; Rhee, C.M.; Chou, J.; Ahmadi, S.F.; Park, J.; Chen, J.L.T.; Amin, A.N. The obesity paradox in kidney disease: How to reconcile it with pbesity management. *Kidney Int. Rep.* **2017**, *2*, 271–281. [CrossRef]
20. Chazot, C.; Gassia, J.P.; Benedetto, A.D.; Cesare, S.; Ponce, P.; Marcelli, D. Is there any survival advantage of obesity in Southern European haemodialysis patient? *Nephrol. Dial. Transplant.* **2009**, *24*, 2871–2876. [CrossRef]
21. Kalantar-Zadeh, K.; Kopple, J.D.; Kilpatrick, R.D.; McAllister, C.J.; Shinaberger, C.S.; Gjertson, D.W.; Greenland, S. Association of morbid obesity and weight change over time with cardiovascular survival in hemodialysis population. *Am. J. Kidney Dis.* **2005**, *46*, 489–500. [CrossRef]
22. Chang, T.I.; Ngo, V.; Streja, E.; Chou, J.A.; Tortorici, A.R.; Kim, T.H.; Kim, T.W.; Soohoo, M.; Gillen, D.; Rhee, C.M.; et al. Association of body weight changes with mortality in incident hemodialysis patients. *Nephrol. Dial. Transplant.* **2017**, *32*, 1549–1558. [CrossRef] [PubMed]
23. Doshi, M.; Streja, E.; Rhee, C.M.; Park, J.; Ravel, V.A.; Soohoo, M.; Moradi, H.; Lau, W.L.; Mehrotra, R.; Kuttykrishnan, S.; et al. Examining the robustness of the obesity paradox in maintenance hemodialysis patients: A marginal structural model analysis. *Nephrol. Dial. Transplant.* **2016**, *31*, 1310–1319. [CrossRef] [PubMed]
24. Stenvinkel, P.; Gillespie, I.A.; Tunks, J.; Addison, J.; Kronenberg, F.; Druke, T.B.; Marcelli, D.; Schernthaner, G.; Eckardt, K.U.; Floege, J.; et al. Inflammation modifies the paradoxical association between body mass index and motality in hemodialysis patients. *J. Am. Soc. Nephrol.* **2016**, *27*, 1479–1486. [CrossRef] [PubMed]
25. Leavey, S.F.; McCullough, K.; Hecking, E.; Goodkin, D.; Port, F.K.; Young, E.W. Body mass index and mortality in 'healthier' as compared with 'sicker' haemodialysis patients: Results from yhe Dialysis Outcomes and Practice Patterns Study (DOPPS). *Nephrol. Dial. Transplant.* **2001**, *16*, 2386–2394. [CrossRef] [PubMed]

26. Cabezas-Rodriguez, I.; Carrero, J.J.; Zoccali, C.; Qureshi, A.R.; Ketteler, M.; Floege, J.; London, G.; Locatelli, F.; Gorriz, J.L.; Rutkowski, B.; et al. Influence of body mass index on the association of weight changes with mortality in hemodialysis patients. *Clin. J. Am. Soc. Nephrol.* **2013**, *8*, 1725–1733. [CrossRef] [PubMed]
27. Rhee, C.M.; Ahmadi, S.F.; Kalantar-Zadeh, K. The dual roles of obesity in chronic kidney disease: A review of the current literature. *Curr. Opin. Nephrol. Hypertens.* **2016**, *25*, 208–216. [CrossRef] [PubMed]
28. Madero, M.; Samak, M.J.; Wang, X.; Sceppa, C.C.; Greene, T.; Beck, G.; Kusek, J.W.; Collins, A.; Levey, A.S.; Menon, V. Body mass index and mortality in CKD. *Am. J. Kidney Dis.* **2007**, *50*, 404–411. [CrossRef] [PubMed]
29. Evans, M.; Fryzek, J.P.; Elinder, C.G.; Cohen, S.S.; McLaughlin, J.K.; Nyren, O.; Fored, C.M. The natural history of chronic renal failure: Results from an unselected, population-based, inception cohort in Sweden. *Am. J. Kidney Dis.* **2005**, *46*, 863–870. [CrossRef]
30. Kovesdy, C.; Anderson, J.E.; Kalantar-Zadeh, K. Paradoxical association between body mass index and mortality in men with CKD not yet on dialysis. *Am. J. Kidney Dis.* **2007**, *49*, 581–591. [CrossRef]
31. Lu, J.L.; Kalantar-Zadeh, K.; Ma, J.Z.; Quarles, L.D.; Kovesdy, C.P. Association of body mass index with outcomes in patients with CKD. *J. Am. Soc. Nephrol.* **2014**, *25*, 2088–2096. [CrossRef]
32. Postorino, M.; Marino, C.; Tripepi, G.; Zoccali, C. Abdominal obesity and all-cause and cardiovascular mortality in end-stage renal disease. *J. Am. Coll. Cardiol.* **2009**, *53*, 1265–1272. [CrossRef] [PubMed]
33. Abramowitz, M.K.; Sharma, D.; Folkert, V.W. Hidden obesity in dialysis patients: Clinical implications. *Semin. Dial.* **2016**, *29*, 391–395. [CrossRef] [PubMed]
34. Fouque, D.; Vennegoor, M.; Wee, P.T.; Wanner, C.; Basci, A.; Canaud, B.; Haage, P.; Konner, K.; Kooman, J.; Martin-Malo, A.; et al. EBPG guideline on nutrition. *Nephrol. Dial. Transplant.* **2007**, *22* (Suppl. 2), ii45–ii87. [CrossRef] [PubMed]
35. Fang, H.; Berg, E.; Cheng, X.; Shen, W. How to best assess abdominal obesity. *Curr. Opin. Clin. Nutr. Metab. Care* **2018**, *21*, 360–365. [CrossRef]
36. Kamimura, M.A.; Santos, N.S.J.D.; Avesani, C.M.; Canziani, M.E.F.; Draibe, S.A.; Cuppari, L. Comparison of three methods for the determination of body fat in patients on long-term hemodialysis therapy. *J. Am. Diet. Assoc.* **2003**, *103*, 195–199. [CrossRef]
37. Oe, B.; de Fijter, C.W.; Oe, P.L.; Stevens, P.; de Vries, P.M. Four-Site skinfold anthropometry (FSA) versus body impedance analysis (BIA) in assessing nutritional status of patients on maintenance hemodialysis: Which method is to be preferred in routine patient care? *Clin. Nephrol.* **1998**, *49*, 180–185.
38. Broers, N.J.H.; Canaud, B.; Dekker, M.J.E.; van der Sande, F.M.; Stuard, S.; Wabel, P.; Kooman, J.P. Three compartment bioimpedance spectroscopy in the nutritional assessment and the outcome of patients with advanced or end stage kidney disease: What have we learned so far? *Hemodial. Int.* **2020**, *24*, 148–161. [CrossRef]
39. Marra, M.; Sammarco, R.; Lorenzo, A.D.; Iellamo, F.; Siervo, M.; Pietrobelli, A.; Donini, L.M.; Santarpia, L.; Cataldi, M.; Pasanisi, F.; et al. Assessment of body composition in health and disease using bioelectrical impedance analysis (BIA) and dual energy X-ray absorptiometry (DXA): A critical overview. *Contrast Media Mol. Imaging* **2019**, *2019*, 3548284. [CrossRef]
40. Horber, F.F.; Thomi, F.; Casez, J.P.; Fonteille, J.; Jaeger, P. Impact of hydration status on body composition as measured by dual energy X-ray absorptiometry in normal volunteers and patients on haemodialysis. *Br. J. Radiol.* **1992**, *65*, 895–900. [CrossRef]
41. Stenver, D.I.; Gotfredsen, A.; Hilsted, J.; Nielsen, B. Body composition in hemodialysis patients measured by dual-energy X-ray absorptiometry. *Am. J. Nephrol.* **1995**, *15*, 105–110. [CrossRef]
42. Nishizawa, Y.; Shoji, T.; Tanaka, S.; Yamashita, M.; Morita, A.; Emoto, M.; Tabata, T.; Inoue, T.; Morii, H. Serum leptin level and its relationship with body composition in hemodialysis patients. *Am. J. Kidney Dis.* **1998**, *31*, 655–661. [CrossRef] [PubMed]
43. Cheung, A.S.; de Rooy, C.; Hoermann, R.; Gianatti, E.J.; Hamilton, E.J.; Roff, G.; Zajac, J.D.; Grossmann, M. Correlation of visceral adipose tissue measured by Lunar Prodigy dual X-ray absorptiometry with MRI and CT in older men. *Int. J. Obes.* **2016**, *40*, 1325–1328. [CrossRef]
44. Ikizler, T.A. Resolved: Being fat is good for dialysis patients: The Godzilla effect: Pro. *J. Am. Soc. Nephrol.* **2008**, *19*, 1059–1064. [CrossRef]
45. Hill, J.O.; DiGirolamo, M. Preferential loss of body fat during starvation in dietary obese rats. *Life Sci.* **1991**, *49*, 1907–1914. [CrossRef]
46. Anton-Perez, G.; Santana-Del-Pino, A.; Henriquez-Palop, F.; Monzon, T.; Sanchez, A.Y.; Valga, F.; Morales-Umpierrez, A.; Garcia-Canton, C.; Rodriguez-Perez, J.C.; Carrero, J.J. Diagnostic usefulness of the protein energy wasting score in prevalent hemodialysis patients. *J. Ren Nutr.* **2018**, *28*, 428–434. [CrossRef] [PubMed]
47. Perez-Torres, A.; Garcia, M.E.G.; Jose-Valiente, B.S.; Rubio, A.B.; Diez, O.C.; Lopez-Sobaler, A.M.; Selgas, R. Protein-Energy wasting syndrome in advanced chronic kidney disease: Prevalence and specific clinical characteristics. *Nefrologia* **2018**, *38*, 141–151. [CrossRef]
48. Cooper, B.A.; Bartlett, L.H.; Aslani, A.; Allen, B.J.; Ibels, L.S.; Pollock, C.A. Validity of subjective global assessment as a nutritional marker in end-stage renal disease. *Am. J. Kidney Dis.* **2002**, *40*, 126–132. [CrossRef]
49. Pieer, T.B.; McCullough, K.P.; Port, F.K.; Goodkin, D.A.; Maroni, B.J.; Held, P.J.; Young, E.W. Mortality risk in hemodialysis patients and changes in nutritional indicators: DOPPS. *Kidney Int.* **2002**, *62*, 2238–2245.
50. Kalantar-Zadeh, K.; Kleiner, M.; Dunne, E.; Lee, G.H.; Luft, F.C. A modified quantitative subjective global assessment of nutrition for dialysis patients. *Nephrol. Dial. Transplant.* **1999**, *14*, 1732–1738. [CrossRef] [PubMed]
51. Paudel, K.; Visser, A.; Burke, S.; Samad, N.; Fan, S.L. Can bioimpedance measurements of lean and fat tissue mass replace subjective global assessments in peritoneal dialysis patients? *J. Ren. Nutr.* **2015**, *25*, 480–487. [CrossRef] [PubMed]

52. Windahl, K.; Irving, G.F.; Almquist, T.; Liden, M.K.; van de Luijtgaarden, M.; Chesnaye, N.C.; Voskamp, P.; Stenvinkel, P.; Klinger, M.; Szymczak, M.; et al. Prevalence and risk of protein-energy wasting assessed by subjective global assessment in older adults with advanced chronic kidney disease: Results from EQUAL study. *J. Ren. Nutr.* **2018**, *28*, 165–174. [CrossRef] [PubMed]
53. Kalantar-Zadeh, K.; Kopple, J.D.; Block, G.; Humphreys, M.H. A malnutrition-inflammation score is correlated with morbidity and mortality in maintenance hemodialysis patients. *Am. J. Kidney Dis.* **2001**, *38*, 1251–1263. [CrossRef]
54. Amparo, F.C.; Kamimura, M.A.; Molnar, M.Z.; Cuppari, L.; Lindholm, B.; Amodeo, C.; Carrero, J.J.; Cordeiro, A.C. Diagnostic validation and prognostic significance of the malnutrition-inflammation score in nondialyzed chronic kidney disease patients. *Nephrol. Dial. Transplant.* **2015**, *30*, 821–828. [CrossRef]
55. Rambod, M.; Bross, R.; Zitterkoph, J.; Benner, D.; Pithia, J.; Colman, S.; Kovesdy, C.P.; Kopple, J.D.; Kalantar-Zadeh, K. Association of malnutrition-inflammation score with quality of life and mortality in hemodialysis patients: A 5-year prospective cohort study. *Am. J. Kidney Dis.* **2009**, *53*, 298–309. [CrossRef]
56. Wang, W.L.; Liang, S.; Zhu, F.L.; Liu, J.Q.; Chen, X.M.; Cai, G.Y. Association of the malnutrition-inflammation score with anthropometry and body composition measurements in patients with chronic kidney disease. *Ann. Palliat. Med.* **2019**, *8*, 596–603. [CrossRef]
57. Arias-Guillen, M.; Perez, E.; Herrera, P.; Romano, B.; Ojeda, R.; Vera, M.; Rios, J.; Fontsere, N.; Maduell, F. Bioimpedance spectroscopy as a practical tool for the early detection aprevention of protein-energy wasting in hemodialysis patients. *J. Ren. Nutr.* **2018**, *28*, 324–332. [CrossRef] [PubMed]
58. Ikizler, T.A.; Cano, N.J.; Franch, H.; Fouque, D.; Himmelfarb, J.; Kalantar-Zadeh, K.; Kuhlmann, M.K.; Stenvinkel, P.; TerWee, P.; Teta, D.; et al. Prevention and treatment of protein energy wasting in chronic kidney disease patients: A consensus statement by the International society of Renal Nutrition and Metabolism. *Kidney Int.* **2013**, *84*, 1096–1107. [CrossRef]
59. Pupim, L.B.; Majchrzak, K.M.; Flakoll, P.J.; Ikizler, T.A. Intradialytic oral nutrition improves protein homeostasis in chronic hemodialysis patients with deranged nutritional status. *J. Am. Soc. Nephrol.* **2006**, *17*, 3149–3157. [CrossRef] [PubMed]
60. Fouque, D.; McKenzie, J.; de Mutsert, R.; Azar, R.; Teta, D.; Plauth, M.; Cano, N.; Multicentre Trial Study Group. Use of a renal-specific oral supplement by haemodialysis patients with low protein intake does not increase the need for phosphate binders and may prevent a decline in nutritional status and quality of life. *Nephrol. Dial. Transplant.* **2008**, *23*, 2902–2910. [CrossRef]
61. Caetano, C.; Valente, A.; Silva, F.J.; Antunes, J.; Garagarza, C. Effect of intradialytic protein-rich meal intake in nutritional and body composition parameters on hemodialysis patients. *Clin. Nutr. ESPEN* **2017**, *20*, 29–33. [CrossRef]
62. Martin-Alemany, G.; Valdez-Ortiz, R.; Olvera-Soto, G.; Gomez-Guerrero, I.; Aguire-Esquivel, G.; Cantu-Quintanilla, G.; Lopez-Alvarenga, J.C.; Miranda-Alatriste, P.; Espinosa-Cuevas, A. The effect of resistance exercise and oral nutritional supplementation during hemodialysis on indicators of nutritional status and quality of life. *Nephrol. Dial. Transplant.* **2016**, *31*, 1712–1720. [CrossRef]
63. Weiner, D.E.; Tighiouart, H.; Ladik, V.; Meyer, K.B.; Zager, P.; Johnson, D.S. Oral intradialytic nutritional supplement use and mortality in hemodialysis patients. *Am. J. Kidney Dis.* **2014**, *63*, 276–285. [CrossRef] [PubMed]
64. Lacson, E., Jr.; Wang, W.; Zebrowski, B.; Wingard, R.; Hakim, R.M. Outcomes associated with intradialytic oral nutritional supplements in patients undergoing maintenance hemodialysis: A quality improvement report. *Am. J. Kidney Dis.* **2012**, *60*, 591–600. [CrossRef] [PubMed]
65. Goldwasser, P.; Kaldas, A.I.; Barth, R.H. Rise in serum albumin and creatinine in the first half year on hemodialysis. *Kidney Int.* **1999**, *56*, 2260–2268. [CrossRef]
66. Ishimura, E.; Okuno, S.; Kim, M.; Yamamoto, T.; Izumotani, T.; Otoshi, T.; Shoji, T.; Inaba, M.; Nishizawa, Y. Increasing body fat mass in the first year of hemodialysis. *J. Am. Soc. Nephrol.* **2001**, *12*, 1921–1926. [CrossRef]
67. Marcelli, D.; Brand, K.; Ponce, P.; Milkowski, A.; Marelli, C.; Ok, E.; Godino, J.I.M.; Gurevich, K.; Jirka, T. Longitudinal changes in body composition in patients after initiation of hemodialysis therapy: Results from an international cohort. *J. Ren. Nutr.* **2016**, *26*, 72–80. [CrossRef]
68. Keane, D.; Gardiner, C.; Lindley, E.; Lines, S.; Woodrow, G.; Wright, M. Changes in body composition in the two years after initiation of haemodialysis: A retrospective cohort study. *Nutrients* **2016**, *8*, 702. [CrossRef]
69. Ishimura, E.; Okuno, S.; Marukawa, T.; Katoh, Y.; Hiranaka, T.; Yamakawa, T.; Morii, H.; Kim, M.; Matsumoto, N.; Shoji, T.; et al. Body fat mass in hemodialysis patients. *Am. J. Kidney Dis.* **2003**, *41* (Suppl. 1), S137–S141. [CrossRef]
70. Fujino, Y.; Ishimura, E.; Okuno, S.; Tsuboniwa, N.; Maekawa, K.; Izumotani, T.; Yamakawa, T.; Inaba, M.; Nishizawa, Y. C-Reactive protein is a significant predictor of decrease in fat mass in hemodialysis patients. *Biomed. Pharmacother.* **2005**, *59*, 264–268. [CrossRef]
71. Qureshi, A.R.; Alvestrand, A.; Danielsson, A.; Divino-Filho, J.C.; Gutierrez, A.; Lindholm, B.; Berastrom, J. Factor predicting malnutrition in hemodialysis patients: A cross-sectional study. *Kidney Int.* **1998**, *53*, 773–782. [CrossRef] [PubMed]
72. Okuno, S.; Ishimura, E.; Kim, M.; Izumotani, T.; Otoshi, T.; Maekawa, K.; Morii, H.; Inaba, M.; Nishizawa, Y. Changes in body fat mass in male hemodialysis patient: A comparison between diabetics and nondiabetics. *Am. J. Kidney Dis.* **2001**, *38* (Suppl. 1), S208–S211. [CrossRef] [PubMed]
73. Bigaard, J.; Frederiksen, K.; Tjonneland, A.; Thomsen, B.L.; Overvad, K.; Heitmann, B.L.; Sorensen, T.I.A. Body fat and fat-free mass and all-cause mortality. *Obes. Res.* **2004**, *12*, 1042–1049. [CrossRef] [PubMed]

74. Kakiya, R.; Shoji, T.; Tsujimoto, Y.; Tatsumi, N.; Hatsuda, S.; Shinohara, K.; Kinoto, E.; Tahara, H.; Koyama, H.; Emoto, M.; et al. Body fat mass and lean mass as predictors of survival in hemodialysis patients. *Kidney Int.* **2006**, *70*, 549–556. [CrossRef] [PubMed]
75. Honda, H.; Qureshi, A.R.; Axelsson, J.; Heimburger, O.; Suliman, M.E.; Barany, P.; Stenvinkel, P.; Lindholm, B. Obese sarcopenia in patients with end-stage renal disease is associated with inflammation and increased mortality. *Am. J. Clin. Nutr.* **2007**, *86*, 633–638. [CrossRef]
76. Yajima, T.; Arao, M.; Yajima, K.; Takahashi, H.; Yasuda, K. The association of fat tissue and muscle mass indices with all-cause motality in patients undergoing hemodialysis. *PLoS ONE* **2019**, *14*, e0211988. [CrossRef]
77. Noori, N.; Kovesdy, C.P.; Dukkipati, R.; Kim, Y.; Duong, U.; Bross, R.; Oreopoulos, A.; Luna, A.; Benner, D.; Kopple, J.D.; et al. Survival predictability of lean and fat mass in men and women undergoing maintenance hemodialysis. *Am. J. Clin. Nutr.* **2010**, *92*, 1060–1070. [CrossRef]
78. Marcelli, D.; Usvyat, L.A.; Kotanko, P.; Bayh, I.; Canaud, B.; Etter, M.; Gatti, E.; Grassmann, A.; Wang, Y.; Marelli, C.; et al. Body composition and survival in dialysis patients: Results from an international cohort study. *Clin. J. Am. Soc. Nephrol.* **2015**, *10*, 1192–1200. [CrossRef]
79. Caetano, C.; Valente, A.; Oliveira, T.; Garagarza, C. Body composition and mortality predictors in hemodialysis patients. *J. Ren. Nutr.* **2016**, *26*, 81–86. [CrossRef]
80. Duong, T.V.; Wong, T.C.; Chen, H.H.; Chen, T.H.; Hsu, Y.H.; Peng, S.J.; Kuo, K.L.; Liu, H.C.; Lin, E.T.; Yang, S.H. Impact of percent body fat on all-cause mortality among adequate dialysis patients with and without insulin resistance: A multi-center prospective cohort study. *Nutrients* **2019**, *11*, 1304. [CrossRef]
81. Fujino, Y.; Ishimura, E.; Okuno, S.; Ysuboniwa, N.; Maekawa, K.; Izumotani, T.; Yamakawa, T.; Inaba, M.; NIshizawa, Y. Annual fat mass change is a significant predictor of mortality in female hemodialysis patients. *Biomed. Pharmacother.* **2006**, *60*, 253–257. [CrossRef] [PubMed]
82. Kalantar-Zadeh, K.; Kuwae, N.; Wu, D.Y.; Shantouf, R.S.; Fouque, D.; Anker, S.D.; Block, G.; Kopple, J.D. Association of body fat and its changes over time with quality life and prospective mortality in hemodialysis patients. *Am. J. Clin. Nutr.* **2006**, *83*, 202–210. [CrossRef] [PubMed]
83. Vishvanath, L.; Gupta, R.K. Contribution of adipogenesis to healthy adipose tissue expansion in obesity. *J. Clin. Investig.* **2019**, *129*, 4022–4031. [CrossRef]
84. Berg, A.H.; Scherer, P.E. Adipose tissue, inflammation, and cardiovascular disease. *Circ. Res.* **2005**, *96*, 939–949. [CrossRef]
85. Fox, C.S.; Massaro, J.M.; Hoffmann, U.; Pou, K.M.; Maurovich-Horvat, P.; Liu, C.Y.; Vasan, R.S.; Murabito, J.M.; Meigs, J.B.; Cupples, L.A.; et al. Abdominal visceral and subcutaneous adipose tissue compartments: Association with metabolic risk factors in the Framingham Heart Study. *Circulation* **2007**, *116*, 39–48. [CrossRef] [PubMed]
86. Schrager, M.A.; Metter, E.J.; Simonsick, E.; Ble, A.; Bandinelli, S.; Lauretani, F.; Ferrucci, L. Sarcopenic obesity and inflammation in the InCHIANTI study. *J. Appl. Physiol.* **2007**, *102*, 919–925. [CrossRef] [PubMed]
87. Brinkley, T.E.; Hsu, F.C.; Beavers, K.M.; Church, T.S.; Goodpaster, B.H.; Stafford, R.S.; Pahor, M.; Kritchevsky, S.B.; Nicklas, B.J. Total and abdominal adiposity are associated with inflammation in older adults using a factor analysis approach. *J. Gerontol. A Biol. Sci. Med. Sci.* **2012**, *67*, 1099–1106. [CrossRef] [PubMed]
88. Stenvinkel, P.; Zoccali, C.; Ikizler, T.A. Obesity in CKD—What should nephrologists know? *J. Am. Soc. Nephrol.* **2013**, *24*, 1727–1736. [CrossRef]
89. Delgado, C.; Chertow, G.M.; Kaysen, G.A.; Dalrymple, L.S.; Komak, J.; Grimes, B.; Johansen, K.L. Association of body mass index and body fat with markers of inflammation and nutrition among patients receiving hemodialysis. *Am. J. Kidney Dis.* **2017**, *70*, 817–825. [CrossRef]
90. Beddhu, S.; Kimmel, P.L.; Ramkumar, N.; Cheung, A.K. Association of metabolic syndrome with inflammation in CKD: Results from the Third National Health and Nutrition Examination Survey (NHANES III). *Am. J. Kidney Dis.* **2005**, *46*, 577–586. [CrossRef]
91. Ishimura, E.; Okuno, S.; Tsuboniwa, N.; Shoji, S.; Yamakawa, T.; Nishizawa, Y.; Inaba, M. Relationship between fat mass and serum high-sensitivity C-reactive protein levels in prevalent hemodialysis patients. *Nephron. Clin. Pract.* **2011**, *119*, c283–c288. [CrossRef]
92. Axelsson, J.; Qureshi, A.R.; Suliman, M.E.; Honda, H.; Pecolits-Filho, R.; Heimburger, O.; Lindholm, B.; Cederholm, T.; Stenvinkel, P. Truncal fat mass as a contributor to inflammation in end-stage renal disease. *Am. J. Clin. Nutr.* **2004**, *80*, 1222–1229. [CrossRef]
93. Kaysen, G.A.; Kotanko, P.; Zhu, F.; Sarkar, S.R.; Heymsfield, S.B.; Kuhlmann, M.K.; Dwyer, T.; Usvyat, L.; Havel, P.; Levin, N.W. Relationship between adiposity and cardiovascular risk factors in prevalent hemodialysis patients. *J. Ren. Nutr.* **2009**, *19*, 357–364. [CrossRef]
94. Gohda, T.; Gotoh, H.; Tanimoto, M.; Sato, M.; Io, H.; Kaneko, K.; Harada, C.; Tomino, Y. Relationship between abdominal fat accumulation and insulin resistance in hemodialysis patients. *Hypertens. Res.* **2008**, *31*, 83–88. [CrossRef]
95. Canoy, D.; Boekholdt, S.M.; Wareham, N.; Luben, R.; Welch, A.; Bingham, S.; Buchan, I.; Day, N.; Khaw, K.T. Body fat distribution and risk of coronary heart disease in men and women in the European Prospective Investigation Into Cancer and Nutrition in Norfolk cohort: A population-based prospective study. *Circulation* **2007**, *116*, 2933–2943. [CrossRef]
96. Johansen, K.L.; Lee, C. Body composition in chronic kidney disease. *Curr. Opin. Nephrol. Hypertens.* **2015**, *24*, 268–275. [CrossRef]
97. Wu, C.C.; Liou, H.H.; Su, P.F.; Chang, M.Y.; Wang, H.H.; Chen, M.J.; Hung, S.Y. Abdominal obesity is the most significant metabolic syndrome component predictive of cardiovascular events in chronic hemodialysis patients. *Nephrol. Dial. Transplant.* **2011**, *26*, 3689–3695. [CrossRef]

98. Kittiskulnam, P.; Johansen, K.L. The obesity paradox: A further consideration in dialysis patients. *Semin. Dial.* **2019**, *32*, 485–489. [CrossRef]
99. Sanches, F.R.M.; Avesani, C.M.; Kamimura, M.A.; Lemos, M.M.; Axelsson, J.; Vasselai, P.; Draibe, S.A.; Cuppari, L. Waist circumference and visceral fat in CKD: A cross-sectional study. *Am. J. Kidney Dis.* **2008**, *52*, 66–73. [CrossRef]
100. Elsayed, E.F.; Tighiouart, H.; Weiner, D.E.; Griffith, J.; Salem, D.; Levey, A.S.; Sarna, M.J. Waist-To-Hip ratio and body mass index as risk factors for cardiovascular events in CKD. *Am. J. Kidney Dis.* **2008**, *52*, 49–57. [CrossRef]
101. Hamdy, O.; Porramatikul, S.; Al-Ozairi, E. Metabolic obesity: The paradox between visceral and subcutaneous fat. *Curr. Diabetes Rev.* **2006**, *2*, 367–373.
102. McLaughlin, T.; Lamendola, C.; Liu, A.; Abbasi, F. Preferential fat deposition in subcutaneous versus visceral depots is associated with insulin sensitivity. *J. Clin. Endocrinol. Metab.* **2011**, *96*, E1756–E1760. [CrossRef] [PubMed]
103. Tanko, L.B.; Bagger, Y.Z.; Alexandersen, P.; Larsen, P.J.; Christiansen, C. Peripheral adiposity exhibits an independent dominant antiatherogenic effect in elderly women. *Circulation* **2003**, *107*, 1626–1631. [CrossRef]
104. Hocking, S.L.; Stewart, R.L.; Brandon, A.E.; Suryana, E.; Stuart, E.; Baldwin, E.M.; Kolumam, G.A.; Modrusan, Z.; Junutula, J.R.; Gunton, J.E.; et al. Subcutaneous fat transplantation alleviates diet-induced glucose intolerance and inflammation in mice. *Diabetologia* **2015**, *58*, 1587–1600. [CrossRef]
105. Elsayed, E.F.; Sarnak, M.J.; Tighiouart, H.; Griffith, J.L.; Kurth, T.; Dalem, D.N.; Levey, S.; Weiner, D.E. Waist to hip ratio, body mass index and subsequent kidney disease and death. *Am. J. Kidney Dis.* **2008**, *52*, 29–38. [CrossRef]
106. Leitzmann, M.F.; Moore, S.C.; Koster, A.; Harris, T.B.; Park, Y.; Hollenbeck, A.; Schatzkin, A. Waist circumference as compared with body-mass index in predicting mortality from specific causes. *PLoS ONE* **2011**, *6*, e18582. [CrossRef] [PubMed]
107. Lahmann, P.H.; Lissner, L.; Gullberg, B.; Berglund, G. A prospective study of adiposity and all-cause mortality: The Malmo diet and cancer study. *Obes. Res.* **2002**, *10*, 361–369. [CrossRef]
108. Guallar-Castillon, P.; Balboa-Castillo, T.; Lopez-Garcia, E.; Leon-Munoz, L.M.; Gutierrez-Fisac, J.L.; Banegas, J.R.; Rodriguez-Artalejo, F. BMI, waist circumference, and mortality according to health status in the older adult population of Spain. *Obesity* **2009**, *17*, 2232–2238. [CrossRef]
109. Kovesdy, C.P.; Czira, M.E.; Rudas, A.; Ujszaszi, A.; Rosivall, L.; Novak, M.; Kalantar-Zadeh, K.; Molnar, M.Z.; Mucsi, I. Body mass index, waist circumference and mortality in kidney transplant recipients. *Am. J. Transplant.* **2010**, *10*, 2644–2651. [CrossRef]
110. Xuong, Y.; Yu, Y.; Jiang, H.; Yang, Q.; Liao, R.; Wang, L.; Zhang, Z.; Fu, C.; Su, B. Visceral fat area is better predictor than coronary artery calcification score for cardiovascular outcome and all-cause death in patients on hemodialysis. *J. Ren. Nutr.* **2021**, *31*, 306–312. [CrossRef] [PubMed]
111. Okamoto, T.; Morimoto, S.; Ikenoue, T.; Furumatsu, Y.; Ichihara, A. Visceral fat is an independent risk factor for cardiovascular mortality in hemodialysis patients. *Am. J. Nephrol.* **2014**, *39*, 122–129. [CrossRef] [PubMed]
112. Kramer, H.; Shoham, D.; McClure, L.A.; Durazo-Arvizu, R.; Howard, G.; Judd, S.; Muntner, P.; Safford, M.; Warnock, D.G.; McClellan, W. Association of waist circumference and body mass index with all-cause mortality in CKD: The REGARDS (Reasons for Geographic and Racial Differences in Stroke) study. *Am. J. Kidney Dis.* **2011**, *58*, 177–185. [CrossRef]
113. Lee, S.W.; Son, J.Y.; Kim, J.M.; Hwang, S.S.; Han, J.S.; Heo, N.J. Body fat distribution is more predictive of all-cause mortality than overall adiposity. *Diabetes Obes. Metab.* **2018**, *20*, 141–147. [CrossRef]
114. Caan, B.J.; Feliciano, E.M.C.; Kroenke, C.H. The importance of body composition in explaining the overweight paradox in cancer. *Cancer Res.* **2018**, *78*, 1906–1912. [CrossRef] [PubMed]
115. Ebadi, M.; Bhanji, R.A.; Tandon, P.; Mazurak, V.; Baracos, V.E.; Montano-Loza, A.J. Review article: Prognostic significance of body composition abnormalities in patients with cirrhosis. *Aliment. Pharmacol. Ther.* **2020**, *52*, 600–618. [CrossRef]
116. Ebadi, M.; Martin, L.; Ghosh, S.; Field, C.J.; Lehner, R.; Baracos, V.E.; Mazurak, V.C. Subcutaneous adiposity is an independent predictor of motality in cancer patient. *Br. J. Cancer* **2017**, *117*, 148–155. [CrossRef] [PubMed]
117. Antoun, S.; Bayar, A.; Ileana, E.; Laplanche, A.; Fizazi, K.; di Palma, M.; Escudier, B.; Albiges, L.; Maddard, C.; Loriot, Y. High subcutaneous adipose tissue predicts the prognosis in metastatic castration-resistant prostate cancer patients in post chemotherapy setting. *Eur. J. Cancer* **2015**, *51*, 2570–2577. [CrossRef]
118. Huang, C.X.; Tighiouart, H.; Beddhu, S.; Cheung, A.K.; Dwyer, J.T.; Eknoyan, G.; Beck, G.J.; Levey, A.S.; Sarnak, M.J. Both low muscle mass and low fat are associated with higher all-cause mortality in hemodialysis patients. *Kidney Int.* **2010**, *77*, 624–629. [CrossRef]
119. Mohamed-Ali, V.; Goodrick, S.; Bulmer, K.; Holly, J.M.; Yudkin, J.S.; Coppack, S.W. Production of soluble tumor necrosis factor receptors by human subcutaneous adipose tissue in vivo. *Am. J. Physiol.* **1999**, *277*, E971–E975. [CrossRef]
120. Khoramipour, K.; Chamari, K.; Hekmatikar, A.A.; Ziyaiyan, A.; Taherkhani, S.; Elguindy, N.M.; Bragazzi, N.L. Adiponectin: Structure, physiological functions, role in diabetes, and effects on nutrition. *Nutrients* **2021**, *13*, 1180. [CrossRef]
121. Beddhu, S. The body mass index paradox and an obesity, inflammation, and atherosclerosis syndrome in chronic kidney disease. *Semin. Dial.* **2004**, *17*, 229–232. [CrossRef] [PubMed]
122. Greenberg, A.S.; Obin, M.S. Obesity and the role of adipose tissue in inflammation and metabolism. *Am. J. Clin. Nutr.* **2006**, *83*, 461S–465S. [CrossRef] [PubMed]
123. Demas, G.E.; Drazen, D.L.; Nelson, R.J. Reductions in total body fat decrease humoral immunity. *Proc. Biol. Sci.* **2003**, *270*, 905–911. [CrossRef] [PubMed]

Review

Methods and Nutritional Interventions to Improve the Nutritional Status of Dialysis Patients in JAPAN—A Narrative Review

Yoshihiko Kanno [1,*], Eiichiro Kanda [2] and Akihiko Kato [3]

1. Department of Nephrology, Tokyo Medical University, Shinjuku, Tokyo 160-0023, Japan
2. Medical Science, Kawasaki Medical School, Kurashiki, Okayama 701-0192, Japan; kms.cds.kanda@gmail.com
3. Blood Purification Unit, Hamamatsu University Hospital, Hamamatsu, Shizuoka 431-3192, Japan; a.kato@hama-med.ac.jp
* Correspondence: kannoyh@tokyo-med.ac.jp

Abstract: Patients receiving dialysis therapy often have frailty, protein energy wasting, and sarcopenia. However, medical staff in Japan, except for registered dietitians, do not receive training in nutritional management at school or on the job. Moreover, registered dietitians work separately from patients and medical staff even inside a hospital, and there are many medical institutions that do not have registered dietitians. In such institutions, medical staff are required to manage patients' nutritional disorders without assistance from a specialist. Recent studies have shown that salt intake should not be restricted under conditions of low nutrition in frail subjects or those undergoing dialysis, and protein consumption should be targeted at 0.9 to 1.2 g/kg/day. The Japanese Society of Dialysis Therapy suggests that the Nutritional Risk Index-Japanese Hemodialysis (NRI-JH) is a useful tool to screen for older patients with malnutrition.

Keywords: frailty; sarcopenia; protein energy wasting; hypercatabolism

1. Introduction

Hemodialysis (HD) therapy, which has been clinically applied in Japan from about 50 years ago, has since undergone various improvements with the use of various new technologies and drugs, and is now one of the world's leading therapies. HD is now also safely used in older patients and patients with various complications, in whom such treatment was once considered impossible, and it has hence substantially helped to extend their lifespan. At the end of 2018, 339,841 patients in Japan were reported to be receiving some form of dialysis therapy [1]. Previously, patients with end-stage kidney disease (ESKD) died because they were unable to excrete water and potassium from the body. On the other hand, peritoneal dialysis therapy is expected to become more commonly used in the future, as it plays an important role in home care. However, at present, the number of patients using this method is only 9445, because it must be performed by the patients themselves or by family members. However, owing to the small number of patients, there is a lack of data in Japan, and evidence-based criteria for food intake have not been established to date [2]. The number of patients undergoing renal transplantation therapy has increased in recent years. The number is thought to be approximately 10,000 people, but diet therapy for this group of patients has not been discussed sufficiently [3]. In any case, it has become possible for humans to avoid death by ESKD using these three methods. Although various problems remain with each type of treatment, the quality of these treatments provided in Japan is high, and they have greatly benefited ESKD patients.

A characteristic feature of dialysis medicine in Japan is that the proportion of patients undergoing hemodialysis is overwhelmingly high [1]. There may be various reasons for this [4], but patients in Japan generally undergo HD 3 times a week for about 4 h at a time, which was the standard decided 50 years ago. Furthermore, patients receive guidance that eating more than the amount that can be removed by the 12 h a week of HD is life threatening. This was guidance that began in the early years of HD therapy, when patients were generally younger and hence found it more difficult to suppress their food intake owing to their appetite, and when the efficiency of dialysis was lower than at present. Specifically, patients were encouraged to reduce dietary intake if excessive weight gain between dialysis, hyperkalemia, or hyperphosphatemia was observed. However, many dialysis facilities do not have a registered dietitian, and as other medical staff do not study nutrition during their training period, specific advice regarding actual meals that take into account adequate nutrition cannot be provided to the patients. As a result, many doctors will just look at the laboratory test results, and if there is a value that is above the criteria, they just tell the patients "You are eating too much!" as a caution. If patients who lack knowledge or elderly patients receive this caution, they will feel guilty about eating, and reduce their overall food intake. This may result in many patients with insufficient energy intake, because patients should actually increase their energy intake to compensate for the reduced protein intake. In the past, the average age of HD patients was low, and hence the patients' body reserves had the capacity to compensate for the lack of energy intake, but as the age of starting dialysis is increasing and dialysis patients are generally aging, it has become necessary to introduce new ideas about nutritional management. That is, it is important to reconsider the guidance that assumes that all patients should follow dietary restrictions.

2. Assessment of Nutritional Status of HD Patients

In Japan, as a large proportion of HD patients are older patients, there are more patients who have low nourishment who require an increase in their food intake than patients who require dietary restrictions. Then, how can we identify patients with low nourishment during general clinical practice?

In recent years, the words frailty, sarcopenia, and protein-energy wasting (PEW) [5] have been attracting attention. The 2014 edition of the Sarcopenia Diagnostic Algorithm created by the Asian Sarcopenia Working Group stated that it is necessary to measure the grip strength and walking speed of elderly patients to diagnose these conditions [6]. However, it is difficult to routinely perform such measurements during daily practice in dialysis facilities in Japan, and hence it was difficult to use these measurements as indices of a patient's nutrition status, resulting in a delay in the identification of patients with low nutrition status. In November 2019, the Asian Sarcopenia Frail Society published the Sarcopenia Diagnostic Criteria 2019 [7]. This new standard states a simple algorithm that enables the identification of patients with a low nutrition status by family doctors and in community medical settings without the need for skeletal muscle mass measurement devices. If family doctors measure the muscle strength or physical function of patients, and if either value does not meet the criteria, they are asked to diagnose the patient as having "possible sarcopenia" and to begin nutritional or exercise therapy interventions. If there is a specialized facility nearby, doctors are recommended to introduce the patient to the facility to receive a definite diagnosis. Muscle strength is measured by grip strength, and the cutoff value is less than 28 kg for men and less than 18 kg for women. Physical function is evaluated by performing the 5-times chair stand-up test, and the cutoff value is 12 s or more. In acute-to-chronic-stage medical settings and in clinical research facilities, the diagnosis of sarcopenia is based on grip strength, physical function, and skeletal muscle mass, as stated in the criteria of the 2014 edition. However, as a new measurement method of physical function, in addition to the 5-times chair stand-up test, a simple physical performance battery (Short Physical Performance Battery) consisting of a balance test, a walking test, and a chair stand-up test has been added, which has increased the choice of measurement methods. As a result, it is expected that diagnoses including possible sarcopenia will become easier, and opportunities for intervention will increase. As an international standard for the diagnosis of low nutritional status, the GLIM criteria were announced in 2018. According to this criteria, after judging that a patient is at risk in the screening, if a patient shows signs of either (1) weight loss, (2) a low body mass index (BMI), or (3) low muscle mass, and if the cause is identified as (1) a decrease in dietary intake or digestive function, or (2) inflammation, the patient is diagnosed as having a low nutritional status. However, owing to differences in physique among individuals of various races, specific numerical values to be used as criteria have not been established, even for weight loss, and hence this is not yet a suitable evaluation method.

3. The Impact of Serum Albumin in Malnourished HD Patients

On the other hand, serum albumin level is useful as a daily indicator of low nutrition [8] and predictor of mortality [9] in HD patients. Figure 1 shows serum albumin levels and protein intake (normalized protein catabolism rate: nPCR) of Japanese HD patients from a statistical survey of the Japanese Society of Dialysis Therapy (JSDT) [10]. For example, because the simple standard of low nutrition is a serum albumin level of below 3.5 g/dL, most of the older patients meet this criteria, and hence the possibility of low nutrition in patients is high. In addition, the standard recommended protein intake for HD patients in Japan is 0.9 to 1.2 g/kg/day, but few patients achieve this level (Figure 1). In other words, it is clear that older HD patients have a high possibility of low nutrition, and that their protein intake, which is one of the solutions, is also insufficient. Regarding serum albumin level, specialists in Japan have discussed whether it should be measured in a state close to overflow before dialysis or measured in a concentrated state after dialysis to obtain a proper index for evaluation.

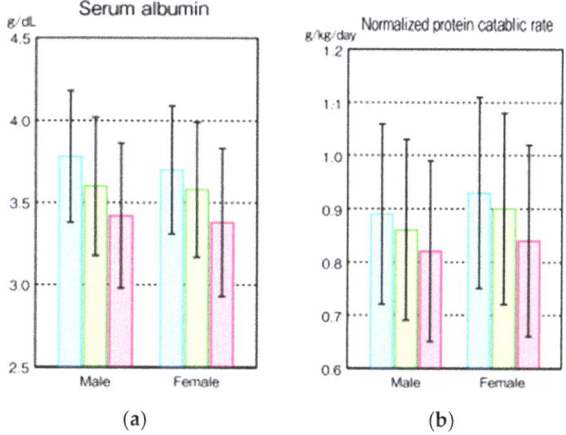

Figure 1. Nutritional status in Japanese HD patients in 2015. (Masakane, I. et al. [10]). (**a**) Serum albumin level (**b**) Normalized protein catabolic rate, of Japanese HD patients. Data are expressed as Mean ± SD. Blue column expresses patients below 60 years old, green column 60–74 years old, and red column over 75 years old.

The basis of this discussion is the old idea of deciding on a particular numerical value and providing guidance based on it. However, the correct approach is to follow the changes in albumin levels of the patient over time, and to change the diet accordingly. However, to establish a conclusion to these discussions, we analyzed statistical survey data (n = 96,700; men, 61.5%) from the JSDT [11] using the outcome event of 1.5-year mortality. Laboratory data included BMI, serum albumin, creatinine, and blood urea nitrogen (BUN) levels, which are generally measured monthly in dialysis units in Japan. Bootstrap resampling was used to compare the accuracy in predicting mortalities between pre-HD and post-HD levels using area under the receiver operating characteristic curves (AUCs) adjusted for baseline characteristics. A total of 6442 (6.7%) patients died within a year, and 30,965 (32.0%) of the patients died within 5 years. The adjusted AUCs for predicting the 1-year and 5-year mortalities showed that pre-HD albumin, creatinine, and BUN levels, and pre-HD BMI were more accurate than the post-HD levels ($p < 0.0001$ for each). Pre-HD albumin and creatinine levels showed the highest adjusted AUCs for predicting 1-year mortality (0.613 [95% CI: 0.598, 0.629]) and 5-year mortality (0.591 [95% CI; 0.586, 0.595]).

4. Methods to Evaluate and Improve Low Nutritional Status

If most older HD patients are likely to be at risk of low nutrition, establishing adequate interventions is crucial. However, at present, professional evaluation methods are very difficult to use for the evaluation of nutritional status. In general medical care, the only way to evaluate a patient is by routine evaluation methods, such as blood tests and weight measurement. In this situation, patients who show, for example, a high serum phosphorus level and a lot of weight gain would be conspicuous. However, it is necessary to look carefully at patients who are not so conspicuous, to identify those with low nourishment, including patients who are thought to have "good self-management". For example, it is necessary to consider that patients who have unconsciously lost dry weight during a 6-month period are at risk of low nutrition.

The difficulty of intervening in and preventing low nutrition is caused by the difficulty in identifying patients at risk, as a low nutritional state does not immediately cause any particular symptoms. It is difficult to recover after becoming undernourished, and it is hence important to intervene beforehand. For this reason, the Nutrition Risk Index-Japanese Hemodialysis shown in Table 1 was created as a screening tool for low nutrition. This is based on statistical survey data of the JSDT for assessing nutritional risks regarding life prognoses after 1 year (Table 2). BMI, serum albumin levels, serum total cholesterol levels, and serum creatinine levels can be used in daily practice to assess low nutritional risk [12]. This index can be used not only as a screening tool, but also as an explanation tool for patients. To treat patients with low nutrition who also have frailty or sarcopenia, it is necessary to switch ideas from the previous ways of nutritional guidance to identifying inconspicuous cases of low nourishment.

Table 1. Parameter estimates of the initial sarcopenia model and risk scores (Kanda E., et al. [12]).

	Parameter Estimate	Ratio	Score
Low BMI (≤ 20 kg/m^2)	0.51798	3.2555279035	3
Low serum albumin level (age < 65, <3.7 g/dL; age $\geq$ 65, <3.5 g/dL	0.68025	4.275075415	4
Low serum total cholesterol level (<130 mg/dL)	0.15912	1	1
High serum total cholesterol level ($\geq$220 mg/dL)	0.24819	1.559766214	2
Low serum creatinine level (age < 65, male < 11.6 mg/dL, female < 9.7 mg/dL; age $\geq$ 65, male < 9.7 mg/dL, female < 8.0 mg/dL)	0.65957	4.145110608	4

Each parameter estimate in a Cox proportional hazards model adjusted for baseline characteristics was compared with the smallest parameter estimate (low serum total cholesterol level). Then, the risk scores were determined. Abbreviations: BMI, body mass index.

Table 2. Risk groups and risk of all-cause deaths among HD patients (Kanda E, et al. [12]). Medium-risk and high-risk groups (total score of 8 to 10 and 11 or more, respectively) showed a higher risk of all-cause death than the low-risk group (score: 0 to 7).

	HR	aHR
Low-risk group	Reference	Reference
Medium-risk group	2.94 (2.68, 3.24)	1.96 (1.77, 2.16)
High-risk group	6.99 (6.45, 7.56)	3.91 (3.57, 4.29)

Values are HRs with 98% Cis of medium- and high-risk groups compared with the low-risk group. Abbreviations: aHR, adjusted hazard ratio; CI, confidence interbval.

5. Methods to Improve Low Nutritional Status

Usually, an increase or decrease in body weight is proportional to the increase or decrease in dietary intake, and thus the increase or decrease in salt intake. In 2019, the Guidelines for the Treatment of Hypertension issued by the Japanese Society of Hypertension set a target salt intake value of less than 6 g/day. Older individuals, people with renal dysfunction, and metabolic syndrome patients are highly salt-sensitive and a reduction in salt intake is often effective, but for individuals who are frail or receiving dialysis therapy, it is desirable to adjust target salt intake appropriately in consideration of their physique, nutritional status, physical activity, etc. [13]. That is, in frail older persons and the chronic dialysis patients, if low nutrition occurs owing to a low salt intake, the amount of salt intake should be increased. It has been shown in Asians that the intake of other nutrients increases with the increase in salt intake [14], and thus adsorption drugs should be used if the problem of hyperkalemia or hyperphosphatemia appears with increased food intake [15]. The most important point in the management of low nutrition is not to give guidance that limits food intake, which should be increased with great care without being caught up in the laboratory data or traditional dietary standards. There are no fatal or urgent side effects associated with increased dietary intake other than hyperkalemia, and this can be improved over time. Moreover, how much protein intake is necessary for HD patients with frailty or sarcopenia remains unknown, although HD patients without frailty or sarcopenia are recommended to take 0.9 to 1.2 g/kg/day of protein, as shown in Table 3. Even though older adults have been found to have a weaker synthetic response to proteins owing to anabolic resistance compared with younger people [16–18], HD patients should still take protein to combat frailty and sarcopenia. Although there are few reports from Japan [19,20], both sarcopenia and frailty are more frequently observed in dialysis patients than non-dialysis patients [21,22]. In addition, if non-diabetic HD patients consume enough energy, skeletal muscle mass is not reduced by the currently recommended amount of protein intake [23]. Therefore, it is first necessary to comply with the current standard intake of 0.9 to 1.2 g/kg/day. In addition, because muscle loss occurs not only by protein deficiency but also by energy deficiency [24], if weight loss occurs despite the intake of the currently recommended amount of protein, it is necessary to consider increasing energy and lipid intake and to reconsider the amount of protein intake. Furthermore, to prevent sarcopenia, it is necessary to perform a combination of exercise therapy and dietary intervention. On the other hand, what are the risks of protein intake of more than 1.2 g/kg/day? Although there was no difference in the muscle area of the abdomen and thighs in patients taking more than 1.2 g/kg/day of protein compared with those taking less, it has been reported that the risk of increase in visceral fat and hyperkalemia increases, and the risk of total death may also be higher in such patients [25]. However, it has also been pointed out that an increase in visceral fat in older HD patients with frailty or sarcopenia may not necessarily be a risk of death [26]. In Japan, according to a survey conducted at the end of fiscal year 2015, the protein intake of dialysis patients was substantially lower than the recommended amount of 0.9 to 1.2 g/kg/day [10], and we hence believe it is important to target the protein consumption of HD patients to the present standard of 0.9 to 1.2 g/kg/day.

Table 3. Standard nutrient intake of patients receiving dialysis and healthy subjects in Japan. The standards for HD patients are from the recommendations of JSDT published in Japanese in 2014. The standards for healthy subjects were calculated from the National Institute of Nutrition (Reference 30), using the mean age and mean body weight of Japanese HD patients. Standard body weight is selected and used as body weight. RDA: recommended dietary allowance, DG: tentative dietary goal for preventing lifestyle-associated diseases.

	Energy (kcal/kgBW/day)	Protein (g/kgBW/day)	Salt (g/day)	Potassium (mg/day)	Phosphate (mg/day)	Calcium (mg/day)
Patients (HD 3 times/wk)	30–35	0.9–1.2	<6	≤2000	≤protein (g) × 15	
Healthy men (66 years old)	35–42 (2100–2450 kcal/day)	1.0 (RDA 60 g/day)	<8 (DG)	2500 (adequate intake) –3000 (DG)	1000 (796.5–1062) (adequate intake)	700 (RDA)
Healthy women (68 years old)	34–40 (1650–1900 kcal/day)	1.0 (RDA 50 g/day)	<7 (DG)	2000 (adequate intake) –2600 (DG)	800 (648–864) (adequate intake)	650 (RDA)

5.1. Meals for Dialysis Patients

Dietary guidance for dialysis patients is provided in accordance with the dietary standards for chronic kidney disease patients proposed in 2014 by the Japanese Society of Nephrology and JSDT [27]. Facilities with registered dietitians can evaluate patient diets according to the nutritional care process and provide correct guidance following this standard. Of course, more accurate assessments of nutritional status using various specialized techniques are also possible [28], and many reports state that individual guidance by registered dietitians is effective in increasing protein intake [29]. On the other hand, many institutions do not have a registered dietitian, and medical professionals who have not studied nutrition are required to provide dietary guidance. However, guidance centered on conventional food restrictions is not necessarily effective, and on the contrary, it has the risk of causing frailty and sarcopenia.

In Japan, the National Institute of Nutrition and Health issues dietary intake standards every 5 years for healthy people to maintain healthy lives [30]. Table 3 compares the standards of healthy individuals and dialysis patients. Dialysis patients have a slightly lower energy setting than healthy people, but they have almost the same settings for protein and salt. Restrictions are necessary only for potassium, and otherwise they should be recommended to eat similar meals as healthy people of the same age range. When a patient's routine laboratory data changes to an abnormal value while following the above diet, the diet can be adjusted with trial and error to gradually reach a balance. The idea of letting dialysis patients eat the same meals as healthy people is quite the opposite of the idea of dietary restriction that has been the standard in the daily care of HD patients. In the absence of a nutrition specialist, it is also important to manage patients by such a "think as you go" type strategy.

5.2. Medical Interventions

The discussion to this point has been about the intake of appropriate meals by patients at their homes. However, for many older dialysis patients in Japan, even though they are provided an ideal menu by a registered dietitian, and this ideal menu is prepared by the family, it is often not possible for the patient to eat a sufficient amount of it owing to old age and a decreased appetite. Therefore, to improve the nutritional status of these patients, supplements may be used to overcome the deficiency of nutrients. Many oral nutritional supplements are available worldwide, and the effective use of these can increase protein intake. Furthermore, oral nutritional support during HD sessions is recommended, as it is generally considered to improve the nutritional status of patients [31], although there are some contradicting reports [32]. The benefits and risks of this type of support varies with the status of the patient, the type of dialysis session, and institute, and hence it is still difficult at present to come to a general conclusion [33].

Parenteral nutrition during HD is another method to increase the nutritional intake of patients with low nutrition. There is more evidence that parenteral nutrition is effective for improving nutritional status in HD patients than oral support. A prospective, multicenter, randomized, open-label, controlled, parallel-group phase IV clinical trial in 107 maintenance hemodialysis patients with PEW was conducted by Marsen et al. [34]. Patients were randomized into 2 groups receiving standardized nutritional counseling with or without intradialytic parenteral nutrition. Prealbumin levels were significantly increased to over baseline levels after 4 weeks of treatment in patients receiving parenteral nutrition compared with the control group. More patients receiving parenteral nutrition therapy achieved an increase in prealbumin level to greater than 30 mg/L after 16 weeks of treatment (48.7% vs. 31.8%). The increase in prealbumin levels as a result of parenteral nutrition therapy was more prominent in patients with moderate malnutrition (SGA score B) compared with patients with severe malnutrition (SGA score C). Unfortunately, we have no clear data at present regarding the effects of parenteral nutrition on HD patients with low nutrition in Japan, and JSDT is currently considering a prospective study to investigate this point.

6. Conclusions

Although high-quality dialysis treatments are available in Japan, with the aging of patients, it is necessary to reconsider the current treatment policies. Nutritional management is at the center of this theme, and it is hence necessary to perform research towards the establishment of intervention methods that are suitable for current dialysis patients in Japan.

Author Contributions: Writing—original draft preparation, Y.K.; writing—review and editing, E.K.; supervision, A.K. All authors have read and agreed to the published version of the manuscript.

Funding: This research received no external funding.

Conflicts of Interest: The authors declare no conflict of interest.

References

1. Nitta, K.; Goto, S.; Masakane, I.; Hanafusa, N.; Taniguchi, M.; Hasegawa, T.; Nakai, S.; Wada, A.; Hamano, T.; Hoshino, J.; et al. Annual dialysis data report for 2018, JSDT Renal Data Registry: Survey methods, facility data, incidence, prevalence, and mortality. *Ren. Replace. Ther.* **2020**, *6*, 41. [CrossRef]
2. Ito, Y. Peritoneal Dialysis Guidelines 2019 Part 1 (Position paper of Japanese Society of Dialysis Therapy). *Ren. Replace. Ther.* in press.
3. Nagaoka, Y.; Onda, R.; Sakamoto, K.; Izawa, Y.; Kono, H.; Nakagawa, K.; Shinoda, K.; Morita, S.; Kanno, Y. Dietary intake in Japanese patients with kidney transplantation. *Clin. Exp. Nephrol.* **2016**, *20*, 972–981. [CrossRef] [PubMed]
4. Kanno, H.; Kanno, Y. Chapter 10—Ethnicity and Chronic Kidney Disease in Japan. In *Chronic Renal Disease*, 2nd ed.; Kimmel, P.L., Rosenberg, M.E., Eds.; Academic Press: London, UK, 2020; pp. 139–148.
5. Carrero, J.J.; Nakashima, A.; Qureshi, A.R.; Lindholm, B.; Heimbürger, O.; Bárány, P.; Stenvinkel, P. Protein-energy wasting modifies the association of ghrelin with inflammation, leptin, and mortality in hemodialysis patients. *Kidney Int.* **2011**, *79*, 749–756. [CrossRef]
6. Chen, L.K.; Liu, L.K.; Woo, J.; Assantachai, P.; Auyeung, T.W.; Bahyah, K.S.; Chou, M.Y.; Chen, L.Y.; Hsu, P.S.; Krairit, O.; et al. Sarcopenia in Asia: Consensus report of the Asian Working Group for Sarcopenia. *J. Am. Med. Dir. Assoc.* **2014**, *15*, 95–101. [CrossRef] [PubMed]
7. Chen, L.K.; Woo, J.; Assantachai, P.; Auyeung, T.W.; Chou, M.Y.; Iijima, K.; Jang, H.C.; Kang, L.; Kim, M.; Kim, S.; et al. Asian Working Group for Sarcopenia: 2019 Consensus Update on Sarcopenia Diagnosis and Treatment. *J. Am. Med. Dir. Assoc.* **2020**, *21*, 300–307. [CrossRef] [PubMed]
8. Gama-Axelsson, T.; Heimbürger, O.; Stenvinkel, P.; Bárány, P.; Lindholm, B.; Qureshi, A.R. Serum albumin as predictor of nutritional status in patients with ESRD. *Clin. J. Am. Soc. Nephrol.* **2012**, *7*, 1446–1453. [CrossRef]
9. Alves, F.C.; Sun, J.; Qureshi, A.R.; Dai, L.; Snaedal, S.; Bárány, P.; Heimbürger, O.; Lindholm, B.; Stenvinkel, P. The higher mortality associated with low serum albumin is dependent on systemic inflammation in end-stage kidney disease. *PLoS ONE* **2018**, *13*, e0190410. [CrossRef]
10. Masakane, I.; Taniguchi, M.; Nakai, S.; Tsuchida, K.; Goto, S.; Wada, A.; Ogata, S.; Hasegawa, T.; Hamano, T.; Hanafusa, N.; et al. Annual Dialysis Data Report 2015, JSDT Renal Data Registry. *Ren. Replace. Ther.* **2018**, *4*, 19. [CrossRef]
11. Kanno, Y.; Kanda, E. Comparison of accuracy between pre-hemodialysis and post-hemodialysis levels of nutritional factors for prediction of mortality in hemodialysis patients. *Clin. Nutr.* **2019**, *38*, 383–388. [CrossRef]
12. Kanda, E.; Kato, A.; Masakane, I.; Kanno, Y. A new nutritional risk index for predicting mortality in hemodialysis patients: Nationwide cohort study. *PLoS ONE* **2019**, *14*, e0214524. [CrossRef] [PubMed]
13. Umemura, S.; Arima, H.; Arima, S.; Asayama, K.; Dohi, Y.; Hirooka, Y.; Horio, T.; Hoshide, S.; Ikeda, S.; Ishimitsu, T.; et al. The Japanese Society of Hypertension Guidelines for the Management of Hypertension (JSH 2019). *Hypertens. Res.* **2019**, *42*, 1235–1481. [CrossRef] [PubMed]
14. Yoon, C.Y.; Noh, J.; Lee, J.; Kee, Y.K.; Seo, C.; Lee, M.; Cha, M.U.; Kim, H.; Park, S.; Yun, H.R.; et al. High and low sodium intakes are associated with incident chronic kidney disease in patients with normal renal function and hypertension. *Kidney Int.* **2018**, *93*, 921–931. [CrossRef]
15. Rhee, C.M.; You, A.S.; Koontz Parsons, T.; Tortorici, A.R.; Bross, R.; St-Jules, D.E.; Jing, J.; Lee, M.L.; Benner, D.; Kovesdy, C.P.; et al. Effect of high-protein meals during hemodialysis combined with lanthanum carbonate in hypoalbuminemic dialysis patients: Findings from the FrEDI randomized controlled trial. *Nephrol. Dial. Transplant.* **2016**, *32*, 1233–1243. [CrossRef] [PubMed]
16. Arentson-Lantz, E.; Clairmont, S.; Paddon-Jones, D.; Tremblay, A.; Elango, R. Protein: A nutrient in focus. *Appl. Physiol. Nutr. Metab.* **2015**, *40*, 755–761. [CrossRef]
17. Moore, D.R.; Churchward-Venne, T.A.; Witard, O.; Breen, L.; Burd, N.A.; Tipton, K.D.; Phillips, S.M. Protein Ingestion to Stimulate Myofibrillar Protein Synthesis Requires Greater Relative Protein Intakes in Healthy Older Versus Younger Men. *J. Gerontol. Ser. A* **2014**, *70*, 57–62. [CrossRef]

18. Morton, R.W.; Traylor, D.A.; Weijs, P.J.M.; Phillips, S.M. Defining anabolic resistance: Implications for delivery of clinical care nutrition. *Curr. Opin. Crit. Care* **2018**, *24*, 124–130. [CrossRef] [PubMed]
19. Mori, K.; Nishide, K.; Okuno, S.; Shoji, T.; Emoto, M.; Tsuda, A.; Nakatani, S.; Imanishi, Y.; Ishimura, E.; Yamakawa, T.; et al. Impact of diabetes on sarcopenia and mortality in patients undergoing hemodialysis. *BMC Nephrol.* **2019**, *20*, 105. [CrossRef]
20. Yasui, S.; Shirai, Y.; Tanimura, M.; Matsuura, S.; Saito, Y.; Miyata, K.; Ishikawa, E.; Miki, C.; Hamada, Y. Prevalence of protein-energy wasting (PEW) and evaluation of diagnostic criteria in Japanese maintenance hemodialysis patients. *Asia Pac. J. Clin. Nutr.* **2016**, *25*, 292–299. [CrossRef]
21. Lee, H.; Kim, K.; Ahn, J.; Lee, D.R.; Lee, J.H.; Hwang, S.D. Association of nutritional status with osteoporosis, sarcopenia, and cognitive impairment in patients on hemodialysis. *Asia Pac. J. Clin. Nutr.* **2020**, *29*, 712–723. [CrossRef] [PubMed]
22. Slee, A.; McKeaveney, C.; Adamson, G.; Davenport, A.; Farrington, K.; Fouque, D.; Kalantar-Zadeh, K.; Mallett, J.; Maxwell, A.P.; Mullan, R.; et al. Estimating the Prevalence of Muscle Wasting, Weakness, and Sarcopenia in Hemodialysis Patients. *J. Ren. Nutr.* **2020**, *30*, 313–321. [CrossRef]
23. Ohkawa, S.; Kaizu, Y.; Odamaki, M.; Ikegaya, N.; Hibi, I.; Miyaji, K.; Kumagai, H. Optimum dietary protein requirement in nondiabetic maintenance hemodialysis patients. *Am. J. Kidney Dis.* **2004**, *43*, 454–463. [CrossRef]
24. Ikizler, T.A. Protein and energy: Recommended intake and nutrient supplementation in chronic dialysis patients. *Semin Dial.* **2004**, *17*, 471–478. [CrossRef] [PubMed]
25. Shinaberger, C.S.; Kilpatrick, R.D.; Regidor, D.L.; McAllister, C.J.; Greenland, S.; Kopple, J.D.; Kalantar-Zadeh, K. Longitudinal associations between dietary protein intake and survival in hemodialysis patients. *Am. J. Kidney Dis.* **2006**, *48*, 37–49. [CrossRef] [PubMed]
26. Machiba, Y.; Inaba, M.; Mori, K.; Kurajoh, M.; Nishide, K.; Norimine, K.; Yamakawa, T.; Shoji, S.; Okuno, S. Paradoxical positive association of serum adiponectin with all-cause mortality based on body composition in Japanese haemodialysis patients. *Sci. Rep.* **2018**, *8*, 14699. [CrossRef] [PubMed]
27. Japanese Society of Nephrology. Dietary recommendations for chronic kidney disease 2014. *Jpn. J. Nephrol.* **2014**, *56*, 553–599.
28. Marcelli, D.; Wabel, P.; Wieskotten, S.; Ciotola, A.; Grassmann, A.; Di Benedetto, A.; Canaud, B. Physical methods for evaluating the nutrition status of hemodialysis patients. *J. Nephrol.* **2015**, *28*, 523–530. [CrossRef] [PubMed]
29. Jo, I.Y.; Kim, W.J.; Park, H.C.; Choi, H.Y.; Lee, J.E.; Lee, S.M. Effect of Personalized Nutritional Counseling on the Nutritional Status of Hemodialysis Patients. *Clin. Nutr. Res.* **2017**, *6*, 285–295. [CrossRef]
30. The Minister of Health. *Overview of Dietary Reference Intakes for Japanese*; The Minister of Health, Labour and Welfare: Tokyo, Japan, 2015.
31. Ikizler, T.A.; Cano, N.J.; Franch, H.; Fouque, D.; Himmelfarb, J.; Kalantar-Zadeh, K.; Kuhlmann, M.K.; Stenvinkel, P.; TerWee, P.; Teta, D.; et al. Prevention and treatment of protein energy wasting in chronic kidney disease patients: A consensus statement by the International Society of Renal Nutrition and Metabolism. *Kidney Int.* **2013**, *84*, 1096–1107. [CrossRef]
32. Beddhu, S.; Filipowicz, R.; Chen, X.; Neilson, J.L.; Wei, G.; Huang, Y.; Greene, T. Supervised oral protein supplementation during dialysis in patients with elevated C-reactive protein levels: A two phase, longitudinal, single center, open labeled study. *BMC Nephrol.* **2015**, *16*, 87. [CrossRef] [PubMed]
33. Kistler, B.; Benner, D.; Burgess, M.; Stasios, M.; Kalantar-Zadeh, K.; Wilund, K.R. To Eat or Not to Eat—International Experiences With Eating During Hemodialysis Treatment. *J. Ren. Nutr.* **2014**, *24*, 349–352. [CrossRef] [PubMed]
34. Marsen, T.A.; Beer, J.; Mann, H. Intradialytic parenteral nutrition in maintenance hemodialysis patients suffering from protein-energy wasting. Results of a multicenter, open, prospective, randomized trial. *Clin. Nutr.* **2017**, *36*, 107–117. [CrossRef] [PubMed]

Review

The Importance of Phosphate Control in Chronic Kidney Disease

Ken Tsuchiya [1],* and Taro Akihisa [2]

1 Department of Blood Purification, Tokyo Women's Medical University, Tokyo 162-8666, Japan
2 Department of Nephrology, Tokyo Women's Medical University, Tokyo 162-8666, Japan; taro09071031@gmail.com
* Correspondence: tsuchiya@twmu.ac.jp

Abstract: A series of problems including osteopathy, abnormal serum data, and vascular calcification associated with chronic kidney disease (CKD) are now collectively called CKD-mineral bone disease (CKD-MBD). The pathophysiology of CKD-MBD is becoming clear with the emerging of αKlotho, originally identified as a progeria-causing protein, and bone-derived phosphaturic fibroblast growth factor 23 (FGF23) as associated factors. Meanwhile, compared with calcium and parathyroid hormone, which have long been linked with CKD-MBD, phosphate is now attracting more attention because of its association with complications and outcomes. Incidentally, as the pivotal roles of FGF23 and αKlotho in phosphate metabolism have been unveiled, how phosphate metabolism and hyperphosphatemia are involved in CKD-MBD and how they can be clinically treated have become of great interest. Thus, the aim of this review is reconsider CKD-MBD from the viewpoint of phosphorus, its involvement in the pathophysiology, causing complications, therapeutic approach based on the clinical evidence, and clarifying the importance of phosphorus management.

Keywords: CKD-MBD; FGF23; aKlotho; phosphate-binder

1. Introduction

The series of changes that occur in renal dysfunction, including decreases in serum calcium levels due to impairment in vitamin D activation, hypersecretion of parathyroid hormone (PTH; i.e., secondary hyperparathyroidism), bone decalcification, and weak bones (osteomalacia), were collectively regarded as renal osteodystrophy. Following the introduction of the term "chronic kidney disease" (CKD), which expands the prior concept of renal dysfunction or renal failure, CKD-associated metabolic disorders of minerals (e.g., calcium) are now defined as CKD-mineral bone disease (CKD-MBD). As if coinciding with these changes, αKlotho was first reported in 1997, a deficiency of which results in an aging phenotype [1], and fibroblast growth factor 23 (FGF23), which causes a form of rickets and hypophosphatemia in bone metastasis, was identified in the early 2000s [2,3]. Phenotypical similarities between αKlotho-deficient mice and FGF23-deficient mice indicated an association between these two molecules, and their considerable involvement in the regulation of phosphate metabolism was subsequently revealed [4]. Given the significance of phosphate metabolism in CKD, and that αKlotho and FGF23 are involved in the pathophysiology as well as the onset of complications and survival in CKD, the importance of the αKlotho/FGF23 regulatory system in CKD-MBD is becoming clearer. This article reviews phosphate metabolism in CKD-MBD and its clinical significance, with a particular focus on the role of αKlotho/FGF23.

2. Basics of Phosphate Metabolism

Phosphate, along with calcium, is abundant in bone and as a component of hydroxyapatite, is essential for bone formation. It also has a variety of roles in cell biology (both in cell functions and maintaining life), including being a component of cell membranes and nucleic acids, being a component of ATP (the cell's energy source), and regulating intracellular signaling via phosphorylation to control the function of enzymes and adjust pH. Phosphate ions are the most abundant intracellular anions, and its intracellular concentration is higher than that of serum. The metabolic balance of phosphate is regulated mainly by maintenance of the phosphate pool in bone and soft tissues, through phosphate absorption in the intestinal tract, osteogenesis, bone resorption, and excretion and reabsorption in the kidneys. Vitamin D and PTH have long been known to play major roles in the regulation [5]. The largest quantity of phosphate is stored in the bones, but the mechanism by which the phosphate pool is maintained in the bones has not yet been fully elucidated, and this is why many aspects of phosphate storage and its control in renal dysfunction or during dialysis remain unknown. Recently, sodium–phosphate cotransporters have been explored, and their critical role in phosphate reabsorption and excretion in the kidney was demonstrated [6]. The movement of phosphate in and out of the body basically relies on phosphate transporters. Sodium-dependent phosphate transporters (Na/Pi) that localize on proximal tubular epithelial cells and small intestinal epithelial cells are important for phosphate homeostasis in blood because they are responsible for excretion and reabsorption of phosphate in the kidney as well as phosphate absorption in the intestinal tract [7]. Approximately 80% of filtered phosphate in urine is reabsorbed in the kidney; of this, 60% is reabsorbed by the proximal convoluted tubules, 10 to 20% by the proximal straight tubule, whereas less than 10% is reabsorbed by the distal convoluted tubules.

Phosphate uptake can be roughly classified into intercellular transport and Na/Pi-mediated cellular transport. Na/Pi are proteins essential for phosphate uptake into cells via the plasma membrane. Three Na/Pi families have been identified. Type I includes gene, SLC17 A1 (Na/Pi-I), and Type II includes the gene, SLC34 family (Na/Pi-I). Both types are expressed in the kidney and small intestine and are responsible for epithelial phosphate transport. Na/Pi-II is further classified into IIa, IIb, and IIc. In proximal tubular epithelial cells, Na/Pi-IIa and Na/Pi-IIc are localized on the brush border membrane and play a pivotal role in phosphate reabsorption. Type III includes the gene, SLC20 family (PiT1, PiT2), which are expressed in various organs and are responsible for high-affinity phosphate transport. With advances in the cloning of genes that encode these sodium-dependent phosphate transporters and the elucidation of phosphate transport kinetics and related molecular mechanisms (e.g., molecular structures), regulatory factors such as FGF23 and associated small molecules have been identified and their functions have been clarified. These molecules are becoming the targets of new drugs [8]. It was long thought that PTH (a hormone that regulates calcium and phosphate levels) and 1,25-dihydroxyvitamin D (1,25(OH)2D) control Na/Pi to maintain the phosphate balance. Furthermore, the FGF23-mediated regulatory mechanism secreted from bone cells, which has recently emerged, is also affecting Na/Pi transport activity, that connects the kidney and bone in which αKlotho is expressed. Taken together, it is clear that many organs are involved in the maintenance of phosphorus homeostasis.

3. The αKlotho/FGF23 Axis

Since the phosphate-related molecules αKlotho and FGF23 were identified in the 1990s, powerful phosphate regulatory mechanisms have been revealed. In patients with abnormal laboratory test results indicative of hyperphosphatemia or secondary hyperparathyroidism, soft tissue calcification (e.g., vascular calcification) can occur in addition to renal osteopathy, and this can lead to fracture, cardiovascular event, and death. This systemic condition is now understood as a disorder of mineral and bone metabolism resulting from CKD, and the term CKD-MBD was proposed [9]. αKlotho is a factor that supports this disease concept. The aklotho gene attracted attention for its characteristic aging phenotype, consisting of a short life span, arterial calcification, pulmonary emphysema, and osteoporosis, in mice carrying an insertion mutation. Furthermore, the high mRNA expression level in the kidney and the development of hyperphosphatemia in insertion mutants suggested the possible involvement in the pathophysiology of kidney diseases [1]. αKlotho protein is composed of domains that show similarities to a carbohydrate-degrading enzyme (i.e., β-glucosidase), and exists in 2 forms (membrane-bound or secreted). The membrane-bound form is involved in the signal transduction of phosphaturic FGF23 by serving as a cofactor of the FGF23 receptor. More precisely, membrane-bound αKlotho acts as a co-replicator of the FGF23 receptor to enhance the specificity of the receptor and FGF23 actions [10,11]. FGF receptors are tyrosine kinase receptors encoded by 4 genes and make a complex with αKlotho to form the high-affinity FGF23 binding site [12]. However, αKlotho was originally recognized as a protein with multipotency, and various mechanisms of action were speculated, including the action of secreted αKlotho. Meanwhile, it was recently reported that the structure of αKlotho was not compatible with its glycosidase activity, suggesting that shed αKlotho functions as an on-demand non-enzymatic scaffold to promote FGF23 signaling [13].

The role of secreted aKlotho remains largely unknown. Secreted aKlotho has sialidase activity and cleaves sialic acids from N-linked glycans of glycoproteins, thereby contributing to the stability of glycoproteins in the membrane [14]. One possible role is preventing endocytosis of cation channels such as TRPV5 and ROMK1, thereby stabilizing them and establishing their calcium channel functions [15,16]. The regulation of TRPC6 channel by secreted αKlotho is reported to be a direct channel-gating action, independent of FGF23 receptors [17,18]. The inhibition of sodium-dependent phosphate transporters (Na/Pi-II), which are located in proximal tubules, inhibits the reabsorption of phosphate in the kidney, resulting in phosphate diuresis. However, given that αKlotho is localized mainly in the distal tubules [19], whereas Na/Pi-II is localized in the proximal tubules, it is possible that FGF23 interacts with the αKlotho–FGF complex to exert a paracrine action on adjacent proximal tubules; alternatively, the secreted form of αKlotho, which has glucuronidase activity, modifies Na/Pi-II glycans to decrease enzymatic activity or enhance the internalization of transporters, thereby modulating the inhibitory regulation [20]. Despite the several reported functions described above, many aspects of the mechanism by which αKlotho and FGF23 regulate Na/Pi-II remain to be elucidated [11], particularly, the mode of action of the secreted form of αKlotho and how it works in distant organs.

FGF23, a member of the fibroblast growth factor family, was identified as a phosphate diuretic factor. Around the same time, the FGF23 gene was identified as a causative gene of autosomal dominant hypophosphatemic rickets [2] and as a humoral factor in tumor-induced osteomalacia [3]. FGF23 is a 26-kDa protein comprising 251 amino acids and is produced and secreted mainly by osteocytes [21]. Phenotypic similarities between FGF23-knockout mice and αKlotho-knockout mice indicated an association between FGF23 and αKlotho, which were shown to be components of the same signal transduction system [4]. FGF family members (22 humoral factors) interact with FGF receptors and are involved in embryogenesis and organ development. Although FGF23 has a low affinity for FGF, the formation of a complex between αKlotho and FGF receptor 1c, 3c, or 4 creates a high-affinity binding site that exert actions in the kidney. The basic biological and physiological actions of FGF23 in calcium/phosphate metabolism is becoming clear. Shimada et al. administered synthetic FGF23 to experimental animals that had undergone parathyroidectomy and examined the effect of FGF23 without PTH action. The administration of synthetic FGF23 decreased serum phosphate levels, likely due to decreased phosphate reabsorption, which was indicated by the suppressed expression of Na/Pi-II in the proximal tubules. In addition, FGF23 decreased the expression of 1α-hydroxylase mRNA and increased the expression of 25-hydroxyvitamin D-24 hydroxylase mRNA, indicating that FGF23 suppresses the active form of vitamin D [22].

4. Phosphate-αKlotho/FGF23 Axis

It has been reported that the renal expression of αKlotho is reduced in CKD [23]. Sakan et al. examined biopsy specimens and showed progressive reduction in αKlotho immunostaining and in αKlotho mRNA expression from the early stage of CKD [24]. The expression of αKlotho is known to be decreased due to various types of stress and ischemia. For example, experiments using αKlotho-expressing cultured cells showed that oxidative stress decreased αKlotho expression [25]. These results indicated that decreased αKlotho expression not only causes metabolic disorders but may also elicit distinctive pathologies. αKlotho is reported to inhibit aging, increase lifespan, and prevent tissue damage, and thus it is easy to imagine an association between decreased expression of αKlotho and progression of CKD [26–28]. An experimental CKD model using *klotho* (+/−) mice with ureteral obstruction showed aggravation of interstitial fibrosis in mice with reduced αKlotho expression, probably due to impaired suppression of TGFβ [29], suggesting that decreases in αKlotho expression weaken the mechanism that suppresses fibrosis. This further suggests a vicious cycle in which stress and ischemia lead to decreased expression of αKlotho in the renal tissue, which accelerates tissue damage during the progression of CKD (Figure 1).

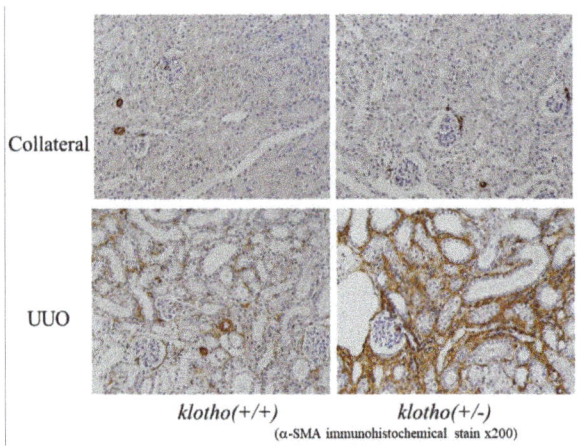

Figure 1. Representative sections immunohistochemically stained for α-SMA in the renal tubules in the reduced Klotho expression mice treated by unilateral ureteral obstruction. Renal fibrosis was induced by unilateral ureteral obstruction (UUO) in mice with reduced αKlotho expression *αkl* (+/−) mice and compared them with wild-type mice. The UUO kidneys from *αkl* (+/−) mice expressed significantly higher levels of fibrosis marker, α-smooth muscle actin (α-SMA), than those from wild-type *αkl* (+/+) mice. Adapted from reference [29].

αKlotho levels in serum and urine have been reported in many studies. The secreted form of αKlotho can be measured, but the correlations of serum αKlotho level with the degree of renal dysfunction and serum phosphate level remain controversial. Decreased urinary excretion of αKlotho and severe renal impairment have been reported in acute kidney injury [30], and its negative correlation with renal function has also been reported [31]. However, Seiler et al. showed that serum αKlotho was correlated with age but not with glomerular filtration rate (GFR), serum calcium level, or serum phosphate level and, compared with FGF23, it was not strongly associated with outcomes in CKD [32]. Whether αKlotho level can be a predictor of outcomes in CKD has not been well studied. In dialysis patients, rates of coronary artery diseases and left ventricular dysfunction were high when the serum αKlotho level was low, but a low serum αKlotho level was not necessarily correlated with cardiovascular disease or aortic calcification score [33]. Also, the association of secreted αKlotho with renal function and prognosis in CKD patients was questioned in a meta-analysis [34]. The measurement system is an important component in the testing of clinical specimens, but there are several limitations in αKlotho measurement that need to be addressed before the significance of αKlotho can be determined [35]. In addition, Ref. [36] summarized important measurement points and soluble αKlotho measurement methods to date. After all, establishment of new reproducible measurement methods, sample management, etc. are indispensable for clarifying the significance of human soluble αKlotho and its relationship with prognosis and pathophysiology. Taken together, it seems certain that αKlotho expression decreases in the renal parenchyma, but many issues still need to be addressed including analysis of the secreted form of αKlotho; investigation of the mode of action of the secreted form of αKlotho and its actions in distant organs; measurement of serum αKlotho level in renal failure with decreased renal αKlotho expression; and development of reproducible measurement techniques. Nevertheless, αKlotho has many potential implications for diagnosis, physiological action, and pathophysiology [36,37].

However, in pre-dialysis CKD, increases in serum phosphate level occur at later stages and therefore hyperphosphatemia is not always detected early. As renal dysfunction progresses, renal αKlotho expression decreases while FGF23 and PTH increase, leading to increased phosphate excretion per nephron to compensate for the decreased GFR [38,39] (Figure 2). It should be noted that FGF23 increases in the early stage of CKD, but at present it is unclear whether αKlotho decreases [40]. FGF23 is likely to have a suppressive effect on phosphate storage attributed to clearance impairment, but early increases in FGF23 level, even when the serum phosphate level is in the normal range, could suggest the presence of other stimulatory factors. A prospective and cohort study involving 3879 patients with a mean eGFR of 42.8 mL/min showed that an increased FGF23 level predicted the prognosis of CKD, specifically, a significantly high mortality and disease progression to end-stage kidney disease [41]. Prognosis was poor in the group with hyperphosphatemia at the initiation of dialysis, and an increased FGF23 level was a risk factor of mortality [42]. FGF23 was also reported to be a predictor of cardiovascular events in predialysis CKD patients but did not predict events at the initiation of dialysis and during maintenance dialysis [43]. The significance of these reported high levels of FGF23 during maintenance dialysis remains inconclusive.

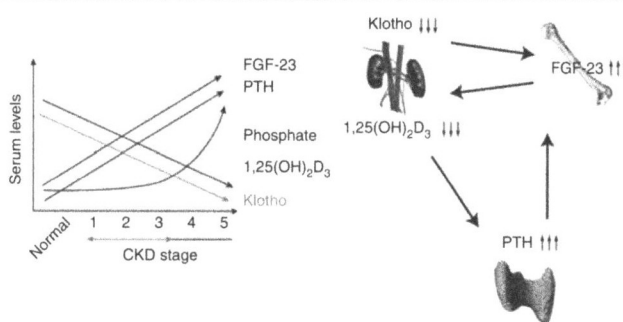

Figure 2. Changes in Klotho protein, FGF-23, PTH, 1,25(OH)2D3, and phosphate as CKD progresses. When Klotho expression first decreases, FGF-23 increases, lowering circulating 1,25(OH)2D3, which depresses Klotho expression further and increases PTH expression. Increased PTH induces further FGF-23 increases, causing large decreases in 1,25(OH)2D3 and large increases in PTH. This cycle results in hyperphosphatemia in late stages of CKD. CKD, chronic kidney disease; FGF-23, fibroblast growth factor-23; PTH, parathyroid hormone. Adapted from reference [38].

αKlotho and FGF23 have been reported to exert physiological activities and direct biological actions, respectively. Also, the multipotency of αKlotho is of great interest. Transgenic mice overexpressing αKlotho protein are reported to have a 20–30% longer lifespan, possibly through a mechanism involving the suppression of insulin/insulin-like growth factor 1 (IGF1) signaling by αKlotho [26]. Generally, intracellular insulin/IGF1 signaling is involved in the activation of redox signaling, the cytotoxicity of which induces aging. It has also been suggested that αKlotho influences Wnt signaling [27] and induces enzymes that scavenge reactive oxygen species to regulate apoptosis, thereby protecting proteins and DNA from damage by oxidative stress as well as suppressing tissue damage [28].

Meanwhile, several studies have reported the activities of FGF23. FGF23 was reported to induce cardiac hypertrophy in an animal model and to enhance sodium reabsorption in humans, thereby inducing hypertension [44,45]. These reports are in good agreement with the association between FGF23 and the risk of chronic heart failure [46]. However, a meta-analysis compared participants in the top third with those in the bottom third of FGF23 concentration and showed that the summary relative ratios (95% confidence intervals [CI]) were 1.33 (1.12–1.58) for myocardial infarction, 1.26 (1.13–1.41) for stroke, 1.48 (1.29–1.69) for heart failure, 1.42 (1.27–1.60) for cardiovascular mortality, and 1.70 (1.52–1.91) for all-cause mortality. For non-cardiovascular mortality, the summary relative ratio was 1.52 (95% CI, 1.28–1.79). These results suggest no causal relationship between FGF23 and cardiovascular disease risk [47]. In the above studies, the FGF level in CKD was measured at a single point in time, rather than over a given period. A prospective and case-cohort study involving chronic renal insufficiency patients monitored the FGF23 level at 2–5 years (mean, 4.0 ± 1.2 years) in a randomly selected sub-cohort of 1135 participants. The median FGF23 level was stable for 5 years of follow-up, but the distribution gradually skewed to the right, suggesting a subpopulation with a markedly elevated FGF23 level. Compared with participants with stable FGF23 levels, those with slowly increasing FGF23 levels had a 4.49-fold higher risk of death (95% CI, 3.17–6.35), whereas those with rapidly increasing FGF23 levels had a 15.23-fold higher risk of death (95% CI, 8.24–28.14). Conclusively, FGF23 levels are stable over time in the majority of CKD patients, but monitoring can identify subpopulations with elevated FGF23 levels and an extremely high risk of death [48]. The biological activities and clinical significance of soluble αKlotho and FGF23 remain largely unknown and further studies are anticipated [49,50].

5. Phosphate Metabolism in CKD

As described earlier, CKD-MBD develops in the early stage of CKD and persists in the dialysis stage after renal function is abolished. The pathophysiology of CKD-MBD has traditionally included vitamin D activation disorder and hypocalcemia due to renal dysfunction; hyperparathyroidism secondary to those stimuli; and bone changes due to elevated PTH levels. Phosphate metabolism disorders and complications such as vascular lesions are also attracting attention. In pre-dialysis CKD, the serum phosphate level starts rising at the late stage, and thus hyperphosphatemia is unlikely to be detected at the early stage. Decreases in GFR lead to increases in phosphate excretion per nephron, as well as increases in the serum level of phosphaturic factors (i.e., PTH and FGF23). These changes are likely caused by the decreased expression of αKlotho in the kidney. However, it remains unclear how the membrane-bound form and the soluble form of αKlotho are involved. Compensatory increases in PTH and FGF23 when serum phosphate levels are within the normal range are reported to be predictors of high mortality [39].

In the dialysis stage, hyperphosphatemia also influences outcomes, for example, by causing vascular calcification. Another cause of hyperphosphatemia is secondary hyperparathyroidism. The serum phosphate level increases due to PTH-dependent bone resorption. In addition, ectopic calcification progresses in the early stage of CKD, suggesting possible phosphate accumulation in soft tissue as well as in bone. When renal function is impaired, excessive phosphate increases PTH secretion and decreases the active form of vitamin D, which in turn induces secondary hyperparathyroidism.

6. Outcomes and Complications in Hyperphosphatemia

6.1. Effect on Renal Function Impairment and on Survival

Generally, in pre-dialysis CKD, the serum phosphate level remains within the normal range until reaching stage 4 or 5. Therefore, it is unclear what kind of prognostic role the serum phosphate level plays. Meanwhile, the significance of the serum phosphate level in a population without kidney disease was reported in a study examining the relationship between phosphate level and the onset of renal failure. Although the phosphate level was thought to be unrelated to the onset and progression of CKD in healthy individuals, a retrospective longitudinal cohort study was performed in the period 1 January 1998 through 31 December 2008 of adults within a vertically integrated health plana. A total of 94,989 individuals within the health plan showed that the risk of end-stage renal disease was significantly higher (the hazard ratio, 1.48) in patients in the 4th (highest) phosphate quartile compared with those in the 1st (lowest) phosphate quartile, suggesting that a relatively high phosphate level within the normal range can be a risk factor for CKD in healthy individuals [51].

Several studies have investigated the relationship of serum phosphate level with renal prognosis and mortality. In post hoc analysis of outcome data retrieved from the cohort of 331 patients with chronic proteinuric nephropathies included in the REIN trial, which is a study examined the progression of renal dysfunction and responses to angiotensin-converting enzyme inhibitor, the proportion of patients who progressed to end-stage renal diseases and a group of faster serum creatinine doubling time was significantly higher in patients with serum phosphate levels in higher quartiles. Also, responsiveness to ramipril, a renin-angiotensin converting inhibitor, was decreased, suggesting the possible influence of serum phosphate level on responsiveness to drugs [52]. A prospective cohort study involving 6730 patients with CKD (defined by elevated serum creatinine level) showed that among the 3490 patients in whom phosphate measurements were performed, a serum phosphate level ≥ 3.5 mg/dL was associated with significantly increased mortality risk, which increased linearly with each subsequent 0.5 mg/dL increase in serum phosphate level. In addition, the mortality risk nearly doubled in patients with a serum phosphate level ≥ 4.5 mg/dL compared with those with a normal serum phosphate level (2.5–2.99 mg/dL) [53]. Furthermore, when the phosphate level was already high in patients with stage 4–5 CKD, the impairment of renal function progressed more rapidly, and the crude mortality risk was increased to 1.62 for every 1-mg/dL increase in phosphate level [54]. A meta-analysis of 12 cohort studies involving a total of 25,546 patients showed that 8.8% developed kidney failure and 13.6% died, and every 1-mg/dL increase in serum phosphate level was associated with kidney failure (hazard ratio, 1.36) and mortality (hazard ratio, 1.20) [55].

Since the 1990s, phosphate has been shown to be a clear risk factor in the dialysis stage, and this is mentioned in several clinical practice and treatment guidelines [56–58]. A 2011 meta-analysis reported that the mortality risk increased by 18% for every 1-mg/dL increase in the serum phosphate level (relative risk [RR], 1.18; 95% CI, 1.12–1.25). There were no significant association of all-cause mortality with serum PTH level (RR per 100-pg/mL increase, 1.01; 95% CI, 1.00–1.02) or serum calcium level (RR per 1-mg/mL increase, 1.01; 95% CI, 1.00–1.162), indicating the importance of phosphate compared with PTH and calcium [58]. Although the degrees of importance were compared only in a limited number of studies [59], the monitoring of phosphate, calcium, and PTH levels in a 3-year cohort of 128,125 hemodialysis patients in Japan showed that mortality was lowest in patients who achieved the phosphate target compared with those who achieved the targets of other markers, indicating that the phosphate level was the strongest predictor of mortality, followed by calcium and PTH [60].

6.2. Hyperphosphatemia and Vascular Calcification

Vascular calcification has been regarded as an aging-associated phenomenon, and conventional risk factors include aging, diabetes, lipid abnormality, and hypertension. In addition, an association with CKD-MBD was recently revealed. Vascular calcification is an important component in CKD-MBD and influences patients' survival [9,61].

Calcification occurs at the vascular intima and the vascular media, and intimal lesions are associated with atherosclerosis. Intimal lesions are characterized by lipid deposition and infiltration by inflammatory cells such as macrophages, resulting in the formation of protruding lesions called plaques. In dialysis patients, these plaques are often associated with a high degree of calcification. On the other hand, medial calcification is known as Mönchsberg's calcification, which is pathologically characterized by calcium deposition within the medial tissues of muscular arteries, sometimes with osseous metaplasia. Medial calcification is reported to be associated with all-cause and cardiovascular mortality and induces arteriosclerosis [62]. The molecular mechanism underlying vascular calcification is becoming clear. In addition to traditional factors such as phosphate, the involvement of new factors like αKlotho and FGF23 as well as regulatory factors at the cellular level, have been identified [63]. Given that proteins associated with bone (e.g., osteopontin, osteocalcin, osteoprotegerin, and matrix Gla protein), which are produced by osteoblasts and chondrocytes, are present in calcified lesions, the transformation of vascular smooth muscle cells is likely to play a central role [64]. Accordingly, the basic mechanism, which involves cellular phosphate uptake via the phosphate transporter Pit-1, followed by transformation of vascular smooth cells into osteoblasts and chondrocytes and then induction of medial calcification, indicated that phosphate is a strong factor in calcification [65]. Additional details of the pathophysiology have been reported, including the enhancement of osteochondrogenic differentiation, the induction of apoptosis, and the fibrosis and mineralization of extracellular matrix [66]. As the association between vascular calcification and phosphate became clearer, several related factors were reported. The Chronic Renal Insufficiency Cohort (CRIC) study revealed that serum phosphate was associated with the coronary artery calcification score in pre-dialysis CKD patients, but that FGF23, which influences the cardiovascular system, had no association with and no influence on coronary artery calcification [67]. In addition, the associations of serum phosphate concentrations with vascular and valvular calcification in 439 participants from the Multi-Ethnic Study of Atherosclerosis study who had moderate CKD and no clinical cardiovascular disease were examined, and high serum phosphate level within the normal range, after adjustment for PHT and vitamin D, was significantly associated with calcification of the coronary arteries and cardiac valves [68]. These studies suggest that the risk of vascular calcification exists from the pre-dialysis stage and that phosphate has a considerable influence on this risk, although it remains unclear what effect reducing the phosphate level might have.

Vascular calcification is very common in aging, diabetes and especially in CKD. Vascular calcification is a powerful predictor of cardiovascular morbidity and mortality in the CKD population. Elevated serum phosphate is a late symptom of CKD and has been shown to promote mineral deposition in both vascular walls and heart valves. αKlotho and FGF23 are new factors in CKD-MBD and are thought to be involved in the pathogenesis of uremic vascular calcification. There are inconsistent reports on the biomedical effects of FGF23, in contrast, increased evidence supports αKlotho's protective role in vascular calcification.

6.3. Hyperphosphatemia and Fracture

The risks of osteoporosis and fracture are expected to increase with age in CKD patients [69]. In particular, the Dialysis Outcomes and Practice Patterns Study (DOPPS) report, which involved 34,579 dialysis patients in 12 countries, showed that the frequency of femoral neck fracture was higher in dialysis patients than in the general population of each participating country. Decreases in the quality of life and a high mortality rate were also reported. Osteoporosis and bone lesions due to renal dysfunction (traditionally called renal osteodystrophy and now called CKD-MBD) differ in terms of pathophysiology, but both are considered complications of aging [70]. A cohort study of 679,114 participants showed that the risk of fracture during the 3-year observation period was high in both sexes when eGFR was ≤ 15 mL/min and participants were aged ≥ 65 years [71]. A Japanese cohort study of 162,360 participants examined 5-year all-cause mortality and cause-specific mortality and showed that crude mortality rates doubled in participants with hip fracture; this higher mortality persisted during the 5-year period [72].

Several studies have reported a direct association between phosphate and fracture. Experiments using cultured osteoblast-like cells revealed that inorganic phosphate induces apoptosis [73]. In addition, increases in the phosphate concentration of cell culture media inhibited the RANK–RANKL signaling-mediated cell differentiation of cultured osteoclast-like cells [74]. Regarding the association between serum phosphate level and fracture in humans, an increased risk of fracture was reported in healthy individuals when the phosphate level was the mid- to upper normal range, and phosphate level was reported to be a significant risk factor for fracture in men with CKD [75,76].

7. Treatment

Dietary Treatment of Hyperphosphatemia

Dietary treatment of CKD is based on the restriction of dietary protein. The Japanese clinical practice guidelines for CKD recommend restricting dietary protein to limit the progression of CKD (e.g., 0.8–1.0 g protein/kg standard bodyweight/day for stage G3a, and 0.6–0.8 g protein/kg standard bodyweight/day for stage G3b or later). Possible rationales include induction of glomerular hyperfiltration by excessive protein intake, which affects renal function, and the accumulation of uremic protein metabolites when renal function is impaired; however clinical studies have not produced conclusive evidence in support of these.

A meta-analysis of randomized controlled trials (RCTs) involving 779 diabetic kidney disease patients showed that GFR was 5.82 mL/min higher in patients on a protein-restricted diet (0.6–0.8 g protein/kg bodyweight/day) for 18 months compared with those who were not (1.0–1.6 g protein/kg bodyweight/day) [77]. Another meta-analysis showed that the estimated effect of a protein-restricted diet compared with the control diet on annual changes in GFR was −0.95 mL/min. The estimated effect for the non-diabetic and type 1 diabetic patients was −1.50 mL/min, whereas that for type 2 diabetic patients was −0.17 mL/min; the estimated effect for type 2 diabetic patients was not significant [78]. The results of a study that searched the Cochrane Kidney and Transplant Specialized Register up to 7 September 2020 were also reported. This study included 17 RCTs involving a total of 2996 non-diabetic pre-dialysis adult CKD patients with renal function impairment and showed that fewer patients progressed to the stage requiring dialysis when a very-low-protein diet (0.3–0.4 g protein/kg bodyweight/day) was provided than when an ordinary low-protein diet (0.5–0.6 g protein/kg bodyweight/day) or a normal-protein diet (0.8 g protein/kg bodyweight/day) was provided for 12 months. There was little difference in the number of patients with non-severe kidney failure who progressed to the stage requiring dialysis between the low-protein diets and normal diet. These results indicate that very low protein intake may delay the progression of kidney failure, but more information, including adverse effects, adherence difficulties, and the impact on quality of life, is needed [79].

Protein restriction has been a clinical proposition for a very long time, but the present situation is as described above. The difficulty of strictly adhering to the protocol, which makes comparisons inaccurate, may be the reason for the inconclusive effect. In addition, the concept of nutritional management changes with the age of the CKD patient. Possible impairments in physical and mental function (e.g., frailty) resulting from drastic protein restriction are of concern. Meanwhile, a study focusing on phosphorus as a harmful substance was also reported [80]. As described earlier, it should be noted that, in pre-dialysis CKD, the serum phosphate level is maintained for a long time because the phosphate excretion per nephron increases as the number of nephrons decreases. FGF23 from the bone is implicated in this, but high FGF23 levels are associated with poor prognosis. The question then arises as to whether restricting phosphorus intake in order to suppress FGF23 would be effective. However, this question remains unanswered. Also, as will be discussed later in this article, an attempt to use phosphate binders to reduce the level of FGF23 in patients with a normal serum phosphate level was unsuccessful.

Then, is protein restriction equal to phosphorus restriction? As the features of phosphorus, especially its role as a nutrient, have attracted increasing attention, the management of phosphorus, rather than protein, has become more important. A study (The NHANES is an ongoing series of the surveys of the non-institutionalized civilian population in the USA conducted by the National Center for Health Statistics. From 1988 to 1994, NHANES III, a cross-sectional survey of the US population was carried out.) examining the effect of dietary phosphorus intake in 1105 patients with stage 3 CKD (eGFR 49.3 ± 9.5 mL/min) showed that dietary phosphorus intake did not influence mortality when the serum phosphate level was in the normal range [81]. Also, analysis of the data from the Modification of Diet in Renal Disease (MDRD) study showed no association of 24-h urine phosphate excretion with progression to end-stage renal disease, all-cause mortality, and cause-specific mortality [82]. Meanwhile, a follow-up of 95 patients with stage 2–3 CKD for 2.7 ± 1.6 years showed a decline in eGFR of 0.5 mL/min/year and a correlation between the rate of eGFR decline and the degree of phosphaturia. In the same study, phosphate load caused renal toxicity in an animal model, suggesting that phosphorus directly damages renal tubules [83]. In addition, a study of patients on maintenance dialysis using the Food Frequency Questionnaire, which was developed to simultaneously obtain information about food intake habits and nutrient intake, showed that dietary phosphorus intake and the phosphorus-to-protein ratio were associated with mortality [84]. Taken together, the significance of phosphorus restriction in the pre-dialysis stage remains inconclusive.

The importance of phosphorus restriction has been reported in hyperphosphatemia, and the phosphorus-to-protein ratio and the characteristics of phosphorus itself, in addition to the absolute amount of dietary phosphorus, are considered important [85]. Dietary phosphorus can largely be classified as organic or inorganic, both of which have different absorption rates in the body. Organic phosphorus binds to proteins and phytic acid and is absorbed at a rate of about 50%. Organic phosphorus can be further classified by source, namely, plant or animal proteins. The organic phosphorus in animal-derived foods is readily digestible, so its absorption rate is relatively high, whereas that in plant-derived foods is often phytate-based, so its absorption is limited. Indeed, compared with animal-derived dietary protein, plant-derived dietary protein led to lower serum phosphate levels and FGF23 levels [86] indicating the usefulness of plant-derived dietary protein in the restriction of dietary phosphorus intake [87]. Meanwhile, inorganic phosphorus is a main component of food additives (e.g., acidifiers, emulsifiers, baking powder, and pH stabilizers) which are a recent cause of concern and are used in many processed foods.

As described earlier, the toxicity of phosphorus itself is considered a problem. The number of studies reporting an association of excessive phosphorus intake with CKD, cardiovascular disease, and bone lesions has been increasing, which likely reflects the excessive consumption of processed foods [88]. Given that calcium contents vary but phosphorus is present in all commonly eaten foods, food additives are likely to increase the phosphate load [89]. Given that dietary phosphorus intake has been increasing, and the harmful nature of phosphate especially in CKD and CKD-MBD has become a cause for concern, the use of phosphorus binders has become central to the management of dietary phosphorus intake. Several systematic reviews conducted in different years reported the effect of dietary educational interventions on the reduction of phosphate levels [90,91]. Dietary educational interventions had a suppressive effect on hyperphosphatemia, as shown in the latest review. Statistical significance was confirmed in some studies, but their reliability was questioned because of the randomization process and deviations from protocol. Monthly dietary educational interventions (20–30 min) reduced phosphate levels without compromising the nutrition status of patients with persistent hyperphosphatemia, but the effect did not persist when the interventions were discontinued. Nevertheless, trials varied widely in terms of design, approach, and so on, and thus the evidence obtained was very much limited [92].

The protein and phosphate contents as well as the phosphate-to-protein ratio are higher in processed foods than in fresh foods. Knowing the phosphate content of foods, especially processed foods, might contribute to better phosphate management in CKD patients with hyperphosphatemia [93]. Phosphorus-containing food additives are becoming a social problem. Given the high levels of such additives among the most popular foods sold in grocery stores as well as the low price of such foods, it is likely that CKD patients often purchase these products [94]. An RCT involving 279 dialysis patients with a high baseline serum phosphate level ($\geq$5.5 mg/dL) examined the effect of dietary education. After 3 months, approximately 1.0-mg/dL or 0.4-mg/mL decreases in serum phosphate level were seen in those who received or did not receive the dietary educational intervention, respectively [95]. The effect of such educational programs on reducing phosphate levels was confirmed in another RCT study [96]. As pointed out, an administrative approach may be important for the management of dietary phosphate intake and, indeed, the restriction of dietary phosphate intake might be achieved through regulatory actions implemented by US Food and Drug Administration. Mandatory labeling of phosphate content on all packaged food and drugs would make it easier to quickly identify healthy low-phosphate food and drugs, which would in turn make it easier for individuals to control their total phosphate intake. Simple changes in regulatory policies and labeling are warranted to enable better management of dietary phosphate intake in all stages of kidney diseases as well as potentially reduce health risks in the general population [97].

8. Aging and Frailty

As described earlier in this article, a certain amount of protein intake is required for aging CKD patients to prevent malnutrition caused by protein-restricted diets. Protein-restricted diets may induce or aggravate impairment in physical function, sarcopenia, and frailty. Indeed, such problems and their outcomes in elderly patients with end-stage kidney disease have been reviewed [98]. Patients with frailty often have CKD. In such cases, the eGFR, which is used as a diagnosis criterion for CKD, should be carefully calculated because estimations based on creatinine level, which reflect the muscle mass, differ from those based on cystatin C level [99]. The prevalence of frailty is high in pre-dialysis CKD patients, and the presence of frailty was associated with the risk of progression to end-stage CKD [100]. A systematic review reported that the prevalence rates of frailty and impaired physical function were high in patients with CKD and that the rate of disease progression to end-stage CKD and mortality were $\geq$2-fold higher when frailty was present [101]. Similar trends were shown in a Japanese study [102]. The prevalence rates of conditions such as frailty and cognitive impairment were also high in elderly dialysis patients, and complications were seen in many patients [103,104]. The prevalence of frailty in 117 patients aged $\geq$69 years (mean age, 78.1 years) was high, and the HR for 12-month mortality was 2.6 in frail participants compared with non-frail participants [105]. Japanese clinical practice guidelines for CKD recommend appropriate management of CKD-MBD in elderly CKD patients aged $\geq$75 years. Restriction of dietary phosphate intake and administration of phosphate binders are recommended for the management of hyperphosphatemia, and care should be taken to avoid decline in appetite and nutritional status, especially in elderly patients. A cohort study (historical cohort) including pre-dialysis CKD patients showed an approximately 40% lower risk of all-cause mortality in those who received oral phosphate binders compared with those who did not. This association was also seen in a subgroup aged $\geq$71 years, suggesting that administration of phosphate binders might improve outcomes in elderly patients [106]. A cohort study of dialysis patients also showed an association between serum phosphate level and risk of mortality in elderly patients. In this study, 107,817 hemodialysis patients in the US were followed for 6 years and increases in all-cause mortality risk were associated with elevated serum phosphate level in subgroups of those aged 70–74 years, $\geq$75 years, and in the younger subgroup [107]. These results indicate that, even when a certain degree of protein intake is ensured in elderly patients, phosphate management should not be neglected; rather, adequate management is required. A RCT of hemodialysis patients demonstrated the superiority of the phosphate-binding medication sevelamer to calcium-based phosphate binders in lowering the mortality only in the subgroups aged $\geq$65 years, indicating that calcium loading should also be avoided in elderly patients [108].

9. The Significance of Phosphate Binders

Ensuring a certain amount of calories and protein intake and protecting against increases in phosphate level are likely to affect the prognosis of CKD, especially in elderly patients (as described earlier). Protein restriction, which is central to the dietary treatment of CKD, may lead to the impairment of physical function, including frailty, especially in elderly patients. Thus, the recent trend in therapy is to use two conflicting strategies, namely, ensuring sufficient protein intake and restricting phosphate intake. If dietary therapy, as described earlier, is not satisfactory, then the use of phosphate binders needs to be considered.

9.1. Administration of Phosphate Binders in Pre-Dialysis and Dialysis Stages

When the serum phosphate level does not increase in pre-dialysis CKD patients, it is likely that the pathophysiology of CKD-MBD described earlier, which includes increases in FGF23 level and downregulation of αKlotho (although it is difficult to prove clinically), has already begun. If phosphate binders (e.g., sevelamer and lanthanum carbonate) can reduce the FGF23 level by decreasing the phosphate load, parameters indicative of poor outcomes may improve. In a study involving CKD patients without hyperphosphatemia (eGFR, 20–45 mL/min/1.73 m^2) (RCT study) who were randomly assigned to receive placebo (58 patients), lanthanum carbonate (30 patients), sevelamer carbonate (30 patients), or calcium acetate (30 patients), those who received phosphate binders showed significant decreases in serum phosphate level (from 4.2 mg/dL to 3.9 mg/dL on average) and urinary phosphate level. In addition, the attenuation of secondary hyperparathyroidism was significantly higher in the groups receiving phosphate binders compared with the placebo group, but phosphate binders did not affect the FGF23 level. Taken together, the effect of phosphate binders on FGF23 levels cannot be expected in pre-dialysis CKD patients without hyperphosphatemia, and thus a dietary therapy-based strategy was recommended [109]. Meanwhile, an observational study demonstrated the usefulness of phosphate binders in CKD complicated by hyperphosphatemia. This study examined the association of using an oral phosphate binder (sevelamer or a calcium-based phosphate binder) with mortality and the eGFR slope in 1188 veterans with CKD. The mean eGFR was 38 ± 17 mL/min/1.73 m^2, and the majority of participants had stage 3 (57%) or stage 4 (30%) CKD. The analysis revealed an association between the use of oral phosphate binders and low mortality (adjusted HR, 0.61; 95% CI, 0.45–0.81) [106].

In dialysis patients, the administration of phosphate binders led to favorable outcomes. The DOPPS, which was a prospective cohort study involving 23,898 dialysis patients from 12 countries, showed that 88% of patients were prescribed phosphate binders and that the mortality rate was 25% lower in those patients than in those without prescription, but only when the phosphate level was ≥ 3.5 mg/dL [110]. In the COSMOS trial (a 3-year follow-up, multicenter, open-cohort, observational prospective study) involving 6797 patients, phosphorus binding prescriptions also associated with the risk of total and cardiovascular mortality by 29% and 22%, respectively [111]. Intention-to-treat analyses (analyzed a prospective cohort study of 10,044 incident hemodialysis patients using Cox proportional hazards analyses to compare 1-year all-cause mortality among patients who were or were not treated with phosphate binders) also revealed the effect of phosphate binders on survival in dialysis patients [112]. Meanwhile, a meta-analysis of studies selected by a recent search of the Cochrane Kidney and Transplant Register of Studies showed that the use of sevelamer during dialysis was more effective in lowering the mortality compared with calcium-based phosphate binders, and that use of any of phosphate binders did not have a significant effect on myocardial infarction, stroke, fracture, or coronary artery calcification [113].

9.2. Types of Phosphate Binders and Their Characteristics
Calcium-Based Preparations

The state of using phosphate binders in pre-dialysis CKD was explained earlier in this article. Several studies have reported the effects of calcium-based preparations. Although the number of participants was limited, the comparison of calcium carbonate (1500 mg/day) and placebo showed that administration of calcium carbonate produced a positive calcium balance but did not affect the phosphate balance in patients with stage 3 or 4 CKD [114].

This means that administration of calcium carbonate has no influence on phosphate balance but does increase the calcium load. Meanwhile, a RCT of pre-dialysis CKD patients with hyperphosphatemia showed that administration of calcium acetate caused decreases in phosphate and PTH levels and increases in the calcium level [115].

Subsequently, calcium loading resulting from administration of phosphate binders became a problem, especially in Japan, where the use of these binders increased because aluminum-based binders were contraindicated for CKD patients. Calcium carbonate preparations were approved for the treatment of hyperphosphatemia, but given the clinical use of activated vitamin D (intravenous injection), problems arose, including hypercalcemia, excessive suppression of the parathyroid, adynamic bone disease, and calcification of soft tissues and blood vessels. For this reason, although calcium carbonate became the standard phosphate binder because of low cost, widespread use is to be avoided.

As a result, clinical studies comparing calcium-based agents and new resin-based alternatives were conducted. Sevelamer is a cationic polymeric resin that binds to free phosphate derived from food within the gastrointestinal tract and is excreted in the stool without being degraded or absorbed, thereby suppressing phosphate absorption in the body. A RCT study of pre-dialysis patients with stage 3 or 4 CKD showed that all-cause mortality, the rate of dialysis inception, and composite endpoint (mortality plus dialysis inception) were significantly lower in the group that received sevelamer compared with the group that received calcium carbonate [116].

The negative influence of a calcium-based phosphate binder compared with a non-calcium-based phosphate binder on survival was also shown in a RCT study of dialysis patients [117]. A 2013 meta-analysis also showed a more favorable effect on survival by using a non-calcium-based phosphate binder compared with a calcium-based phosphate binder [118]. Although the superiority of resin-based phosphate binders to conventional calcium-based phosphate binders was reported [119], the results of a more recent meta-analysis were inconclusive [120]. Furthermore, there are emerging problems related to resin-based phosphate binders, including a high pill burden, non-adherence, and consequent poor control of serum phosphate level [121].

9.3. Metal-Based Phosphate Binders

9.3.1. Lanthanum Carbonate Preparations

More recently, metal-based phosphate binders have been launched. Lanthanum carbonate was introduced in 2004, and its characteristics, which include better phosphate binding efficacies and lower pill burden compared with those of resin-based phosphate binders, are of great interest in the treatment of CKD, where polypharmacy is a considerable challenge. A study examining lanthanum carbonate in pre-dialysis patients (RCT) and a study comparing lanthanum carbonate with calcium carbonate in dialysis patients (a crossover study) showed that lanthanum carbonate successfully decreased the phosphate level and allowed for increased dose of vitamin D analogue without causing hypercalcemia [122,123]. A systematic review of RCTs and quasi-RCTs showed similar results, reporting that heavy metal accumulation in blood and bone was below toxic levels, albeit with a higher rate of vomiting compared with other agents [124]. Based on the experience with aluminum-based preparations, accumulation of heavy metals in the body is a cause of concern. However, paired bone biopsies confirmed no accumulation of lanthanum in patients treated with lanthanum carbonate over a long period of time [125]. On the other hand, whereas aluminum is excreted via renal pathway, lanthanum is predominantly via the hepatobiliary pathway [126]. The subcellular localization of lanthanum in liver tissue was determined using microscopy and spectroscopy techniques [127]. Lanthanum is present in the lysosomes of hepatocytes, and there are no reports of cells or tissue damage in the liver. Moreover, there was no evidence of an increase in the incidence or severity of liver-related adverse effects in patients who received lanthanum for up to 6 years [128].

Meanwhile, a meta-analysis of RCTs showed significantly lower mortality in the lanthanum carbonate-treated group compared with groups that received other agents, but no significant difference in the rate of cardiovascular events was observed between the groups [129]. Recently, lanthanum has attracted attention not only for its effect on phosphate levels but also on nutritional status. As mentioned earlier in this article, lowering the serum phosphate level without drastically restricting protein intake is considered beneficial in aging patients, and indeed, patients who received lanthanum carbonate showed improved mortality and nutritional status [130]. In addition, the proportion of hypoalbuminemic dialysis patients who achieved a ≥ 0.2 g/dL increase in serum albumin level and maintained their serum phosphate level within a range of 3.5–5.5 mg/dL was significantly higher when they consumed a high-protein diet containing 400–500 mg phosphorus with lanthanum carbonate compared with a low-protein diet containing ≤ 200 mg phosphorus with a conventional phosphate binder (27% vs. 12%) in RCT study [131]. Lanthanum carbonate has an inhibitory effect on calcium absorption [132] and so does not have a suppressive effect on PTH in pre-dialysis patients. In addition, lanthanum carbonate, in RCT of CKD stage 3b/4 patients without hyperphosphatemia, did not significantly affect on arterial stiffness, aortic calcification, and serum phosphorus, PTH, and FGF23 levels for 96 weeks [133].

9.3.2. Ferric Citrate Preparations and Sucroferric Oxyhydroxide

Ferric citrate is a new type of phosphate binder, the active ingredient of which is ferric citrate hydrate. Ferric iron inhibits phosphorus absorption by binding to phosphorus in the gastrointestinal tract, thereby lowering the serum phosphate level. Its effective in lowering phosphorus is expected to be similar to that of other phosphate binders. It is classified as a metal-based agent, and in addition to its role as a phoshpate binder, it is expected to provide the beneficial activities of iron itself.

Iron is expected to inhibit the osteochondrogenic transformation of vascular smooth muscle cells induced by high phosphate in cultured cells. It binds to phosphorus to inhibit phosphate transport and suppresses calcification by directly controlling transformation [134]. Furthermore, a RCT study involving 203 pre-dialysis CKD patients with eGFR ≤ 20 mL/min showed that compared with conventional phosphate binders, ferric iron significantly extended the time to hospitalization, death, dialysis inception, and transplantation. In addition, the FGF23 level in the group treated with ferric iron was half of that in the group treated with a conventional binder [135]. An RCT involving 441 dialysis patients showed a significant decrease in the phosphate level, significant increases in iron-related test parameters, and a significant reduction in the usage of iron and erythropoietin-simulating agent [136]. A meta-analysis confirmed that calcium levels were lower in patients who received ferric citrate compared with those who received other phosphate binders. In addition, ferric citrate had an additive effect on iron repletion and anemia control, which was predominantly associated with gastrointestinal side effects [137].

Give its nature as an iron agent, the risk of iron overload should be taken into account when administering ferric citrate. However, it is beneficial as iron replacement because it can be administered orally instead of intravenously. In addition, ferric citrate reduced FGF23 levels by more than half and also lowered the intact PTH (iPTH) level, thereby exerting effect on secondary hyperparathyroidism [138].

Meanwhile, sucroferric oxyhydroxide is a stable mixture of polynuclear iron (III)-oxyhydroxide, sucrose, and starch. After oral administration, the sucrose is broken down into glucose and fructose, and the starch into maltose and glucose, and finally the polynuclear iron (III)-oxyhydroxide is released. The phosphorous is bound via ligand exchange between a hydroxyl group and the hydrated water molecule of polynuclear iron (III)-oxyhydroxide and a phosphate ion. Iron, a biological element present in the body, is the key component of sucroferric oxyhydroxide. Phosphate binding occurs through ion exchange and iron ions are not expected to be released in the gastrointestinal tract. Nevertheless, it is not known whether the structure of sucroferric oxyhydroxide remains unaltered. If part of the structure is disturbed, some iron ions might be released and absorbed.

Sucroferric oxyhydroxide is indicated for use in dialysis patients. A phase 3 clinical study involving 644 patients compared the sucroferric oxyhydroxide treated group and the sevelamer treated group and showed significant decreases in the serum phosphate level in both groups, and a significantly smaller tablet number in the sucroferric oxyhydroxide treated group compared with the sevelamer treated group; the ferritin level was increased slightly, but transferrin saturation (TSAT), iron, and hemoglobin levels were stable [139]. A study (post hoc analysis of a randomized, 24-week Phase 3 study and its 28-week extension) that focused on iron-related parameters showed that changes in several parameters occurred within the first 24 weeks in both sucroferric oxyhydroxide- and sevelamer-treated groups, but to a lesser extent in longer-term observation. When sucroferric oxyhydroxide was compared with sevelamer, there were significantly greater increases in TSAT (+4.6% vs. +0.6%, $p = 0.003$) and hemoglobin levels (+1.6 g/L vs. -1.1 g/L during the first 24 weeks from baseline; the mean serum ferritin level was increased, although the difference between the groups was not significant (+119 ng/mL vs. +56.2 ng/mL) [140]. A different observational study also reported no significant changes in iron-related parameters in the 6-month observation period, indicating that, although both are iron-based, sucroferric oxyhydroxide appears to exert different effects compared with ferric citrate [141]. Also, in another study, 1059 patients were randomized 2:1 to sucroferric oxyhydroxide 1.0–3.0 g/day (n = 719) or sevelamer 2.4–14.4 g/day (n = 349) for 24 weeks. Sucroferric oxyhydroxide caused significant and sustained 30% reductions in serum phosphate level ($p < 0.001$) and significant 64% decreases in FGF23 level ($p < 0.001$). The iPTH level was decreased significantly at week 24 ($p < 0.001$) but returned to nearly the baseline level at week 52. Among bone resorption makers, tartrate-resistant acid phosphatase 5b decreased significantly ($p < 0.001$), whereas both bone formation markers, namely, bone-specific alkaline phosphatase and osteocalcin, increased [142].

After all, since both ferric citrate and sucroferric oxyhydroxide are based on iron. It can be said that there is a sense of security that iron is metal that has been used in the past, and there is less resistance to use with other heavy metals. However, the premise is different between the two that the iron is absorbed or not absorbed. Therefore, ferric citrate has medicinal property as an iron preparation, whereas sucroferric oxyhydroxide is not suitable for it. Ferric citrate can also be supplemented as iron, but conversely, decreasing or increasing the amount of ferric citrate only with respect to the phosphorus level may affect the decrease or otherwise overload of iron. On the other hand, sucroferric oxyhydroxide is not approved for use during the non-dialysis period in Japan, but it is not expected to play a role in iron supplementation, so on the contrary, iron may be absorbed in case, and along with the phosphorus level, iron dynamics need to be confirmed during administration.

10. Conclusions

The concept of CKD-MBD has been established, and several attempts have been made to address phosphate-associated toxicity and complications in CKD-MBD. Meanwhile, the αKlotho/FGF23 axis has been discovered and the phosphate metabolism mechanism, which involves the phosphate transporter Na/Pi, is becoming clear. Against this backdrop, dietary therapy and the use of a phosphate binders have become the basic approaches in managing phosphate levels in CKD patients. Unfortunately, both types of renal replacement therapy (hemodialysis and peritoneal dialysis) have limited phosphate excretion capacity, and so the phosphate balance tends to be positive even with a restricted diet. Despite the marked aging observed in CKD patients, extreme dietary restriction can cause both physical and mental functional impairments, and thus realistically there is a limit to protein restriction. In addition, phosphate intake is increasing due to the widespread use of phosphate-containing food additives. To address this situation, there is a movement to regulate the use of inorganic phosphate in foods, and development of new drugs that prevent phosphate absorption is under way. Phosphate absorption and excretion do not occur independently but are regulated by a network involving calcium, vitamin D, and PTH.

Phosphate control requires continuous daily management, and further multidisciplinary studies are anticipated.

Author Contributions: Conceptualization, K.T.; methodology, K.T.; software, K.T.; validation, K.T.; formal analysis, K.T.; investigation, K.T.; resources, K.T.; data curation, K.T.; writing—original draft preparation, K.T.; writing—review and editing, K.T., T.A.; visualization, K.T.; supervision, K.T.; project administration, K.T.; funding acquisition, K.T., T.A. All authors have read and agreed to the published version of the manuscript.

Funding: This review article received no external funding.

Institutional Review Board Statement: Not applicable.

Informed Consent Statement: Not applicable.

Data Availability Statement: Not applicable.

Acknowledgments: A.T. is supported by the Grant-in-Aid for Young Scientists B (20K17261) of the Japan Science and Technology Agency (JST), Japan.

Conflicts of Interest: The authors declare no conflict of interest.

References

1. Kuro-o, M.; Matsumura, Y.; Aizawa, H.; Kawaguchi, H.; Suga, T.; Utsugi, T.; Ohyama, Y.; Kurabayashi, M.; Kaname, T.; Kume, E.; et al. Mutation of the mouse klotho gene leads to a syndrome resembling ageing. *Nature* **1997**, *390*, 45–51. [CrossRef]
2. ADHR Consortium. Autosomal dominant hypophosphataemic rickets is associated with mutations in FGF23. *Nat. Genet.* **2000**, *26*, 345–348. [CrossRef]
3. Shimada, T.; Mizutani, S.; Muto, T.; Yoneya, T.; Hino, R.; Takeda, S.; Takeuchi, Y.; Fujita, T.; Fukumoto, S.; Yamashita, T. Cloning and characterization of FGF23 as a causative factor of tumor-induced osteomalacia. *Proc. Natl. Acad. Sci. USA* **2001**, *98*, 6500–6505. [CrossRef]
4. Kurosu, H.; Ogawa, Y.; Miyoshi, M.; Yamamoto, M.; Nandi, A.; Rosenblatt, K.P.; Baum, M.G.; Schiavi, S.; Hu, M.C.; Moe, O.W.; et al. Regulation of fibroblast growth factor-23 signaling by klotho. *J. Biol. Chem.* **2006**, *281*, 6120–6123. [CrossRef]
5. Jacquillet, G.; Unwin, R.J. Physiological regulation of phosphate by vitamin D, parathyroid hormone (PTH) and phosphate (Pi). *Pflug. Arch.* **2019**, *471*, 83–98. [CrossRef] [PubMed]
6. Murer, H.; Hernando, N.; Forster, I.; Biber, J. Proximal tubular phosphate reabsorption: Molecular mechanisms. *Physiol. Rev.* **2000**, *80*, 1373–1409. [CrossRef]
7. Tatsumi, S.; Miyagawa, A.; Kaneko, I.; Shiozaki, Y.; Segawa, H.; Miyamoto, K. Regulation of renal phosphate handling: Inter-organ communication in health and disease. *J. Bone Min. Metab.* **2016**, *34*, 1–10. [CrossRef] [PubMed]
8. Levi, M.; Gratton, E.; Forster, I.C.; Hernando, N.; Wagner, C.A.; Biber, J.; Sorribas, V.; Murer, H. Mechanisms of phosphate transport. *Nat. Rev. Nephrol.* **2019**, *15*, 482–500. [CrossRef]
9. Moe, S.; Drüeke, T.; Cunningham, J.; Goodman, W.; Martin, K.; Olgaard, K.; Ott, S.; Sprague, S.; Lameire, N.; Eknoyan, G. Definition, evaluation, and classification of renal osteodystrophy: A position statement from kidney disease: Improving global outcomes (KDIGO). *Kidney Int.* **2006**, *69*, 1945–1953. [CrossRef]
10. Urakawa, I.; Yamazaki, Y.; Shimada, T.; Iijima, K.; Hasegawa, H.; Okawa, K.; Fujita, T.; Fukumoto, S.; Yamashita, T. Klotho converts canonical FGF receptor into a specific receptor for FGF23. *Nature* **2006**, *444*, 770–774. [CrossRef]
11. Hu, M.C.; Shi, M.; Moe, O.W. Role of αKlotho and FGF23 in regulation of type II Na-dependent phosphate co-transporters. *Pflug. Arch.* **2019**, *471*, 99–108. [CrossRef]
12. Goetz, R.; Beenken, A.; Ibrahimi, O.A.; Kalinina, J.; Olsen, S.K.; Eliseenkova, A.V.; Xu, C.; Neubert, T.A.; Zhang, F.; Linhardt, R.J.; et al. Molecular insights into the klotho-dependent, endocrine mode of action of fibroblast growth factor 19 subfamily members. *Mol. Cell Biol.* **2007**, *27*, 3417–3428. [CrossRef]
13. Chen, G.; Liu, Y.; Goetz, R.; Fu, L.; Jayaraman, S.; Hu, M.C.; Moe, O.W.; Liang, G.; Li, X.; Mohammadi, M. α-Klotho is a non-enzymatic molecular scaffold for FGF23 hormone signalling. *Nature* **2018**, *553*, 461–466. [CrossRef]
14. Cha, S.K.; Ortega, B.; Kurosu, H.; Rosenblatt, K.P.; Kuro-o, M.; Huang, C.L. Removal of sialic acid involving Klotho causes cell-surface retention of TRPV5 channel via binding to galectin-1. *Proc. Natl. Acad. Sci. USA* **2008**, *105*, 9805–9810. [CrossRef]
15. Chang, Q.; Hoefs, S.; van der Kemp, A.W.; Topala, C.N.; Bindels, R.J.; Hoenderop, J.G. The β-glucuronidase klotho hydrolyzes and activates the TRPV5 channel. *Science* **2005**, *310*, 490–493. [CrossRef]
16. Wolf, M.T.; An, S.W.; Nie, M.; Bal, M.S.; Huang, C.L. Klotho up-regulates renal calcium channel transient receptor potential vanilloid 5 (TRPV5) by intra- and extracellular n-glycosylation-dependent mechanisms. *J. Biol. Chem.* **2014**, *289*, 35849–35857. [CrossRef]
17. Wright, J.D.; An, S.W.; Xie, J.; Lim, C.; Huang, C.L. Soluble klotho regulates TRPC6 calcium signaling via lipid rafts, independent of the FGFR-FGF23 pathway. *FASEB J.* **2019**, *33*, 9182–9193. [CrossRef]

18. Huang, C.L. Regulation of ion channels by secreted Klotho: Mechanisms and implications. *Kidney Int.* **2010**, *77*, 855–860. [CrossRef]
19. Farrow, E.G.; Davis, S.I.; Summers, L.J.; White, K.E. Initial FGF23-mediated signaling occurs in the distal convoluted tubule. *J. Am. Soc. Nephrol.* **2009**, *20*, 955–960. [CrossRef]
20. Hu, M.C.; Shi, M.; Zhang, J.; Pastor, J.; Nakatani, T.; Lanske, B.; Razzaque, M.S.; Rosenblatt, K.P.; Baum, M.G.; Kuro-o, M.; et al. Klotho: A novel phosphaturic substance acting as an autocrine enzyme in the renal proximal tubule. *FASEB J.* **2010**, *24*, 3438–3450. [CrossRef]
21. Liu, S.; Zhou, J.; Tang, W.; Jiang, X.; Rowe, D.W.; Quarles, L.D. Pathogenic role of Fgf23 in Hyp mice. *Am. J. Physiol. Endocrinol. Metab.* **2006**, *291*, E38–E49. [CrossRef]
22. Shimada, T.; Hasegawa, H.; Yamazaki, Y.; Muto, T.; Hino, R.; Takeuchi, Y.; Fujita, T.; Nakahara, K.; Fukumoto, S.; Yamashita, T. FGF23 is a potent regulator of the vitamin D metabolism and phosphate homeostasis. *J. Bone Min. Res.* **2004**, *19*, 429–435. [CrossRef] [PubMed]
23. Koh, N.; Fujimori, T.; Nishiguchi, S.; Tamori, A.; Shiomi, S.; Nakatani, T.; Sugimura, K.; Kishimoto, T.; Kinoshita, S.; Kuroki, T.; et al. Severely reduced production of klotho in human chronic renal failure kidney. *Biochem. Biophys. Res. Commun.* **2001**, *280*, 1015–1020. [CrossRef] [PubMed]
24. Sakan, H.; Nakatani, K.; Asai, O.; Imura, A.; Tanaka, T.; Yoshimoto, S.; Iwamoto, N.; Kurumatani, N.; Iwano, M.; Nabeshima, Y.; et al. Reduced renal α-Klotho expression in CKD patients and its effect on renal phosphate handling and vitamin D metabolism. *PLoS ONE* **2014**, *9*, e86301. [CrossRef]
25. Mitobe, M.; Yoshida, T.; Sugiura, H.; Shirota, S.; Tsuchiya, K.; Nihei, H. Oxidative stress decreases klotho expression in a mouse kidney cell line. *Nephron. Exp. Nephrol.* **2005**, *101*, e67–e74. [CrossRef]
26. Kurosu, H.; Yamamoto, M.; Clark, J.D.; Pastor, J.V.; Nandi, A.; Gurnani, P.; McGuinness, O.P.; Chikuda, H.; Yamaguchi, M.; Kawaguchi, H.; et al. Suppression of aging in mice by the hormone Klotho. *Science* **2005**, *309*, 1829–1833. [CrossRef]
27. Liu, H.; Fergusson, M.M.; Castilho, R.M.; Liu, J.; Cao, L.; Chen, J.; Malide, D.; Rovira, I.I.; Schimel, D.; Kuo, C.J.; et al. Augmented Wnt signaling in a mammalian model of accelerated aging. *Science* **2007**, *317*, 803–806. [CrossRef] [PubMed]
28. Sugiura, H.; Yoshida, T.; Mitobe, M.; Yoshida, S.; Shiohira, S.; Nitta, K.; Tsuchiya, K. Klotho reduces apoptosis in experimental ischaemic acute kidney injury via HSP-70. *Nephrol. Dial. Transpl.* **2010**, *25*, 60–68. [CrossRef]
29. Sugiura, H.; Yoshida, T.; Shiohira, S.; Kohei, J.; Mitobe, M.; Kurosu, H.; Kuro-o, M.; Nitta, K.; Tsuchiya, K. Reduced Klotho expression level in kidney aggravates renal interstitial fibrosis. *Am. J. Physiol. Ren. Physiol.* **2012**, *302*, F1252–F1264. [CrossRef]
30. Neyra, J.A.; Li, X.; Mescia, F.; Ortiz-Soriano, V.; Adams-Huet, B.; Pastor, J.; Hu, M.C.; Toto, R.D.; Moe, O.W. Urine klotho is lower in critically ill patients with versus without acute kidney injury and associates with major adverse kidney events klotho and acute kidney injury (KLAKI) study group. *Crit. Care Explor.* **2019**, *1*, e0016. [CrossRef]
31. Pavik, I.; Jaeger, P.; Ebner, L.; Wagner, C.A.; Petzold, K.; Spichtig, D.; Poster, D.; Wüthrich, R.P.; Russmann, S.; Serra, A.L. Secreted Klotho and FGF23 in chronic kidney disease stages 1 to 5: A sequence suggested from a cross-sectional study. *Nephrol. Dial. Transpl.* **2013**, *28*, 352–359. [CrossRef]
32. Seiler, S.; Wen, M.; Roth, H.J.; Fehrenz, M.; Flügge, F.; Herath, E.; Weihrauch, A.; Fliser, D.; Heine, G.H. Plasma Klotho is not related to kidney function and does not predict adverse outcome in patients with chronic kidney disease. *Kidney Int.* **2013**, *83*, 121–128. [CrossRef]
33. Buiten, M.S.; de Bie, M.K.; Bouma-de Krijger, A.; van Dam, B.; Dekker, F.W.; Jukema, J.W.; Rabelink, T.J.; Rotmans, J.I. Soluble Klotho is not independently associated with cardiovascular disease in a population of dialysis patients. *BMC Nephrol.* **2014**, *15*, 197. [CrossRef]
34. Wang, Q.; Su, W.; Shen, Z.; Wang, R. Correlation between Soluble α-Klotho and renal function in patients with chronic kidney disease: A review and meta-analysis. *BioMed Res. Int.* **2018**. [CrossRef]
35. Hu, M.C.; Kuro-o, M.; Moe, O.W. Secreted klotho and chronic kidney disease. *Adv. Exp. Med. Biol.* **2012**, *728*, 126–157. [PubMed]
36. Neyra, J.A.; Hu, M.C.; Moe, O.W. Klotho in clinical nephrology: Diagnostic and therapeutic implications. *Clin. J. Am. Soc. Nephrol.* **2020**, *16*, 162–176. [CrossRef]
37. John, G.B.; Cheng, C.Y.; Kuro-o, M. Role of Klotho in aging, phosphate metabolism, and CKD. *Am. J. Kidney Dis.* **2011**, *58*, 127–134. [CrossRef]
38. Kuro-o, M. Phosphate and Klotho. *Kidney Int.* **2011**, *79121*, S20–S23. [CrossRef]
39. Nakano, C.; Hamano, T.; Fujii, N.; Matsui, I.; Tomida, K.; Mikami, S.; Inoue, K.; Obi, Y.; Okada, N.; Tsubakihara, Y.; et al. Combined use of vitamin D status and FGF23 for risk stratification of renal outcome. *Clin. J. Am. Soc. Nephrol.* **2012**, *7*, 810–819. [CrossRef]
40. Isakova, T.; Wahl, P.; Vargas, G.S.; Gutiérrez, O.M.; Scialla, J.; Xie, H.; Appleby, D.; Nessel, L.; Bellovich, K.; Chen, J.; et al. Fibroblast growth factor 23 is elevated before parathyroid hormone and phosphate in chronic kidney disease. *Kidney Int.* **2011**, *79*, 1370–1378. [CrossRef] [PubMed]
41. Isakova, T.; Xie, H.; Yang, W.; Xie, D.; Anderson, A.H.; Scialla, J.; Wahl, P.; Gutiérrez, O.M.; Steigerwalt, S.; He, J.; et al. Chronic Renal Insufficiency Cohort (CRIC) Study Group. Fibroblast growth factor 23 and risks of mortality and end-stage renal disease in patients with chronic kidney disease. *JAMA* **2011**, *305*, 2432–2439. [CrossRef]

42. Gutiérrez, O.M.; Mannstadt, M.; Isakova, T.; Rauh-Hain, J.A.; Tamez, H.; Shah, A.; Smith, K.; Lee, H.; Thadhani, R.; Jüppner, H.; et al. Fibroblast growth factor 23 and mortality among patients undergoing hemodialysis. *N. Engl. J. Med.* **2008**, *359*, 584–592. [CrossRef]
43. Nakano, C.; Hamano, T.; Fujii, N.; Obi, Y.; Matsui, I.; Tomida, K.; Mikami, S.; Inoue, K.; Shimomura, A.; Nagasawa, Y.; et al. Intact fibroblast growth factor 23 levels predict incident cardiovascular event before but not after the start of dialysis. *Bone* **2012**, *50*, 1266–1274. [CrossRef]
44. Faul, C.; Amaral, A.P.; Oskouei, B.; Hu, M.C.; Sloan, A.; Isakova, T.; Gutiérrez, O.M.; Aguillon-Prada, R.; Lincoln, J.; Hare, J.M.; et al. FGF23 induces left ventricular hypertrophy. *J. Clin. Investig.* **2011**, *121*, 4393–4408. [CrossRef]
45. Andrukhova, O.; Slavic, S.; Smorodchenko, A.; Zeitz, U.; Shalhoub, V.; Lanske, B.; Pohl, E.E.; Erben, R.G. FGF23 regulates renal sodium handling and blood pressure. *EMBO Mol. Med.* **2014**, *6*, 744–759. [CrossRef]
46. Scialla, J.J.; Xie, H.; Rahman, M.; Anderson, A.H.; Isakova, T.; Ojo, A.; Zhang, X.; Nessel, L.; Hamano, T.; Grunwald, J.E.; et al. Chronic Renal Insufficiency Cohort (CRIC) Study Investigators. Fibroblast growth factor-23 and cardiovascular events in CKD. *J. Am. Soc. Nephrol.* **2014**, *25*, 349–360. [CrossRef]
47. Marthi, A.; Donovan, K.; Haynes, R.; Wheeler, D.C.; Baigent, C.; Rooney, C.M.; Landray, M.J.; Moe, S.M.; Yang, J.; Holland, L.; et al. Fibroblast growth factor-23 and risks of cardiovascular and noncardiovascular diseases: A meta-analysis. *J. Am. Soc. Nephrol.* **2018**, *29*, 2015–2027. [CrossRef]
48. Isakova, T.; Cai, X.; Lee, J.; Xie, D.; Wang, X.; Mehta, R.; Allen, N.B.; Scialla, J.J.; Pencina, M.J.; Anderson, A.H.; et al. Chronic Renal Insufficiency Cohort (CRIC) Study Investigators. Longitudinal FGF23 trajectories and mortality in patients with CKD. *J. Am. Soc. Nephrol.* **2018**, *29*, 579–590. [CrossRef]
49. Smith, E.R.; Holt, S.G.; Hewitson, T.D. alphaKlotho-FGF23 interactions and their role in kidney disease: A molecular insight. *Cell. Mol. Life Sci.* **2019**, *76*, 4705–4724. [CrossRef]
50. Musgrove, J.; Wolf, M. Regulation and effects of FGF23 in chronic kidney disease. *Annu. Rev. Physiol.* **2020**, *82*, 365–390. [CrossRef]
51. Sim, J.J.; Bhandari, S.K.; Smith, N.; Chung, J.; Liu, I.L.; Jacobsen, S.J.; Kalantar-Zadeh, K. Phosphorus and risk of renal failure in subjects with normal renal function. *Am. J. Med.* **2013**, *126*, 311–318. [CrossRef]
52. Zoccali, C.; Ruggenenti, P.; Perna, A.; Leonardis, D.; Tripepi, R.; Tripepi, G.; Mallamaci, F.; Remuzzi, G.; REIN Study Group. Phosphate may promote CKD progression and attenuate renoprotective effect of ACE inhibition. *J. Am. Soc. Nephrol.* **2011**, *22*, 1923–1930. [CrossRef]
53. Kestenbaum, B.; Sampson, J.N.; Rudser, K.D.; Patterson, D.J.; Seliger, S.L.; Young, B.; Sherrard, D.J.; Andress, D.L. Serum phosphate levels and mortality risk among people with chronic kidney disease. *J. Am. Soc. Nephrol.* **2005**, *16*, 520–528. [CrossRef]
54. Voormolen, N.; Noordzij, M.; Grootendorst, D.C.; Beetz, I.; Sijpkens, Y.W.; van Manen, J.G.; Boeschoten, E.W.; Huisman, R.M.; Krediet, R.T.; Dekker, F.W.; et al. High plasma phosphate as a risk factor for decline in renal function and mortality in pre-dialysis patients. *Nephrol. Dial. Transpl.* **2007**, *222*, 909–916. [CrossRef]
55. Da, J.; Xie, X.; Wolf, M.; Disthabanchong, S.; Wang, J.; Zha, Y.; Lv, J.; Zhang, L.; Wang, H. Serum phosphorus and progression of CKD and mortality: A meta-analysis of cohort studies. *Am. J. Kidney Dis.* **2015**, *66*, 258–265. [CrossRef]
56. Block, G.A.; Hulbert-Shearon, T.E.; Levin, N.W.; Port, F.K. Association of serum phosphorus and calcium x phosphate product with mortality risk in chronic hemodialysis patients: A national study. *Am. J. Kidney Dis.* **1998**, *31*, 607–617. [CrossRef]
57. Covic, A.; Kothawala, P.; Bernal, M.; Robbins, S.; Chalian, A.; Goldsmith, D. Systematic review of the evidence underlying the association between mineral metabolism disturbances and risk of all-cause mortality, cardiovascular mortality and cardiovascular events in chronic kidney disease. *Nephrol. Dial. Transpl.* **2009**, *24*, 1506–1523. [CrossRef]
58. Palmer, S.C.; Hayen, A.; Macaskill, P.; Pellegrini, F.; Craig, J.C.; Elder, G.J.; Strippoli, G.F. Serum levels of phosphorus, parathyroid hormone, and calcium and risks of death and cardiovascular disease in individuals with chronic kidney disease: A systematic review and meta-analysis. *JAMA* **2011**, *305*, 1119–1127. [CrossRef]
59. Danese, M.D.; Belozeroff, V.; Smirnakis, K.; Rothman, K.J. Consistent control of mineral and bone disorder in incident hemodialysis patients. *Clin. J. Am. Soc. Nephrol.* **2008**, *3*, 1423–1429. [CrossRef]
60. Taniguchi, M.; Fukagawa, M.; Fujii, N.; Hamano, T.; Shoji, T.; Yokoyama, K.; Nakai, S.; Shigematsu, T.; Iseki, K.; Tsubakihara, Y. Committee of Renal Data Registry of the Japanese Society for Dialysis Therapy. Serum phosphate and calcium should be primarily and consistently controlled in prevalent hemodialysis patients. *Ther. Apher. Dial.* **2013**, *17*, 221–228. [CrossRef]
61. Block, G.A.; Klassen, P.S.; Lazarus, J.M.; Ofsthun, N.; Lowrie, E.G.; Chertow, G.M. Mineral metabolism, mortality, and morbidity in maintenance hemodialysis. *J. Am. Soc. Nephrol.* **2004**, *15*, 2208–2218. [CrossRef] [PubMed]
62. London, G.M.; Guérin, A.P.; Marchais, S.J.; Métivier, F.; Pannier, B.; Adda, H. Arterial media calcification in end-stage renal disease: Impact on all-cause and cardiovascular mortality. *Nephrol. Dial. Transpl.* **2003**, *18*, 1731–1740. [CrossRef] [PubMed]
63. Yamada, S.; Giachelli, C.M. Vascular calcification in CKD-MBD: Roles for phosphate, FGF23, and Klotho. *Bone* **2017**, *100*, 87–93. [CrossRef] [PubMed]
64. Shroff, R.; Long, D.A.; Shanahan, C. Mechanistic insights into vascular calcification in CKD. *J. Am. Soc. Nephrol.* **2013**, *24*, 179–189. [CrossRef] [PubMed]
65. Jono, S.; McKee, M.D.; Murry, C.E.; Shioi, A.; Nishizawa, Y.; Mori, K.; Morii, H.; Giachelli, C.M. Phosphate regulation of vascular smooth muscle cell calcification. *Circ. Res.* **2000**, *87*, E10–E17. [CrossRef]
66. Paloian, N.J.; Giachelli, C.M. A current understanding of vascular calcification in CKD. *Am. J. Physiol. Ren. Physiol.* **2014**, *307*, F891–F900. [CrossRef]

67. Scialla, J.J.; Lau, W.L.; Reilly, M.P.; Isakova, T.; Yang, H.Y.; Crouthamel, M.H.; Chavkin, N.W.; Rahman, M.; Wahl, P.; Amaral, A.P.; et al. Fibroblast growth factor 23 is not associated with and does not induce arterial calcification. *Kidney Int.* **2013**, *83*, 1159–1168. [CrossRef]
68. Adeney, K.L.; Siscovick, D.S.; Ix, J.H.; Seliger, S.L.; Shlipak, M.G.; Jenny, N.S.; Kestenbaum, B.R. Association of serum phosphate with vascular and valvular calcification in moderate CKD. *J. Am. Soc. Nephrol.* **2009**, *20*, 381–387. [CrossRef]
69. Pimentel, A.; Ureña-Torres, P.; Zillikens, M.C.; Bover, J.; Cohen-Solal, M. Fractures in patients with CKD-diagnosis, treatment, and prevention: A review by members of the European Calcified Tissue Society and the European Renal Association of Nephrology Dialysis and Transplantation. *Kidney Int.* **2017**, *92*, 1343–1355. [CrossRef]
70. Tentori, F.; McCullough, K.; Kilpatrick, R.D.; Bradbury, B.D.; Robinson, B.M.; Kerr, P.G.; Pisoni, R.L. High rates of death and hospitalization follow bone fracture among hemodialysis patients. *Kidney Int.* **2014**, *85*, 166–173. [CrossRef]
71. Naylor, K.L.; McArthur, E.; Leslie, W.D.; Fraser, L.A.; Jamal, S.A.; Cadarette, S.M.; Pouget, J.G.; Lok, C.E.; Hodsman, A.B.; Adachi, J.D.; et al. The three-year incidence of fracture in chronic kidney disease. *Kidney Int.* **2014**, *86*, 810–818. [CrossRef]
72. Wakasugi, M.; Kazama, J.J.; Wada, A.; Hamano, T.; Masakane, I.; Narita, I. Long-term excess mortality after hip fracture in hemodialysis patients: A nationwide cohort study in Japan. *J. Bone Min. Metab.* **2020**, *38*, 718–729. [CrossRef]
73. Meleti, Z.; Shapiro, I.M.; Adams, C.S. Inorganic phosphate induces apoptosis of osteoblast-like cells in culture. *Bone* **2000**, *27*, 359–366. [CrossRef]
74. Mozar, A.; Haren, N.; Chasseraud, M.; Louvet, L.; Mazière, C.; Wattel, A.; Mentaverri, R.; Morlière, P.; Kamel, S.; Brazier, M.; et al. High extracellular inorganic phosphate concentration inhibits RANK-RANKL signaling in osteoclast-like cells. *J. Cell. Physiol.* **2008**, *215*, 47–54. [CrossRef]
75. Campos-Obando, N.; Koek, W.N.H.; Hooker, E.R.; van der Eerden, B.C.; Pols, H.A.; Hofman, A.; van Leeuwen, J.P.; Uitterlinden, A.G.; Nielson, C.M.; Zillikens, M.C. Serum phosphate is associated with fracture risk: The Rotterdam study and MrOS. *J. Bone Min. Res.* **2017**, *32*, 1182–1193. [CrossRef]
76. Fusaro, M.; Holden, R.; Lok, C.; Iervasi, G.; Plebani, M.; Aghi, A.; Gallieni, M.; Cozzolino, M. Phosphate and bone fracture risk in chronic kidney disease patients. *Nephrol. Dial. Transpl.* **2021**, *36*, 405–412. [CrossRef]
77. Nezu, U.; Kamiyama, H.; Kondo, Y.; Sakuma, M.; Morimoto, T.; Ueda, S. Effect of low-protein diet on kidney function in diabetic nephropathy: Meta-analysis of randomised controlled trials. *BMJ Open* **2013**, *3*, e002934. [CrossRef] [PubMed]
78. Rughooputh, M.S.; Zeng, R.; Yao, Y. Protein diet restriction slows chronic kidney disease progression in non-diabetic and in type 1 diabetic patients, but not in type 2 diabetic patients: A meta-analysis of randomized controlled trials using glomerular filtration rate as a surrogate. *PLoS ONE* **2015**, *10*, e0145505. [CrossRef]
79. Hahn, D.; Hodson, E.M.; Fouque, D. Low protein diets for non-diabetic adults with chronic kidney disease. *Cochrane Database Syst. Rev.* **2020**, *10*, CD001892. [CrossRef]
80. Shinaberger, C.S.; Greenland, S.; Kopple, J.D.; Van Wyck, D.; Mehrotra, R.; Kovesdy, C.P.; Kalantar-Zadeh, K. Is controlling phosphorus by decreasing dietary protein intake beneficial or harmful in persons with chronic kidney disease? *Am. J. Clin. Nutr.* **2008**, *88*, 1511–1518. [CrossRef]
81. Murtaugh, M.A.; Filipowicz, R.; Baird, B.C.; Wei, G.; Greene, T.; Beddhu, S. Dietary phosphorus intake and mortality in moderate chronic kidney disease: NHANES III. *Nephrol. Dial. Transpl.* **2012**, *27*, 990–996. [CrossRef] [PubMed]
82. Selamet, U.; Tighiouart, H.; Sarnak, M.J.; Beck, G.; Levey, A.S.; Block, G.; Ix, J.H. Relationship of dietary phosphate intake with risk of end-stage renal disease and mortality in chronic kidney disease stages 3–5: The modification of diet in renal disease study. *Kidney Int.* **2016**, *89*, 176–184. [CrossRef] [PubMed]
83. Santamaría, R.; Díaz-Tocados, J.M.; Pendón-Ruiz de Mier, M.V.; Robles, A.; Salmerón-Rodríguez, M.D.; Ruiz, E.; Vergara, N.; Aguilera-Tejero, E.; Raya, A.; Ortega, R.; et al. Increased phosphaturia accelerates the decline in renal function: A search for mechanisms. *Sci. Rep.* **2018**, *8*, 13701. [CrossRef] [PubMed]
84. Noori, N.; Kalantar-Zadeh, K.; Kovesdy, C.P.; Bross, R.; Benner, D.; Kopple, J.D. Association of dietary phosphorus intake and phosphorus to protein ratio with mortality in hemodialysis patients. *Clin. J. Am. Soc. Nephrol.* **2010**, *5*, 683–692. [CrossRef] [PubMed]
85. Kalantar-Zadeh, K.; Gutekunst, L.; Mehrotra, R.; Kovesdy, C.P.; Bross, R.; Shinaberger, C.S.; Noori, N.; Hirschberg, R.; Benner, D.; Nissenson, A.R.; et al. Understanding sources of dietary phosphorus in the treatment of patients with chronic kidney disease. *Clin. J. Am. Soc. Nephrol.* **2010**, *5*, 519–530. [CrossRef]
86. Moe, S.M.; Zidehsarai, M.P.; Chambers, M.A.; Jackman, L.A.; Radcliffe, J.S.; Trevino, L.L.; Donahue, S.E.; Asplin, J.R. Vegetarian compared with meat dietary protein source and phosphorus homeostasis in chronic kidney disease. *Clin. J. Am. Soc. Nephrol.* **2011**, *6*, 257–264. [CrossRef]
87. Garcia-Torres, R.; Young, L.; Murray, D.P.; Kheda, M.; Nahman, N.S., Jr. Dietary protein source and phosphate levels in patients on hemodialysis. *J. Ren. Nutr.* **2020**, *30*, 423–429. [CrossRef]
88. Calvo, M.S.; Uribarri, J. Public health impact of dietary phosphorus excess on bone and cardiovascular health in the general population. *Am. J. Clin. Nutr.* **2013**, *98*, 6–15. [CrossRef] [PubMed]
89. Benini, O.; D'Alessandro, C.; Gianfaldoni, D.; Cupisti, A. Extra-phosphate load from food additives in commonly eaten foods: A real and insidious danger for renal patients. *J. Ren. Nutr.* **2011**, *21*, 303–308. [CrossRef]
90. Caldeira, D.; Amaral, T.; David, C.; Sampaio, C. Educational strategies to reduce serum phosphorus in hyperphosphatemic patients with chronic kidney disease: Systematic review with meta-analysis. *J. Ren. Nutr.* **2011**, *21*, 285–294. [CrossRef]

91. Karavetian, M.; de Vries, N.; Rizk, R.; Elzein, H. Dietary educational interventions for management of hyperphosphatemia in hemodialysis patients: A systematic review and meta-analysis. *Nutr. Rev.* **2014**, *72*, 471–482. [CrossRef]
92. St-Jules, D.E.; Rozga, M.R.; Handu, D.; Carrero, J.J. Effect of phosphate-specific diet therapy on phosphate levels in adults undergoing maintenance hemodialysis: A systematic review and meta-analysis. *Clin. J. Am. Soc. Nephrol.* **2020**, *16*, 107–120. [CrossRef]
93. Watanabe, M.T.; Araujo, R.M.; Vogt, B.P.; Barretti, P.; Caramori, J.C.T. Most consumed processed foods by patients on hemodialysis: Alert for phosphate-containing additives and the phosphate-to-protein ratio. *Clin. Nutr. Espen.* **2016**, *14*, 37–41. [CrossRef]
94. León, J.B.; Sullivan, C.M.; Sehgal, A.R. The prevalence of phosphorus-containing food additives in top-selling foods in grocery stores. *J. Ren. Nutr.* **2013**, *23*, 265–270. [CrossRef]
95. Sullivan, C.; Sayre, S.S.; Leon, J.B.; Machekano, R.; Love, T.E.; Porter, D.; Marbury, M.; Sehgal, A.R. Effect of food additives on hyperphosphatemia among patients with end-stage renal disease: A randomized controlled trial. *JAMA* **2009**, *301*, 629–635. [CrossRef]
96. De Fornasari, M.L.; Dos Santos Sens, Y.A. Replacing phosphorus-containing food additives with foods without additives reduces phosphatemia in end-stage renal disease patients: A randomized clinical trial. *J. Ren. Nutr.* **2017**, *27*, 97–105. [CrossRef]
97. Calvo, M.S.; Sherman, R.A.; Uribarri, J. Dietary phosphate and the forgotten kidney patient: A critical need for FDA regulatory action. *Am. J. Kidney Dis.* **2019**, *73*, 542–551. [CrossRef]
98. Kim, J.C.; Kalantar-Zadeh, K.; Kopple, J.D. Frailty and protein-energy wasting in elderly patients with end stage kidney disease. *J. Am. Soc. Nephrol.* **2013**, *24*, 337–351. [CrossRef]
99. Ballew, S.H.; Chen, Y.; Daya, N.R.; Godino, J.G.; Windham, B.G.; McAdams-DeMarco, M.; Coresh, J.; Selvin, E.; Grams, M.E. Frailty, kidney function, and polypharmacy: The atherosclerosis risk in communities (ARIC) study. *Am. J. Kidney Dis.* **2017**, *69*, 228–236. [CrossRef]
100. Shlipak, M.G.; Stehman-Breen, C.; Fried, L.F.; Song, X.; Siscovick, D.; Fried, L.P.; Psaty, B.M.; Newman, A.B. The presence of frailty in elderly persons with chronic renal insufficiency. *Am. J. Kidney Dis.* **2004**, *43*, 861–867. [CrossRef]
101. Walker, S.R.; Gill, K.; Macdonald, K.; Komenda, P.; Rigatto, C.; Sood, M.M.; Bohm, C.J.; Storsley, L.J.; Tangri, N. Association of frailty and physical function in patients with non-dialysis CKD: A systematic review. *BMC Nephrol.* **2013**, *14*, 228. [CrossRef] [PubMed]
102. Yamada, M.; Arai, H.; Nishiguchi, S.; Kajiwara, Y.; Yoshimura, K.; Sonoda, T.; Yukutake, T.; Kayama, H.; Tanigawa, T.; Aoyama, T. Chronic kidney disease (CKD) is an independent risk factor for long-term care insurance (LTCI) need certification among older Japanese adults: A two-year prospective cohort study. *Arch. Gerontol. Geriatr.* **2013**, *57*, 328–332. [CrossRef]
103. Nitta, K.; Hanafusa, N.; Tsuchiya, K. Role of frailty on outcomes of dialysis patients. *Contrib. Nephrol.* **2018**, *195*, 102–109. [PubMed]
104. Kallenberg, M.H.; Kleinveld, H.A.; Dekker, F.W.; van Munster, B.C.; Rabelink, T.J.; van Buren, M.; Mooijaart, S.P. Functional and cognitive impairment, frailty, and adverse health outcomes in older patients reaching ESRD—A systematic review. *Clin. J. Am. Soc. Nephrol.* **2016**, *11*, 1624–1639. [CrossRef]
105. López-Montes, A.; Martínez-Villaescusa, M.; Pérez-Rodríguez, A.; Andrés-Monpeán, E.; Martínez-Díaz, M.; Masiá, J.; Giménez-Bachs, J.M.; Abizanda, P. Frailty, physical function and affective status in elderly patients on hemodialysis. *Arch. Gerontol. Geriatr.* **2020**, *87*, 103976. [CrossRef] [PubMed]
106. Kovesdy, C.P.; Kuchmak, O.; Lu, J.L.; Kalantar-Zadeh, K. Outcomes associated with phosphorus binders in men with non-dialysis-dependent CKD. *Am. J. Kidney Dis.* **2010**, *56*, 842–851. [CrossRef] [PubMed]
107. Lertdumrongluk, P.; Rhee, C.M.; Park, J.; Lau, W.L.; Moradi, H.; Jing, J.; Molnar, M.Z.; Brunelli, S.M.; Nissenson, A.R.; Kovesdy, C.P.; et al. Association of serum phosphorus concentration with mortality in elderly and nonelderly hemodialysis patients. *J. Ren. Nutr.* **2013**, *23*, 411–421. [CrossRef] [PubMed]
108. Suki, W.N.; Zabaneh, R.; Cangiano, J.L.; Reed, J.; Fischer, D.; Garrett, L.; Ling, B.N.; Chasan-Taber, S.; Dillon, M.A.; Blair, A.T.; et al. Effects of sevelamer and calcium-based phosphate binders on mortality in hemodialysis patients. *Kidney Int* **2007**, *72*, 1130–1137. [CrossRef] [PubMed]
109. Block, G.A.; Wheeler, D.C.; Persky, M.S.; Kestenbaum, B.; Ketteler, M.; Spiegel, D.M.; Allison, M.A.; Asplin, J.; Smits, G.; Hoofnagle, A.N.; et al. Effects of phosphate binders in moderate CKD. *J. Am. Soc. Nephrol.* **2012**, *23*, 1407–1415. [CrossRef]
110. Lopes, A.A.; Tong, L.; Thumma, J.; Li, Y.; Fuller, D.S.; Morgenstern, H.; Bommer, J.; Kerr, P.G.; Tentori, F.; Akiba, T.; et al. Phosphate binder use and mortality among hemodialysis patients in the dialysis outcomes and practice patterns study (DOPPS): Evaluation of possible confounding by nutritional status. *Am. J. Kidney Dis.* **2012**, *60*, 90–101. [CrossRef]
111. Cannata-Andía, J.B.; Fernández-Martín, J.L.; Locatelli, F.; London, G.; Gorriz, J.L.; Floege, J.; Ketteler, M.; Ferreira, A.; Covic, A.; Rutkowski, B.; et al. Use of phosphate-binding agents is associated with a lower risk of mortality. *Kidney Int.* **2013**, *84*, 998–1008. [CrossRef]
112. Isakova, T.; Gutiérrez, O.M.; Chang, Y.; Shah, A.; Tamez, H.; Smith, K.; Thadhani, R.; Wolf, M. Phosphorus binders and survival on hemodialysis. *J. Am. Soc. Nephrol.* **2009**, *20*, 388–396. [CrossRef]
113. Ruospo, M.; Palmer, S.C.; Natale, P.; Craig, J.C.; Vecchio, M.; Elder, G.J.; Strippoli, G.F. Phosphate binders for preventing and treating chronic kidney disease-mineral and bone disorder (CKD-MBD). *Cochrane Database Syst. Rev.* **2018**, *8*, CD006023. [CrossRef] [PubMed]

114. Hill, K.M.; Martin, B.R.; Wastney, M.E.; McCabe, G.P.; Moe, S.M.; Weaver, C.M.; Peacock, M. Oral calcium carbonate affects calcium but not phosphorus balance in stage 3–4 chronic kidney disease. *Kidney Int.* **2013**, *83*, 959–966. [CrossRef]
115. Qunibi, W.; Winkelmayer, W.C.; Solomon, R.; Moustafa, M.; Kessler, P.; Ho, C.H.; Greenberg, J.; Diaz-Buxo, J.A. A randomized, double-blind, placebo-controlled trial of calcium acetate on serum phosphorus concentrations in patients with advanced non-dialysis-dependent chronic kidney disease. *BMC Nephrol.* **2011**, *12*, 9. [CrossRef]
116. Di Iorio, B.; Bellasi, A.; Russo, D.; INDEPENDENT Study Investigators. Mortality in kidney disease patients treated with phosphate binders: A randomized study. *Clin. J. Am. Soc. Nephrol.* **2012**, *7*, 487–493. [CrossRef]
117. Di Iorio, B.; Molony, D.; Bell, C.; Cucciniello, E.; Bellizzi, V.; Russo, D.; Bellasi, A.; INDEPENDENT Study Investigators. Sevelamer versus calcium carbonate in incident hemodialysis patients: Results of an open-label 24-month randomized clinical trial. *Am. J. Kidney Dis.* **2013**, *62*, 771–778. [CrossRef]
118. Jamal, S.A.; Vandermeer, B.; Raggi, P.; Mendelssohn, D.C.; Chatterley, T.; Dorgan, M.; Lok, C.E.; Fitchett, D.; Tsuyuki, R.T. Effect of calcium-based versus non-calcium-based phosphate binders on mortality in patients with chronic kidney disease: An updated systematic review and meta-analysis. *Lancet* **2013**, *382*, 1268–1277. [CrossRef]
119. Patel, L.; Bernard, L.M.; Elder, G.J. Sevelamer versus calcium-based binders for treatment of hyperphosphatemia in CKD: A meta-analysis of randomized controlled trials. *Clin. J. Am. Soc. Nephrol.* **2016**, *11*, 232–244. [CrossRef]
120. Palmer, S.C.; Gardner, S.; Tonelli, M.; Mavridis, D.; Johnson, D.W.; Craig, J.C.; French, R.; Ruospo, M.; Strippoli, G.F. Phosphate-binding agents in adults with CKD: A network meta-analysis of randomized trials. *Am. J. Kidney Dis.* **2016**, *68*, 691–702. [CrossRef]
121. Fissell, R.B.; Karaboyas, A.; Bieber, B.A.; Sen, A.; Li, Y.; Lopes, A.A.; Akiba, T.; Bommer, J.; Ethier, J.; Jadoul, M.; et al. Phosphate binder pill burden, patient-reported non-adherence, and mineral bone disorder markers: Findings from the DOPPS. *Hemodial. Int.* **2016**, *20*, 38–49. [CrossRef] [PubMed]
122. Takahara, Y.; Matsuda, Y.; Takahashi, S.; Shigematsu, T.; Lanthanum Carbonate Study Group. Efficacy and safety of lanthanum carbonate in pre-dialysis CKD patients with hyperphosphatemia: A randomized trial. *Clin. Nephrol.* **2014**, *82*, 181–190. [CrossRef] [PubMed]
123. Toida, T.; Fukudome, K.; Fujimoto, S.; Yamada, K.; Sato, Y.; Chiyotanda, S.; Kitamura, K. Effect of lanthanum carbonate vs. calcium carbonate on serum calcium in hemodialysis patients: A crossover study. *Clin. Nephrol.* **2012**, *78*, 216–223. [CrossRef] [PubMed]
124. Zhang, C.; Wen, J.; Li, Z.; Fan, J. Efficacy and safety of lanthanum carbonate on chronic kidney disease-mineral and bone disorder in dialysis patients: A systematic review. *BMC Nephrol.* **2013**, *14*, 226. [CrossRef]
125. Hutchison, A.J.; Wilson, R.J.; Garafola, S.; Copley, J.B. Lanthanum carbonate: Safety data after 10 years. *Nephrology* **2016**, *21*, 987–994. [CrossRef]
126. Bervoets, A.R.; Behets, G.J.; Schryvers, D.; Roels, F.; Yang, Z.; Verberckmoes, S.C.; Damment, S.J.; Dauwe, S.; Mubiana, V.K.; Blust, R.; et al. Hepatocellular transport and gastrointestinal absorption of lanthanum in chronic renal failure. *Kidney Int.* **2009**, *75*, 389–398. [CrossRef] [PubMed]
127. Yang, Z.; Schryvers, D.; Roels, F.; D'Haese, P.C.; De Broe, M.E. Demonstration of lanthanum in liver cells by energy-dispersive X-ray spectroscopy, electron energy loss spectroscopy and high-resolution transmission electron microscopy. *J. Microsci.* **2006**, *223 Pt 2*, 133–139. [CrossRef]
128. Hutchison, A.J.; Barnett, M.E.; Krause, R.; Kwan, J.T.; Siami, G.A.; SPD405-309 Lanthanum Study Group. Long-term efficacy and safety profile of lanthanum carbonate: Results for up to 6 years of treatment. *Nephron. Clin. Pr.* **2008**, *110*, c15–c23. [CrossRef]
129. Wang, F.; Lu, X.; Zhang, J.; Xiong, R.; Li, H.; Wang, S. Effect of lanthanum carbonate on all-cause mortality in patients receiving maintenance hemodialysis: A meta-analysis of randomized controlled trials. *Kidney Blood Press. Res.* **2018**, *43*, 536–544. [CrossRef]
130. Komaba, H.; Kakuta, T.; Wada, T.; Hida, M.; Suga, T.; Fukagawa, M. Nutritional status and survival of maintenance hemodialysis patients receiving lanthanum carbonate. *Nephrol. Dial. Transpl.* **2019**, *34*, 318–325. [CrossRef]
131. Rhee, C.M.; You, A.S.; Koontz Parsons, T.; Tortorici, A.R.; Bross, R.; St-Jules, D.E.; Jing, J.; Lee, M.L.; Benner, D.; Kovesdy, C.P.; et al. Effect of high-protein meals during hemodialysis combined with lanthanum carbonate in hypoalbuminemic dialysis patients: Findings from the FrEDI randomized controlled trial. *Nephrol. Dial. Transpl.* **2017**, *32*, 1233–1243. [CrossRef]
132. Behets, G.J.; Dams, G.; Damment, S.J.; Martin, P.; De Broe, M.E.; D'Haese, P.C. Differences in gastrointestinal calcium absorption after the ingestion of calcium-free phosphate binders. *Am. J. Physiol. Ren. Physiol.* **2014**, *306*, F61–F67. [CrossRef]
133. Toussaint, N.D.; Pedagogos, E.; Lioufas, N.M.; Elder, G.J.; Pascoe, E.M.; Badve, S.V.; Valks, A.; Block, G.A.; Boudville, N.; Cameron, J.D.; et al. A randomized trial on the effect of phosphate reduction on vascular end points in CKD (IMPROVE-CKD). *J. Am. Soc. Nephrol.* **2020**, *31*, 2653–2666. [CrossRef]
134. Ciceri, P.; Falleni, M.; Tosi, D.; Martinelli, C.; Bulfamante, G.; Block, G.A.; Messa, P.; Cozzolino, M. High-phosphate induced vascular calcification is reduced by iron citrate through inhibition of extracellular matrix osteo-chondrogenic shift in VSMCs. *Int. J. Cardiol.* **2019**, *297*, 94–103. [CrossRef]
135. Block, G.A.; Block, M.S.; Smits, G.; Mehta, R.; Isakova, T.; Wolf, M.; Chertow, G.M. A pilot randomized trial of ferric citrate coordination complex for the treatment of advanced CKD. *J. Am. Soc. Nephrol.* **2019**, *30*, 1495–1504. [CrossRef]
136. Lewis, J.B.; Sika, M.; Koury, M.J.; Chuang, P.; Schulman, G.; Smith, M.T.; Whittier, F.C.; Linfert, D.R.; Galphin, C.M.; Athreya, B.P.; et al. Ferric citrate controls phosphorus and delivers iron in patients on dialysis. *J. Am. Soc. Nephrol.* **2015**, *26*, 493–503. [CrossRef] [PubMed]

137. Choi, Y.J.; Noh, Y.; Shin, S. Ferric citrate in the management of hyperphosphataemia and iron deficiency anaemia: A meta-analysis in patients with chronic kidney disease. *Br. J. Clin. Pharm.* **2021**, *87*, 414–426. [CrossRef]
138. Yokoyama, K.; Hirakata, H.; Akiba, T.; Fukagawa, M.; Nakayama, M.; Sawada, K.; Kumagai, Y.; Block, G.A. Ferric citrate hydrate for the treatment of hyperphosphatemia in nondialysis-dependent CKD. *Clin. J. Am. Soc. Nephrol.* **2014**, *9*, 543–552. [CrossRef] [PubMed]
139. Floege, J.; Covic, A.C.; Ketteler, M.; Mann, J.F.; Rastogi, A.; Spinowitz, B.; Chong, E.M.; Gaillard, S.; Lisk, L.J.; Sprague, S.M.; et al. Long-term effects of the iron-based phosphate binder, sucroferric oxyhydroxide, in dialysis patients. *Nephrol. Dial. Transpl.* **2015**, *30*, 1037–1046. [CrossRef]
140. Covic, A.C.; Floege, J.; Ketteler, M.; Sprague, S.M.; Lisk, L.; Rakov, V.; Rastogi, A. Iron-related parameters in dialysis patients treated with sucroferric oxyhydroxide. *Nephrol. Dial. Transpl.* **2017**, *32*, 1330–1338. [CrossRef]
141. Lioulios, G.; Stangou, M.; Sarafidis, P.A.; Tsouchnikas, I.; Minasidis, I.; Vainas, A.; Faitatzidou, D.; Sampani, E.; Papagianni, A. Chronic therapy with sucroferric oxyhydroxide does not affect iron and anemia markers in dialysis patients. *Blood Purif.* **2020**, *49*, 440–447. [CrossRef] [PubMed]
142. Ketteler, M.; Sprague, S.M.; Covic, A.C.; Rastogi, A.; Spinowitz, B.; Rakov, V.; Walpen, S.; Floege, J. Effects of sucroferric oxyhydroxide and sevelamer carbonate on chronic kidney disease-mineral bone disorder parameters in dialysis patients. *Nephrol. Dial. Transpl.* **2019**, *34*, 1163–1170. [CrossRef] [PubMed]

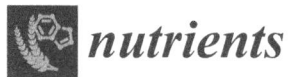

Review

Potassium Metabolism and Management in Patients with CKD

Shinsuke Yamada [1,*] and Masaaki Inaba [2]

1. Department of Metabolism, Endocrinology, and Molecular Medicine, Osaka City University Graduate School of Medicine, 1-4-3, Asahi-machi, Abeno-ku, Osaka 545-8585, Japan
2. Kidney Center, Ohno Memorial Hospital, 1-26-10, Minami-Horie, Nishi-ku, Osaka 550-0015, Japan; inaba-m@med.osaka-cu.ac.jp
* Correspondence: m1265626@med.osaka-cu.ac.jp

Abstract: Potassium (K), the main cation inside cells, plays roles in maintaining cellular osmolarity and acid–base equilibrium, as well as nerve stimulation transmission, and regulation of cardiac and muscle functions. It has also recently been shown that K has an antihypertensive effect by promoting sodium excretion, while it is also attracting attention as an important component that can suppress hypertension associated with excessive sodium intake. Since most ingested K is excreted through the kidneys, decreased renal function is a major factor in increased serum levels, and target values for its intake according to the degree of renal dysfunction have been established. In older individuals with impaired renal function, not only hyperkalemia but also hypokalemia due to anorexia, K loss by dialysis, and effects of various drugs are likely to develop. Thus, it is necessary to pay attention to K management tailored to individual conditions. Since abnormalities in K metabolism can also cause lethal arrhythmia or sudden cardiac death, it is extremely important to monitor patients with a high risk of hyper- or hypokalemia and attempt to provide early and appropriate intervention.

Keywords: potassium; potassium excretion; blood pressure; salt; hypertension; sodium; CKD

1. Introduction

Abnormalities in potassium (K) metabolism are induced by a variety of factors. However, since K metabolism is regulated in a large part by the kidneys, most cases of hyper- and hypokalemia are caused by renal mechanisms [1]. Decreased renal function increases the risk of developing abnormal K metabolism, though aging of affected patients, and the increasing complexity introduced by various medications and dialysis treatments make the pathogenesis more complicated (Figure 1). In this article, the basics of K metabolism, the pathogenesis of abnormal K metabolism, and the relationships among factors related to K and its dynamics are examined, along with a review of relevant literature.

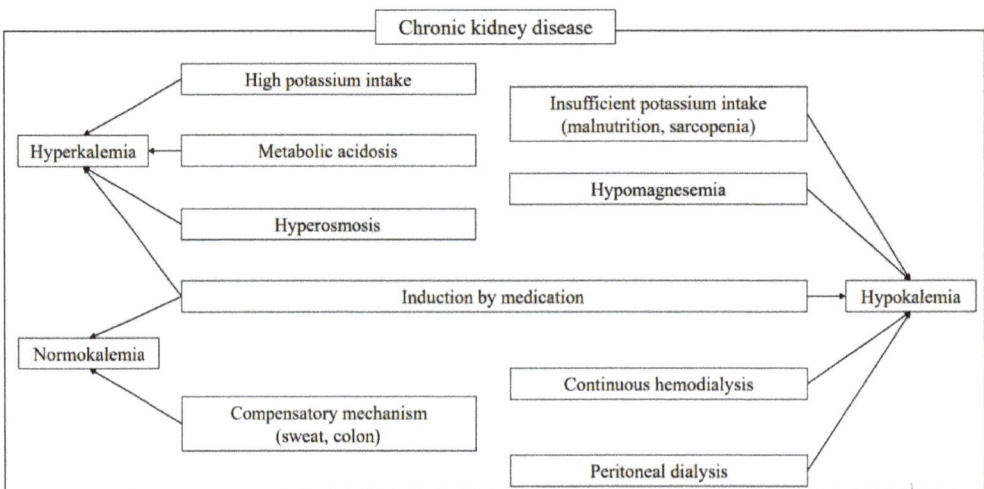

Figure 1. Factors affecting potassium metabolism in chronic kidney disease. Various factors cause abnormal K metabolism in affected patients. Although sweat and the intestinal tract provide compensatory mechanisms, correction with medication is also usually needed.

2. Distribution of K in the Body and Its Roles

Approximately 60% of adult body weight is water, two-thirds of which is intracellular and one-third extracellular. The major cation in intracellular fluid is K, while the major cation in extracellular fluid is sodium (Na). The total amount of K in the body is about 50–55 mEq/kg, about 98% of which is contained in intracellular (skeletal muscle, red blood cells, liver, etc.) and 1–2% in extracellular fluid. This concentration gradient (intracellular concentration: 150 mEq/L, extracellular concentration: 3.5–5.0 mEq/L) regulates excitatory conduction in nerve and muscle cells, as well as maintenance of osmotic pressure in body fluids and acid–base balance [2].

3. Regulatory Mechanisms of K in Kidneys

The normal daily intake of K in adults is 50–100 mEq, most of which is absorbed from the small intestine. Increased K in blood is taken up into cells by active transport through Na-K ATPase, with about 90% of excess K excreted in urine and about 10% in feces. When renal function is normal, serum K does not increase rapidly or significantly after K intake [3].

Of freely filtered K in the glomerulus, approximately 70% is reabsorbed in the proximal tubules and about 20% in the thick ascending limb (TAL) of Henle's loop, with the remaining 10% regularly excreted (secreted) or reabsorbed by the cortical collecting duct (CCD). In the proximal tubules, reabsorption occurs by passive transport along with reabsorption of water and Na, and in the TAL by active transport by Na-K-2Cl cotransporters (NKCCs). In the CCD, several K channels, such as the renal outer medullary potassium channel (ROMK), Maxi-K, and Kv1.3, are expressed in the lumen and on both sides of blood vessels. K secretion is regulated by changes in the amount of K reaching the CCD lumen in response to changes in K concentration in blood, as well as the velocity of flow (urine volume) and negative potential in the lumen [4].

3.1. CCD Intraluminal Flow Velocity and Na Arrival Volume

When serum K concentration is increased, water and Na reabsorption become decreased due to increased K reabsorption in the proximal tubule and TAL, resulting in increases in flow velocity (urine volume) and Na arrival volume due to water diuresis in the CCD. This flow-dependent increase in K secretion is mediated by Maxi-K channels on the luminal side of CCD principal cells (PCs) and intercalated cells (ICs) [5]. When flow velocity in the lumen increases, transient receptor potential vanilloid (TRPV)–4 channels, which are also present in PC and IC cells, release stored intracellular calcium (Ca) and induce Ca influx from the lumen into the cells [6], thereby activating Maxi-K and enhancing K secretion [7]. When Na is reabsorbed in collecting tubules due to an increased amount of Na reaching the lumen, K secretion is enhanced by promotion of exchangeable excretion of K by the same cation.

3.2. ROMK and Maxi-K

A decrease in serum K concentration leads to decreased ROMK expression in PC cells of the CCD, endocytosis of ROMK protein, and degradation of channel protein from the luminal side membrane [8], as well as ROMK translocation into cells by activation of intracellular tyrosine kinase in the luminal side membrane of TAL, resulting in decreased K secretion [9]. Meanwhile, as K intake increases, Maxi-K expression on the luminal side of the collecting duct [10] and renal K excretion mediating Maxi-K [11] increase. In IC cells, K reabsorption by H-K ATPase activation in the luminal membrane is enhanced when serum K concentration is decreased. Although the existence of a K excretory function of IC cells during K ingestion has also been suggested [12], such a mechanism is not clear at present.

3.3. Aldosterone and Kallikrein

An elevated level of K in serum stimulates aldosterone secretion from the globular layer of the adrenal cortex, then aldosterone increases epithelial sodium channel (ENaC) and ROMK expression on the luminal side of PC cells, as well as Na-K ATPase on the vascular side, resulting in K secretion with Na reabsorption as the driving force [13]. In addition, hyperkalemia increases kallikrein production in junctional tubules, which enhances ENaC activity in PC cells, thereby promoting K secretion from ROMK and Maxi-K, and suppresses K reabsorption via H-K ATPase in IC cells.

3.4. Vasopressin (Arginine Vasopressin: AVP), Insulin, and Glucocorticoids

AVP and insulin enhance K secretion by increasing and activating ENaC, respectively [13]. While AVP also directly activates ROMK, K secretion is reduced during antidiuresis due to decreased flow velocity (urine volume); thus, the effects on K secretion are counterbalanced and suppressed. On the other hand, glucocorticoids appear to increase the glomerular filtration rate (GFR) and increase K secretion via increased CCD intraluminal flow velocity and Na arrival.

4. K Transportation in Intestinal Tract

Most ingested K is absorbed in the small intestine, with about 10% excreted in feces. There are two pathways for ion transport in intestinal epithelium; the intercellular collateral pathway, a passive transport pathway through the tight junction, and the transcellular pathway, an active transport pathway. K permeability tends to be greater in the upper small intestine (jejunum > ileum), and most of it is rapidly absorbed by the intercellular collateral pathway. The permeability of the intercellular collateral tracts of the colon is lower than that of the small intestine, though there are regulatory mechanisms in the colon for K absorption via H-K-ATPase in the cellular pathway and K secretion via ROMK on the lumen side. The presence of an enteric-derived factor that increases renal K secretion by K loading to the gastrointestinal tract has also been suggested [14].

In cases of VIPoma and colonic pseudo-obstruction, which cause marked watery diarrhea, K secretion into the stool is abnormally high, suggesting the involvement of vasoactive intestinal peptide (VIP) in intestinal K regulation [15]. Although Maxi-K is involved in K secretion in the colon [16], it has been reported that its expression in colonic cell epithelium and fecal K excretion is increased in patients with end-stage renal failure [17], thus indicating the existence of a compensatory mechanism for K excretion in the colon.

5. Metabolic Regulators of Intracellular K

5.1. Insulin

Since most ingested K is rapidly transferred from extracellular to intracellular fluid after absorption from the small intestine, the concentration of K in extracellular fluid is normally maintained in a range of 3.5–5.0 mEq/L without the appearance of hyperkalemia. Insulin promotes K uptake into skeletal muscle cells and hepatocytes by increasing Na-H exchange transport (NHE1) activity in the plasma membrane and also Na-K ATPase activity. Glucose is administered as glucose–insulin (GI) therapy for hyperkalemia to stimulate endogenous insulin secretion and prevent hypoglycemia. It has also been reported that oral glucose administration can increase endogenous insulin secretion and decrease plasma K concentration, even in hemodialysis patients with impaired renal function [18].

5.2. Catecholamine

Alpha-receptor stimulation inhibits intracellular K transport, while beta-receptor stimulation increases that by increasing intracellular cAMP, and activating protein kinase A and Na-K ATPase. In fact, β2-adrenoceptor agonists have been used for emergency treatment of hyperkalemia in chronic kidney disease (CKD) cases [19].

5.3. Intravascular pH

Under acidosis, H-transfer into cells is decreased, and thus the activity of NHE1 and intracellular Na concentration are decreased. As a result, Na-K ATPase activity and K transport into cells are reduced, resulting in an increase in serum K concentration. Generally, a decrease of 0.1 in intravascular (extracellular fluid) pH is thought to increase serum K concentration by approximately 0.6 mEq/L [20].

In cases of acidosis caused by accumulation of inorganic acids (e.g., HCl), hyperkalemia is exacerbated because K efflux from the cells is enhanced, whereas in acidosis caused by accumulation of organic acids (e.g., lactic acid), the concentration of K in serum remains nearly unchanged because organic acids enter the cells together with H. However, in severe cases of ketoacidosis and lactic acidosis, hyperkalemia is often observed due to the effects of insulin deficiency and hyperosmolarity. In patients with metabolic acidosis, a frequent complication of renal failure, the serum K concentration is more likely to increase as compared to those with respiratory acidosis. Thus, when renal function is impaired, treatment options that take into account regulation of intravascular pH are also necessary.

5.4. Osmotic Pressure

When plasma osmolality increases due to hyperglycemia, hypernatremia, or urea nitrogen accumulation, serum K concentration also increases, because the osmotic difference causes water to move out of cells, which increases intracellular K concentration and induces extracellular K transfer. In general, an increase in plasma osmolality of approximately 10 mOsm/kg is thought to increase serum K concentration in a range of 0.4–0.8 mEq/L. In particular, K control is likely to be difficult in diabetic kidney disease (DKD) patients with inadequate glycemic control; thus, strict glycemic control is important from the viewpoint of K management.

6. Epidemiological Results Showing Serum K Levels in Patients with CKD

An observational retrospective cohort study that used a Japanese hospital claims database (n = 1,022,087) reported that the prevalence of hyperkalemia was significantly higher in CKD patients (227.9; 95% confidence interval (CI): 224.3–231.5) as compared to all enrolled subjects (67.9; 95% CI: 67.1–68.8) (per 1000) [21]. On the other hand, in a study that examined the Japan Chronic Kidney Disease Database (J-CKD-DB) (n = 35,508), the prevalence of hyperkalemia in CKD stage G4 and G5 patients was found to be only 8.3% and 11.6%, respectively. However, though the serum potassium levels in stage G4 and G5 were significantly greater than those in G3 cases, there was little risk of rising above normal [(G3, G4, G5: 4.33 ± 0.44, 4.68 ± 0.73, 4.71 ± 0.76, respectively, (mean $\pm$ SD)] [22]. These

7. Compensatory Mechanism of K Excretion in Renal Failure Patients

Even though urinary excretion of K decreases with a reduction in number of nephrons due to decreased renal function, K secretion per nephron and K excretion in the intestine are increased in a compensatory manner [23–25]. Furthermore, hyperkalemia requiring treatment is rare until the GFR is less than 10 mL/min [23,24]. Intestinal potassium transport mainly occurs by absorption in the jejunum and ileum, and secretion in the colon, though it has been reported that K excretion in the rectum is greater in hemodialysis and peritoneal dialysis patients compared to healthy subjects [26]. It is considered that elevated aldosterone in cases of renal failure increases ROMK in the colonic mucosa [17,27] and promotes K excretion via Na-K ATPase in the colonic mucosa [28]. Suppression of fecal K level by administration of spironolactone in patients with renal failure supports this speculation [29]. It should be noted that constipation and administration of a renin–angiotensin system inhibitor in patients with renal failure may contribute to refractory hyperkalemia and should thus be handled with caution. K is also excreted from the epidermis in the form of sweat, though to a lesser extent, while it has been reported that the concentration of K in sweat is higher in dialysis patients than in healthy subjects [30].

8. Recommended Daily Intake of K

The minimum daily requirement for K intake in adults, estimated based on its unavoidable loss through sweat, stool, urine, and other sources, is considered to be about 1600 mg (40 mEq). On the other hand, the WHO recommends a daily intake of 3510 mg (90 mEq) from the viewpoint of hypertension prevention [31,32]. Based on the above, the target amount of K in the *Dietary Reference Intakes for Japanese* is set at 2700–3000 mg per day, though actual intake is estimated to be around 2200–2400 mg (50–60 mEq).

Approximately 90% of K is excreted by the kidneys, and since healthy individuals can excrete more than 400 mEq per day, there is no upper limit regarding intake, as a normal diet will not result in excess K in the body. However, it takes several hours after ingestion for renal excretion to be completed, and K absorbed from the intestinal tract is first distributed extracellularly (in blood vessels). Thus, even oral intake by healthy individuals can cause transient hyperkalemia if it is rapid and in a large amount [33]. In this regard, cases of fatal arrhythmia due to supplements or salt substitutes containing large amounts of K have been reported [34].

9. Precautions for K Restriction in Elderly Patients with Renal Failure

Presently, Japan is a super-aged society, with more than 25% of the total population over the age of 65. The proportion of CKD patients in the elderly population is also high, with 30% of those over 70 and 40% of those over 80 years old meeting the definition of CKD [35]. While the importance of dietary restriction increases with progression of CKD, excessive restrictions may worsen the general condition of elderly individuals because they tend to have lower cognitive function and activities of daily living and are at higher risk of hyponutrition, frailty, and sarcopenia. Although target values for K restriction are the same for elderly and non-elderly patients, those who are elderly and have a small stature and low muscle mass are more likely to develop hyperkalemia because they generally take up less K intracellularly [36], while elderly patients with a low-K pool due to diuretics use tend to develop hypokalemia. In particular, management of K levels in elderly patients with renal failure must be individually tailored.

10. K Restriction Target Value

10.1. Target Value for Patients with Conservative Renal Failure

For CKD patients, it is recommended that the serum K level should be regulated in the range of 4.0–5.4 mEq/L. However, since renal K excretion decreases as renal function declines, target values for K restriction have been set according to the severity of CKD (CKD stage). In these patients, K restriction starts to become necessary after stage G3b [37] (or eGFR 40 mL/min/1.73 m^2 or lower) [38], while for those in stage G1 or G2, the recommended intake is about the same as that of healthy individuals (2700–3000 mg/day). K-rich fruits and vegetables are also rich in vitamins and dietary fibers and have a protective effect against hypertension and renal disorders due to their alkalinizing effect on body fluids [39]. Therefore, some countries and regions recommend a daily intake of 4000 mg or more for healthy individuals as well as those at high risk of developing kidney disease [40].

Since the risk of developing hyperkalemia (serum K concentration ≥5.5 mEq/L) increases in proportion to decreased renal function in CKD stage G3 and above [37], it is recommended to limit K intake to 2000 mg/day or less in stage G3b and 1500 mg/day or less in stage G4 and G5 patients. It has been reported that hyperkalemia negatively affects not only life prognosis but also renal prognosis [41] and significantly increases the risk of transition to end-stage renal failure [42]. On the other hand, it has also been demonstrated that the risk of death from the same degree of hyperkalemia is reduced as the CKD stage progresses from G3 to G5 [40]. These findings suggest that chronic mild hyperkalemia is protective against cardiotoxicity caused by severe hyperkalemia and that a patient with even mildly impaired renal function requires careful attention in regard to fatal arrhythmia caused by hyperkalemia. In CKD patients without hyperkalemia (serum K concentration ≤5.4 mEq/L), higher levels of K intake, shown by urinary K excretion, indicate better mortality and renal prognosis [43,44]. Therefore, it is important to carefully monitor serum K concentration and encourage consumption of balanced amounts of vitamins and dietary fiber obtained from vegetables, fruits, and other foods.

Meat and fish also contain large amounts of K [45]; thus, reducing protein intake will reduce K intake. However, emaciation and malnutrition tend to become chronic conditions in elderly individuals [46], and thus excessive protein restriction may adversely affect life expectancy [47,48]. With development of medical technology, the number of CKD patients is increasing, though protein intake tends to decrease due to alterations in dietary habits associated with decreased renal function, especially in the elderly [49]. Undernutrition induces chronic inflammation and atherosclerosis caused by increased protein catabolism [50] and significantly worsens the prognosis of CKD patients [51]; thus, it has been suggested that protein intake of approximately 1.3 g/kg has little effect on renal prognosis [52]. In particular, adequate nutritional management for older patients is necessary based on a comprehensive assessment of individual conditions, risks, and adherence.

10.2. Target Value for Hemodialysis Patients

The K concentration in dialysate solutions commercially available in Japan ranges from 2.0 to 2.5 mEq/L, while 40–110 mEq is usually removed during a single dialysis session. As a result, K restriction has been relaxed compared to conservative CKD treatment, with the target K intake for dialysis patients set at less than 2000 mg/day. Nevertheless, potassium poisoning/sudden death still accounts for 2.7–4.7% of deaths among hemodialysis patients in Japan, with the highest serum K levels seen before the start of the week, because of the two-day gap between dialysis treatments [53], and the mortality rate showing a tendency to increase on weekends [54], confirming the difficulty of K control in dialysis patients. On the other hand, a study of elderly dialysis patients reported that the risk of mortality increases with lower levels of albumin, urea nitrogen, phosphate, and K [55]; thus, it is necessary to carefully monitor not only restrictions but also appropriate dietary intake, especially in older patients.

10.3. Target Value for Continuous Hemodialysis Patients

Increases in duration and frequency of hemodialysis have been shown to improve life expectancy [56], and the number of patients undergoing continuous dialysis is increasing. Continuous dialysis is commonly performed at home 5–7 days per week. Since there is no special dialysate used in those cases and dialysis is performed with ordinary dialysate with a K concentration of 2.0–2.5 mEq/L, there is a risk of hypokalemia, hypocalcemia, hypophosphatemia, and excessive alkalinization. At present, only about 0.2% of hemodialysis patients in Japan are receiving daily dialysis; thus, there is no clear target for K intake, and it is necessary to respond to individual conditions.

10.4. Target Value for Peritoneal Dialysis Patients

It is estimated that about 3% of Japanese patients with end-stage renal failure are treated with peritoneal dialysis. Removal of K by peritoneal dialysis is due to diffusion by a concentration gradient between the peritoneal capillaries and peritoneal dialysate. Commercially available peritoneal dialysate does not contain K [57], and since K is continuously removed on a daily basis, the need for K restriction is low unless there is a decline in residual renal or peritoneal function, with an intake of 2000–2500 mg/day recommended, about the same as that for healthy subjects. In these patients, attention should be paid to the appearance of hypokalemia, such as when dietary intake is inadequate.

11. Vegetables with Low K Content

Fruit intake should be minimized in CKD patients, while vegetables should be exposed to water or boiled down, and then the cooking water discarded to remove K. However, restriction of fruits and vegetables can contribute to intractable constipation due to fiber deficiency, with that associated with increased risk of chronic inflammation and mortality [58]. In addition, exposure of vegetables to water or boiling causes leaching and breakdown of minerals and water-soluble vitamins other than K. Above all, daily stress associated with dietary restrictions can significantly reduce the quality of life for these patients. Therefore, development of vegetables with low K content has recently been promoted. Since K is one of the elements essential for plant growth and an excessive decrease in the plant body causes growth disorders [59], low-K-content vegetables are cultivated by adjusting the amount of K fertilization in the nutrient solution during the growth process. Using this method, low-K edible parts have been achieved in leafy greens such as spinach, leaf lettuce, Chinese lettuce, komatsuna, and mesclun [60,61], as well as in fruit vegetables including tomatoes, melons, and strawberries [59–63]. It has also been reported that consumption of low-K-containing melons suppresses the increase in serum K concentration in dialysis patients before and after eating [64]. However, low-K vegetables cannot be cultivated in ordinary outdoor soil because it is necessary to exclude the effect of K contained in soil, which requires a plant factory that can control the cultivation environment, such as hydroponics. Since this requires a great deal of cost and labor, only lettuce, which is relatively easy to cultivate, is currently widely distributed. The effects of low-K-content vegetables on the human body and quality remain unclear and future developments are anticipated in this field.

12. Evaluation of K Kinetics Using Urinary K Measurement

12.1. Fractional Excretion (FE)

Approximately the same amount of K received as intake is reabsorbed, mainly in the small intestine, with about 90% of it then excreted in urine. Thus, the amount of K intake is nearly equal to the amount excreted in urine without taking into account unusual excretion or loss by defecation. In hypokalemia cases, urinary K of 5–25 mEq/day is generally considered to indicate inadequate K intake or extrarenal loss from the intestinal tract (diarrhea, vomiting, ileus, etc.), while more than 25 mEq/day suggests renal K loss (excessive K intake or increased aldosterone action). To accurately determine the amount of K excretion, it is necessary to collect urine throughout an entire day, though that has often been avoided in recent years due to the possibility of nosocomial infection caused by multidrug-resistant *Pseudomonas aeruginosa* (MDRP). Therefore, fractional excretion (FE), which is the ratio of solute clearance according to renal function without urine storage, is often used. The FE value is calculated as (FEK) (%) = (urine K concentration × serum Cr concentration)/(serum K concentration × urine Cr concentration) and used to determine how primary urine filtered by glomeruli is regulated during its passage through the tubules. The standard value is 15–20%. For example, if FEK is more than 10% under hypokalemia, it is considered to indicate sustained K excretion. However, in patients with a markedly reduced GFR, FEK tends to be overestimated beyond the margin of error, and this calculation should only be used in CKD cases up to stage G3. Furthermore, there are diurnal variations in urinary K excretion, with that in the early morning tending to be lower than during the day. This should be kept in mind when evaluating with spot urine so as to avoid over- or underestimation in clinical practice [65].

12.2. Transtubular K Gradient (TTKG)

Since the kidneys are capable of excreting more than 400 mEq/day of K, impaired urinary K excretion is always present in hyperkalemia cases, caused by decreased GFR, or insufficient aldosterone secretion and action. Moreover, renal K excretion is strongly influenced by Na concentration, a major regulator, thus urinary K secretion is enhanced in patients treated with thiazides or loop diuretics, for example, due to the presence of large amounts of Na in the lumen of the cortical collecting ducts. On the other hand, urinary K secretion is suppressed in renal failure patients who have been on a high sodium diet and are suddenly subjected to a strict salt restriction. The transtubular K gradient (TTKG) is used as an index of aldosterone action in the cortical collecting ducts because it is thought that most K excreted into the tubules is due to aldosterone action in the main cells of the cortical collecting ducts. TTKG is calculated as (urine K concentration/serum K concentration)/(urine osmolality/plasma osmolality) and generally decreased (<3) in hypokalemia and increased (>8) in hyperkalemia cases [66]. When TTKG is less than 2 in hypokalemia, it is presumed to indicate non-renal loss of K and when more than 2, renal loss (especially aldosterone action) is presumed, while TTKG less than 6 in spite of hyperkalemia leads to suspicion of adrenal insufficiency [67]. TTKG does not require urine storage as in FEK, though it is not possible to evaluate cases of extreme polyuria (hypotonic urine: urine osmolality < plasma osmolality) with no free water production or extreme dehydration (urinary Na concentration <25 mEq/L), in which free water production in the collecting duct cannot be accurately determined. TTKG was originally based on the assumption that the osmotic pressure ratio is equal to the solvent (free water) ratio, because solutes are neither reabsorbed nor secreted after the collecting duct segment [68]. However, a mechanism of recycling large amounts of urea in the collecting duct (reabsorbed urea circulating in the interstitium) was later found [69], disproving the assumption on which TTKG was based. Nevertheless, TTKG remains important for estimating renal K dynamics, though it is necessary to combine FEK, blood renin/aldosterone levels, blood gas findings, and other factors, including TTKG, to evaluate K dynamics based on measurement of urinary K.

13. Hyperkalemia

13.1. Causes

The normal range of serum K concentration is 3.5–5.0 mEq/L. Hyperkalemia is diagnosed at 5.0 mEq/L or higher, with therapeutic intervention required at 5.5 mEq/L or more. The causes can be broadly classified into pseudohyperkalemia, increased extracellular shift, increased extrarenal K load, and renal K retention. Pseudohyperkalemia and extracellular shift should be ruled out first, and renal K retention can be suspected if a large K load is ruled out. A comprehensive evaluation based on GFR, FEK, TTKG, blood gases, renin–aldosterone levels, and others similar should be performed. Pseudohyperkalemia is often caused by problems during blood collection (hemolysis, over-tightening of the tourniquet, excessive grasping) and, though rare, when thrombocytosis (>1,000,000/mL) or leukocytosis (>100,000/mL) has developed, K in blood cells is released, resulting in high levels of K in measurements. Increased extracellular shift can be seen in crush syndrome, increased catabolism, infection, and severe acidosis. Most chronic hyperkalemia is renal in origin and in the absence of renal failure can be considered a broad form of high-K distal-type acidosis (type IV RTA). Type IV RTA is caused by impaired ENaC due to aldosterone deficiency or insufficiency, which results in decreased excretion of K and H in the distal tubule and hyperkalemia, causing K to move intracellularly and H to move extracellularly, resulting in increased intracellular pH, which then inhibits ammonia production and decreases acid excretion [70]. TTKG can differentiate between decreased flow into the collecting duct and decreased K secretion at the same site, though the majority of cases are the latter and can be determined based on blood renin/aldosterone levels and blood gases. The most common cause is chronic renal failure, with hyperkalemia usually a problem in CKD stage G3b or later [37] (or eGFR 40 mL/min/1.73 m^2 or less) [38]. On the other hand, in patients with cardiac or renal disease, hyperkalemia is often associated with medications that suppress the renin–angiotensin–aldosterone system, such as angiotensin-converting enzyme (ACE) inhibitors, angiotensin receptor blockers (ARBs), and K-retaining diuretics.

13.2. Symptoms

Severe and rapid hyperkalemia of 6.0 mEq/L or more (6.5–7.0 mEq/L or more in patients with end-stage renal failure) causes numbness and muscle weakness in the limbs, starting from the terminal muscles, and also arrhythmia, while 8.0 mEq/L or more results in bradycardia, dyspnea, and loss of consciousness. These symptoms are the result of depolarization of cell membranes due to increased K concentration in extracellular fluid, which enhances and sometimes attenuates excitatory cell functions of the heart, muscles, and nerves that depend on membrane potential. Electrocardiogram results show tent-like T waves, P wave flattening, QRS widening, bradycardia with junctional rhythm, and ventricular fibrillation. Since the rate of increase in serum K concentration is also involved in their appearance, ECG changes are often not seen in patients with end-stage renal failure or persistent hyperkalemia (Table 1).

Table 1. Various diseases/conditions associated with potassium deficiency and toxicity.

Deficiency	Toxicity
Gastrointestinal symptoms	Neuromuscular symptoms
vomiting/anorexia	lip numbness
ileus	muscle weakness
Neuromuscular symptoms	dyspnea due to respiratory paralysis
tetraplegia	Arrhythmia
muscle weakness	bradycardia
dyspnea due to respiratory paralysis	ventricular fibrillation
Impaired insulin secretion	ventricular flutter
Kidney disorders	cardiac arrest
impaired urine concentration	Lassitude
tubulointerstitial changes	Loss of consciousness
Arrhythmia	
extrasystoles	
tachyarrhythmias	
atrioventricular block	
ventricular fibrillation	
Lassitude	
Loss of consciousness	

13.3. Treatment

Because of the possibility of fatal arrhythmia in the acute phase, intravenous Ca (to stabilize myocardial cell membranes), insulin, beta 2 stimulants, bicarbonate (to promote intracellular K shift), fluids (to correct dehydration), diuretics, ion exchange resins, and emergency hemodialysis (to promote extracorporeal K excretion) should be administered in the best combination for each patient's individual condition. Although hemodialysis is the most reliable method, it is necessary to re-measure serum K concentration 1–2 h after completion because even if the concentration becomes normalized by hemodialysis, K may be transferred from the intracellular pool again, resulting in hyperkalemia. Should persistent hyperkalemia be observed in chronic renal failure cases, diet and medications should be checked. K-containing salt substitutes in patients with a salt-restricted diet are easily missed and require attention. When K is difficult to control by dietary K restriction, consider the use of cation exchange resin preparations, such as sodium polystyrene sulfonate (PS-Na), Ca polystyrene sulfonate (PS-Ca), and sodium zirconium cyclosilicate (ZS-9), which chelate K in the intestinal tract and excrete it outside the body. PS is a polymeric adsorbent and may cause side effects, including constipation, abdominal pain, and fullness due to distention in the intestinal tract, and PS-Ca use is contraindicated in patients with an intestinal obstruction due to the risk of intestinal perforation. In salt-restricted patients, K-containing salt substitutes are easily missed and require attention. When control is difficult with dietary K restriction, use of cation exchange resin preparations, such as sodium polystyrene sulfonate (PS-Na), Ca polystyrene sulfonate (PS-Ca), and sodium zirconium cyclosilicate (ZS-9), which chelate K in the intestinal tract and excrete it outside the body, should be considered. PS-Ca is a polymeric adsorbent and may cause side effects including constipation, abdominal pain, and fullness due to distention in the intestinal tract, and its use is contraindicated in patients with an intestinal obstruction due to the risk of intestinal perforation. However, the recently developed ZS-9 has been shown to be associated with a lower risk of intestinal perforation as it is a non-polymeric, while PS-Na has about twice the K adsorption capacity of PS-Ca, though there is a risk of causing intestinal necrosis when used in combination with D-sorbitol, a sugar laxative [71–73]. PS is insoluble in water and when water is absorbed in the colon hard stools are produced, causing an increase in intestinal pressure. Furthermore, the decrease in intestinal blood flow induced by water removal by dialysis is thought to cause ischemic enteritis, which in turn results in intestinal perforation when it becomes severe. ZS-9 adsorbs monovalent K preferentially over divalent cations such as Ca and magnesium (Mg); thus, it is relatively efficient in excreting K [74]. Nevertheless, the maximum amount of K adsorption by these K-adsorbent resin preparations is approximately 1 mEq per gram of active ingredient and dietary therapy must be performed in parallel. It should also be noted that PS-Na is less effective when taken with a Ca preparation and that PS-Ca may contribute to hypercalcemia due to Ca release from the drug.

14. K Dynamics in Diabetic Dialysis Patients

While a function of insulin is translocating K into cells [75], in diabetes mellitus (DM) patients, such translocation tends to be inhibited due to decreased endogenous insulin secretion [76]. In addition, in cases of diabetic nephropathy, there is decreased renin activity and [77] metabolic acidosis due to ketone body accumulation.

We previously investigated the relationship between protein intake and K dynamics in 42 maintenance hemodialysis patients (22 DM, 20 non-DM). Their clinical characteristics are shown in Table 2. In the DM group, the normalized protein catabolism rate (n-PCR) from post-weekend hemodialysis to pre-Monday or pre-Tuesday hemodialysis was significantly and positively correlated with serum K level, as well as interdialytic serum K gain at the pre-hemodialysis examination (Figure 2a,b), whereas there was no such relationship in the non-DM group (Figure 2c,d). These results were similar among the patients, after excluding those using insulin and/or cation exchange resin products, and the relationships did not change after adjusting for age, gender, and hemodialysis duration (unpublished data). Our findings suggest that the defense mechanism against K elevation is weakened in T2DM hemodialysis patients compared to non-DM patients.

Table 2. Baseline clinical characteristics of non-DM and T2DM HD patients at the pre-Monday or pre-Tuesday HD session (data from previous research).

	All HD Patients (n = 42)	Non-DM Group (n = 20)	T2DM Group (n = 22)	p Value
Age, years	65.5 ± 11.1	66.1 ± 10.7	65.0 ± 11.7	0.6960
Gender, male/female	29/13	17/5	12/8	0.2322
BMI, kg/m^2	22.7 ± 4.5	21.3 ± 4.3	24.0 ± 4.3	0.0494
HD duration, years	4.6 (2.8–6.4)	6.1 (3.4–8.0)	4.2 (2.1–5.5)	0.0365
Interdialytic BW gain, %	5.2 (4.3–5.8)	5.3 (4.5–6.9)	5.1 (4.3–5.5)	0.2733
Serum urea nitrogen, mg/dL	61.3 ± 15.3	65.0 ± 17.3	58.0 ± 12.8	0.1511
Cre, mg/dL	10.0 ± 2.5	10.3 ± 2.7	10.5 ± 2.5	0.7818
Alb, g/dL	3.7 (3.4–3.8)	3.5 (3.2–3.7)	3.7 (3.5–4.0)	0.0298
Casual plasma glucose, mg/dL	121.0 (101.0–149.0)	107.0 (93.0–127.5)	141.0 (117.0–162.0)	0.0048
Glycoalbumin, %	16.6 ± 3.0	14.9 ± 2.1	18.1 ± 3.0	0.0004
Na, mEq/L	139.8 ± 3.4	139.3 ± 4.5	140.2 ± 2.2	0.6935
K, mEq/L	4.9 ± 0.7	5.1 ± 0.8	4.8 ± 0.7	0.2775
Cl, mEq/L	105.9 ± 3.3	105.6 ± 4.1	106.2 ± 2.4	0.7039
PCR, g/day	45.72 (42.09–53.29)	45.65 (42.14–52.51)	46.38 (40.88–53.29)	>0.9999
n-PCR, g/kg/day	0.834 ± 0.181	0.911 ± 0.185	0.765 ± 0.149	0.0135
pH	7.34 (7.33–7.36)	7.34 (7.32–7.37)	7.34 (7.33–7.36)	0.5371
HCO$_3$, mEq/L	19.8 ± 2.3	19.2 ± 2.7	20.4 ± 1.8	0.1658
AcAc, μmol/L	25.0 (21.0–44.0)	24.5 (19.0–36.5)	27.0 (22.0–53.0)	0.2360
β-HB, μmol/L	20.5 (15.0–40.0)	17.0 (12.5–33.0)	30.5 (19.0–64.0)	0.0070
AcAc/β-HB ratio, μmol/μmol	1.19 (0.75–1.47)	1.35 (1.07–1.79)	0.97 (0.69–1.24)	0.0136

Values in parentheses show range.

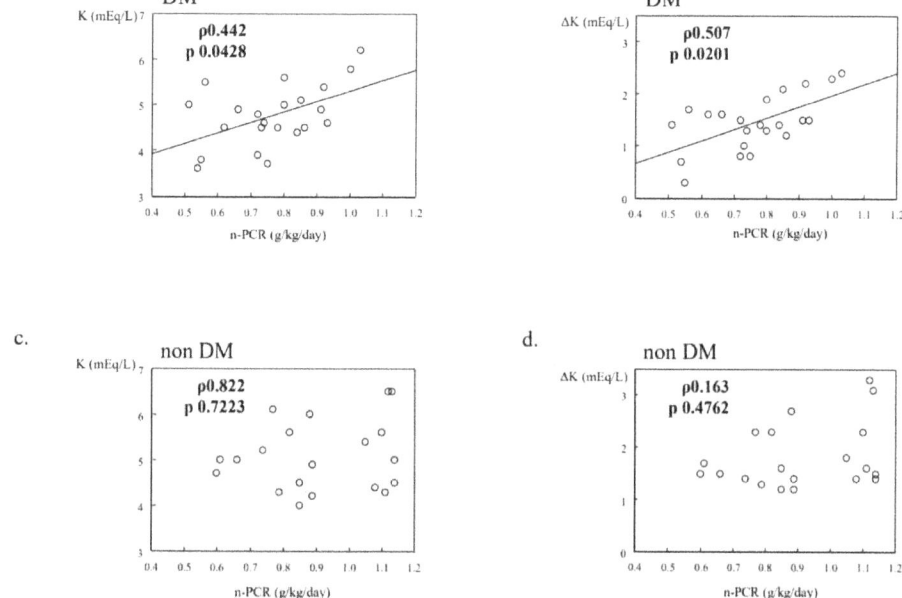

Figure 2. Potassium dynamics in DM/non-DM dialysis patients (data from previous research). N-PCR was significantly and positively correlated with serum K levels at the pre-Monday or pre-Tuesday HD session, and interdialytic serum K gain from post-weekend HD to the next session (**a,b**), whereas no relationship was noted in the non-DM group (**c,d**).

15. Hypokalemia

15.1. Causes

A serum K concentration of 3.5 mEq/L or less is used for diagnosis of hypokalemia, which is the second-most common electrolyte abnormality after abnormal Na concentration. Since 98% of K in the body exists in an intracellular location, with 70–80% in muscle, elderly individuals, especially those with low muscle mass, are prone to K deficiency due to decreased total K in the body. The causes of hypokalemia can be broadly classified into increased intracellular transport, decreased K uptake, and K loss (renal and extrarenal) [78], with renal loss the most frequent.

Increased intracellular transport can be caused by medications (e.g., insulin, beta-stimulants), familial hypokalemic periodic tetraplegia, and hyperthyroidism, as well as others, while renal loss is induced by medications (e.g., diuretics), increased renin–angiotensin system, and tubular dysfunction (Bartter syndrome, Gitelman syndrome, Liddle syndrome, etc.). As for extrarenal K loss, that can be caused by prolonged poor food intake, severe vomiting, and diarrhea. Since renal K excretion persists for approximately one week even after a decrease in serum K concentration, delayed renal adaptation to the disease in the acute phase may contribute to worsening of the disease.

Although hypokalemia is rare in patients with end-stage renal failure due to reduced K excretion, it can occur in individuals with reduced dietary intake because the concentration of K in standard hemodialysis fluid is set at 2–2.5 mEq/L and standard peritoneal dialysis fluid does not contain K. A survey by the Japanese Society of Dialysis Therapy found that hypokalemia can occur in patients with low dietary intake and 8% of patients had a post-dialysis K concentration of less than 3 mEq/L. In addition, the incidence of hypokalemia during CHDF is very high, ranging from 4% to 24% [79,80]. In CKD patients, not only hyperkalemia but also a serum K level below 3.5–4.0 mEq/L [41,81] are significant risk factors for total mortality, and there are several reports of sudden cardiac death of hemodialysis patients due to hypokalemia [82]. In particular, elderly patients should be carefully monitored to ensure that serum K levels are not too low.

15.2. Symptoms

Gastrointestinal symptoms such as vomiting and anorexia, muscular symptoms such as weakness and muscle weakness, impaired urine concentration (polydipsia, polyuria), and impaired insulin secretion (glucose intolerance) are observed when the serum K concentration is 2.5–3.0 mEq/L. When that concentration is lower than 2.5 mEq/L, tetraplegia, respiratory paralysis, ileus, and ventricular arrhythmia appear. The first change observed in ECG results is a decrease in the T wave, then ST depression and T waves become flat or negative as the K concentration decreases further, with U waves becoming apparent below 2.7 mEq/L, and extrasystoles, tachyarrhythmia, and 2–3 degrees of atrioventricular block noted at a concentration below 2.0 mEq/L [83], while torsades de pointes, ventricular fibrillation, and cardiac arrest may also occur. In hemodialysis patients, a sudden change in serum K level associated with dialysis can cause ventricular premature contractions and QT prolongation, thus leading to torsade de pointes and ventricular fibrillation.

Hypokalemia also leads to a variety of tubulointerstitial pathologic and functional changes. As for pathologic changes, those include vacuolar degeneration of the proximal tubules [84,85], interstitial infiltration of mononuclear cells [86], and renal cysts [87] (Figure 3). Chronic hypokalemia due to an eating disorder is a risk factor leading to end-stage renal failure [88]. It has also been reported that hypokalemia predisposes to acute kidney injury from medications such as gentamicin and amphotericin, while impaired NaCl reabsorption due to ROMK suppression in TAL has been speculated to be a factor contributing to impaired urine concentration [78].

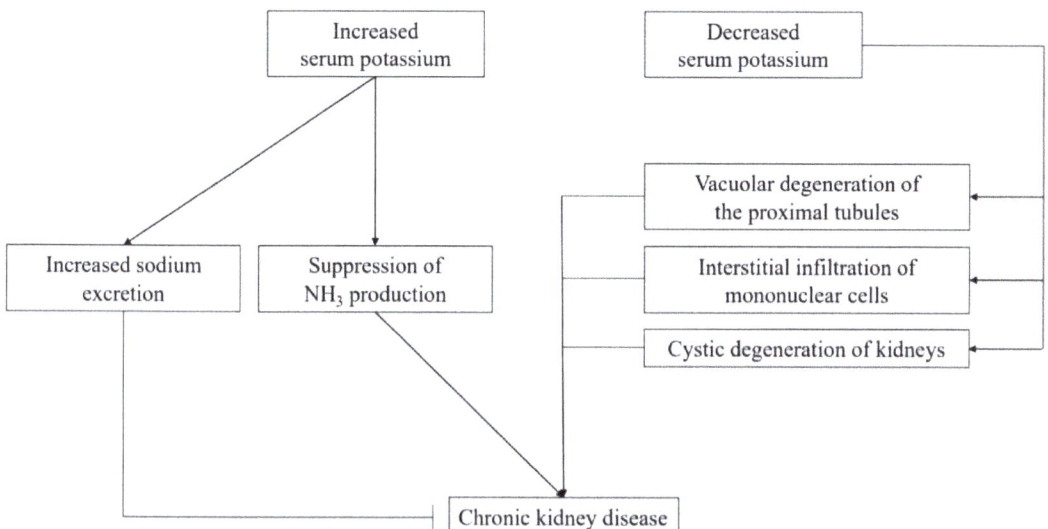

Figure 3. Role of potassium in CKD pathogenesis. Elevated serum K has protective effects on the kidneys by promoting salt excretion and reducing renal function by acidosis due to suppression of NH_3 production. On the other hand, decreased serum K reduces renal function with a direct negative effect on renal tissue.

15.3. Treatment

Hypokalemia associated with muscle paralysis and arrhythmia requires parenteral K replacement. Care should be taken to strictly adhere to the dose given (<60–80 mEq/day), K concentration in the infusion (peripheral vein: <40 mEq/L, central vein: <100 mEq/L), and administration rate (<20 mEq/hour) to avoid the risk of a rapid rise in concentration of K in serum. To avoid such an increase, K supplementation should be given orally, except in emergency cases. KCl is frequently used as an oral drug because it can also correct metabolic alkalosis. However, it is somewhat difficult to absorb and may cause ulcerations in the intestinal tract; thus, organic acid K salts (K aspartate, K gluconate), which are well absorbed and less likely to cause mucosal lesions, are often used. In RTA-induced hypokalemia, organic acid K salts should be used because of acidosis. Moreover, K-retaining diuretics are also effective for chronic hypokalemia, though care should be taken to avoid development of hyperkalemia in CKD patients using ACE, ARB, or NSAID.

16. Relationship between Mg and K

Following Ca, K, and Na, the most abundant cation in the body is Mg. More than 99% of total Mg in the body is distributed intracellularly and it is the second-most abundant electrolyte after K in cells. Hypomagnesemia is diagnosed when the serum Mg concentration is less than 1.5 mg/dL, and it is estimated that about 40% of hypokalemia patients also have hypomagnesemia. Since Mg has an ROMK-mediated inhibitory function toward K secretion, it is thought that K secretion is enhanced in an Mg-deficient state [89]. The decrease in urinary K excretion after Mg supplementation seen in hypokalemic patients being treated with thiazides [90] supports this speculation.

17. Relationship between NH_3 and K

NH_3 is produced not only in the liver but also in the proximal tubules of the kidneys in approximately the same amount as that produced in the liver. Nonvolatile acids produced by the metabolism of ingested proteins are excreted in urine as NH_4, which helps to maintain the acid–base balance in the body [91]. In CKD patients, NH_3 production is reduced due to a decrease in number of functional nephrons, resulting in decreased excretion of nonvolatile acids and metabolic acidosis [92]. Phosphate-dependent glutaminase (PDG) is the key enzyme for NH_3 production, and its activity is increased by acidosis and hypokalemia. Therefore, hyperkalemia acts to suppress NH_3 production and correction of hyperkalemia is important to correct acidosis associated with CKD (Figure 3).

18. Relationship between Na and K

NaCl is regulated by reabsorption via thiazide-sensitive Na-Cl cotransporters (NCCs) in the distal tubule, ENaC in the collecting duct, and pendrin. Under low-K conditions, NaCl reabsorption is enhanced by activation of NCC [93] and pendrin [94], whereas under high-K conditions, urinary Na excretion is enhanced by K influx into cells via K channels in distal tubules [95]. Therefore, K is thought to be a factor that can alleviate the effects of hypertension caused by excessive salt intake and its antihypertensive effect has been known for a long time [96]. Ca and Mg have been reported to have antihypertensive effects by promoting Na excretion and vasodilation, respectively [97], though their effects are not as significant as those of K [98].

Recently, the antihypertensive effect of K was made more apparent in results of a randomized controlled trial of hypertensive patients [99]. A diet rich in fruits and vegetables not only improves salt sensitivity related to high blood pressure [100] and lowers blood pressure [101,102], but also reduces the risk of renal failure and cardiovascular events [103]. Furthermore, in recent years it has been recommended that the optimal serum K concentration be set higher in patients with acute myocardial infarction, heart failure, or hypertension [104] (Figure 3). In CKD patients, it has been observed that blood pressure tends to be higher in those with a low serum K level [105], while it has been reported that a K-rich diet in patients with CKD stage G3 lowers blood pressure without changing serum K level [106]. Thus, it is necessary to constantly monitor for any hyperkalemia development in these patients, while ensuring that the serum K level is not excessively lowered.

The urinary Na/K ratio has been recommended as an indicator of dietary salt and K intake [107]. Both urinary Na and K tend to be low in the early morning, and the urinary Na/K ratio also tends to be low in the early morning due to the larger variation of K than Na [65]. On the other hand, the urinary Na/K ratio in 24 h urine and spot urine has been shown to be strongly correlated in normotensive [108] and hypertensive individuals [109], as well as early renal failure patients (CKD stage 1–3) [110]. However, this relationship is not seen in cases of advanced renal failure (CKD stage 4, 5) and it is difficult to evaluate using urinary Na/K ratio [110].

19. Drug-Induced K Abnormalities

19.1. Hyperkalemia

Elderly individuals are physiologically susceptible to hyperkalemia due to an age-related decline in renin–aldosterone secretion, and this risk is further amplified in those complicated by impaired renal function. Although ACEs and ARBs are being used with increasing frequency for cardio-renal protection, they may cause transient increases in serum Cr and K, especially in cases of renal failure and diabetic nephropathy, and treated patients should be carefully followed after starting administration [111]. K-retaining diuretics are antihypertensive agents that inhibit Na reabsorption and decrease K excretion by inhibiting ENaC in the collecting ducts, though they may sometimes cause fatal arrhythmia due to hyperkalemia. Among available K-retaining diuretics, spironolactone is contraindicated in anuria or acute renal failure cases, and eplerenone is contraindicated for diabetic nephropathy with albuminuria or proteinuria patients, and in those with creatinine clearance less than 30 mL/min. In addition, β-inhibitors and NSAIDs are prone to cause hyperkalemia by altering the distribution of K in and out of cells, and renin secretion, respectively [112].

19.2. Hypokalemia

The causes of drug-induced hypokalemia can be broadly divided into intracellular K shift, enhanced renal K excretion, and enhanced extrarenal K excretion. Beta-stimulants, glucose loading, insulin, xanthines, risperidone, and quetiapine promote intracellular K shift. Loop diuretics inhibit NKCC of the TAL, and thiazide diuretics inhibit NCC of the distal tubule, both of which increase K excretion by increasing the amount of Na reaching the collecting duct. High doses of penicillin, aminoglycoside, or platinum anticancer drugs stimulate K secretion by loading more nonabsorbable anions into the distal tubule. Fludrocortisone is a potent stimulator of Na reabsorption and K excretion, and hypokalemia may occur even at low doses. Most drugs that increase extrarenal K excretion, with the exception of cation exchange resins, are laxatives. In addition to direct K loss, secondary aldosteronism associated with extracellular fluid loss further enhances K excretion [113].

20. Conclusions

K is an electrolyte essential for maintenance of body functions, though its optimal concentration range is narrow, making it extremely vulnerable to metabolic abnormalities, especially when renal function is impaired. When managing K levels in CKD patients, it is extremely important to accurately determine and carefully monitor conditions in individual cases and attempt to appropriately intervene at an early stage.

Author Contributions: S.Y. wrote the manuscript. M.I. critically reviewed and corrected all versions of the manuscript. Both authors have read and agreed to the published version of the manuscript.

Funding: This research received no external funding.

Institutional Review Board Statement: The study was conducted according to the guidelines of the Declaration of Helsinki.

Informed Consent Statement: Not applicable.

Data Availability Statement: Not applicable.

Conflicts of Interest: The authors have no relevant financial interest to declare.

References

1. Gilligan, S.; Raphael, K.L. Hyperkalemia and Hypokalemia in CKD: Prevalence, Risk Factors, and Clinical Outcomes. *Adv. Chronic Kidney Dis.* **2017**, *24*, 315–318. [CrossRef]
2. Seldin, D.W.; Giebisch, G. (Eds.) *The Regulation of Potassium Balance*; Raven Press: New York, NY, USA, 1989; pp. 3–29.
3. Johnson, L.R. (Ed.) Renal regulation of potassium, calcium and magnesium. In *Essential Medical Physiology*, 3rd ed.; Elsevier Academic Press: San Diego, CA, USA, 2003; pp. 437–446.
4. Giebisch, G.; Wang, W. Potassium transport: From clearance to channels and pumps. *Kidney Int.* **1996**, *49*, 1624–1631. [CrossRef] [PubMed]
5. Rieg, T.; Vallon, V.; Sausbier, M.; Kaissling, B.; Ruth, P.; Osswald, H. The role of the BK channel in potassium homeostasis and flow-induced renal potassium excretion. *Kidney Int.* **2007**, *72*, 566–573. [CrossRef]
6. Liu, W.; Xu, S.; Woda, C.; Kim, P.; Weinbaum, S.; Satlin, L.M. Effect of flow and stretch on the [Ca^{2+}] response of principle and intercalated cells in cortical collecting duct. *Am. J. Physiol. Ren. Physiol.* **2003**, *285*, 998–1012. [CrossRef]
7. Taniguchi, J.; Tsuruoka, S.; Mizuno, A.; Sato, J.-I.; Fujimura, A.; Suzuki, M. TRPV4 as a flow sensor in flow-dependent K+ secretion from the cortical collecting duct. *Am. J. Physiol. Physiol.* **2007**, *292*, F667–F673. [CrossRef]
8. Chu, P.-Y.; Quigley, R.; Babich, V.; Huang, C.-L. Dietary potassium restriction stimulates endocytosis of ROMK channel in rat cortical collecting duct. *Am. J. Physiol. Physiol.* **2003**, *285*, F1179–F1187. [CrossRef]
9. Wang, W.-H. Regulation of ROMK (Kir1.1) channels: New mechanisms and aspects. *Am. J. Physiol. Physiol.* **2006**, *290*, F14–F19. [CrossRef] [PubMed]
10. Najjar, F.; Zhou, H.; Morimoto, T.; Bruns, J.B.; Li, H.-S.; Liu, W.; Kleyman, T.R.; Satlin, L.M. Dietary K+ regulates apical membrane expression of maxi-K channels in rabbit cortical collecting duct. *Am. J. Physiol. Physiol.* **2005**, *289*, F922–F932. [CrossRef]
11. Bailey, M.A.; Cantone, A.; Yan, Q.; MacGregor, G.G.; Leng, Q.; Amorim, J.B.O.; Wang, T.; Hebert, S.C.; Giebisch, G.; Malnic, G. Maxi-K channels contribute to urinary potassium excretion in the ROMK deficient mouse model of type II bartter's syndrome and in adaptation to a high-K diet. *Kidney Int.* **2006**, *70*, 51–59. [CrossRef]
12. Rodan, A.R.; Cheng, C.-J.; Huang, C.-L. Recent advances in distal tubular potassium handling. *Am. J. Physiol. Physiol.* **2011**, *300*, F821–F827. [CrossRef] [PubMed]

13. Giebisch, G.H. A trail of research on potassium. *Kidney Int.* **2002**, *62*, 1498–1512. [CrossRef] [PubMed]
14. Lee, F.N.; Oh, G.; McDonough, A.A.; Youn, J.H. Evidence for gut factor in K+ homeostasis. *Am. J. Physiol. Physiol.* **2007**, *293*, F541–F547. [CrossRef] [PubMed]
15. Va Dinter, T.G.; Fuerst, F.C.; Richardson, C.T.; Ana, C.A.S.; Polter, D.E.; Fordtran, J.S.; Binder, H.J. Stimulated active potassium secretion in a patient with colonic pseudo-obstruction: A new mechanism of secretory diarrhea. *Gastroenterology* **2005**, *129*, 1268–1273. [CrossRef]
16. Sausbier, M.; Matos, J.E.; Sausbier, U.; Beranek, G.; Arntz, C.; Neuhuber, W.; Ruth, P.; Leipziger, J. Distal Colonic K$^+$ Secretion Occurs via BK Channels. *J. Am. Soc. Nephrol.* **2006**, *17*, 1275–1282. [CrossRef]
17. Mathialahan, T.; A MacLennan, K.; Sandle, L.N.; Verbeke, C.; Sandle, G.I. Enhanced large intestinal potassium permeability in end-stage renal disease. *J. Pathol.* **2005**, *206*, 46–51. [CrossRef] [PubMed]
18. Muto, S.; Sebata, K.; Watanabe, H.; Shoji, F.; Yamamoto, Y.; Ohashi, M.; Yamada, T.; Matsumoto, H.; Mukouyama, T.; Yonekura, T.; et al. Effect of Oral Glucose Administration on Serum Potassium Concentration in Hemodialysis Patients. *Am. J. Kidney Dis.* **2005**, *46*, 697–705. [CrossRef]
19. Sowinski, K.M.; Cronin, D.; Mueller, B.A.; Kraus, M.A. Subcutaneous terbutamine use in CKD to reduce potassium concentrations. *Am. J. Kidney Dis.* **2005**, *45*, 1040–1045. [CrossRef]
20. Adrogue, H.J.; Masias, N.E. Change in plasma potassium concentration during acute acid-base disturbances. *Am. J. Med.* **1981**, *71*, 456–467. [CrossRef]
21. Kashihara, N.; Kohsaka, S.; Kanda, E.; Okami, S.; Yajima, T. Hyperkalemia in Real-World Patients Under Continuous Medical Care in Japan. *Kidney Int. Rep.* **2019**, *4*, 1248–1260. [CrossRef]
22. Sofue, T.; Nakagawa, N.; Kanda, E.; Nagasu, H.; Matsushita, K.; Nangaku, M.; Maruyama, S.; Wada, T.; Terada, Y.; Yamagata, K.; et al. Prevalences of hyperuricemia and electrolyte abnormalities in patients with chronic kidney disease in Japan: A nationwide, cross-sectional cohort study using data from the Japan Chronic Kidney Disease Database (J-CKD-DB). *PLoS ONE* **2020**, *15*, 0240402. [CrossRef] [PubMed]
23. Hayes, C.P.; McLeod, M.L.; Robinson, R.R. An extrarenal mechanism for the maintenance of potassium balance in sever chronic renal failure. *Trans. Assoc. Am. Phys.* **1967**, *80*, 207–216.
24. Sandle, G.I.; Gaiger, E.; Tapster, S.; Goodshep, T.H.J. Enhanced rectal potassium secretion in chronic renal insufficiency: Evidence for large intestinal potassium adaptation in man. *Clin. Sci.* **1986**, *71*, 393–401. [CrossRef] [PubMed]
25. Panese, S.; Mártin, R.S.; Virginillo, M.; Litardo, M.; Siga, E.; Arrizurieta, E.; Hayslett, J.P. Mechanism of enhanced transcellular potassium–secretion in man with chronic renal failure. *Kidney Int.* **1987**, *31*, 1377–1382. [CrossRef]
26. Sandle, G.I.; Gaiger, E.; Tapster, S.; Goodship, T.H.J. Evidence for large intestinal control of potassium homoeostasis in uraemic patients undergoing long-term dialysis. *Clin. Sci.* **1987**, *73*, 247–252. [CrossRef]
27. Sandle, G.I.; Hunter, M. Apical potassium (BK) channels and enhanced potassium secretion in human colon. *Qjm: Int. J. Med.* **2009**, *103*, 85–89. [CrossRef] [PubMed]
28. Unwin, R.J.; Luft, F.C.; Shirley, D.G. Pathophysiology and management of hypokalemia: A clinical perspective. *Nat. Rev. Nephrol.* **2011**, *7*, 75–84. [CrossRef] [PubMed]
29. Wilson, H.E.; Ing, T.S.; Metcalfe-Gibson, A.; Wrong, O.M. The chemical composition of faeces in uraemia, as revealed by in-vivo faecal dialysis. *Clin. Sci.* **1968**, *35*, 35.
30. Yosipovitch, G.; Reis, J.; Tur, E.; Blau, H.; Harell, D.; Morduchowicz, G.; Boner, G. Sweat electrolytes in patients with advanced renal failure. *J. Lab. Clin. Med.* **1994**, *124*, 808–812.
31. Joint National Committee on Prevention, Detection, Evaluation, and Treatment of High Blood Pressure. The sixth report of the joint national committee on prevention, detection, evaluation, and treatment of high blood pressure. *Arch. Intern. Med.* **1997**, *157*, 2413–2446.
32. WHO. *Guideline: Potassium Intake for Adults and Children*; WHO: Geneva, Switzerland, 2012.
33. Rabelink, T.; Koomans, H.A.; Hené, R.J.; Mees, E.J.D. Early and late adjustment to potassium loading in humans. *Kidney Int.* **1990**, *38*, 942–947. [CrossRef] [PubMed]
34. Hultgren, H.N.; Swenson, K.; Settach, G. Cardiac arrest due to oral potassium administration. *Am. J. Med.* **1975**, *58*, 139–142. [CrossRef]
35. Imai, E.; Horio, M.; Watanabe, T.; Iseki, K.; Yamagata, K.; Hara, S.; Ura, N.; Kiyohara, Y.; Moriyama, T.; Ando, Y.; et al. Prevalence of chronic kidney disease in the Japanese general population. *Clin. Exp. Nephrol.* **2009**, *13*, 621–630. [CrossRef]
36. Takaichi, K.; Takemoto, F.; Ubara, Y.; Mori, Y. Analysis of Factors Causing Hyperkalemia. *Intern. Med.* **2007**, *46*, 823–829. [CrossRef] [PubMed]
37. Einhorn, L.M.; Zhan, M.; Hsu, V.D.; Walker, L.D.; Moen, M.F.; Seliger, S.L.; Weir, M.R.; Fink, J.C. The Frequency of Hyperkalemia and Its Significance in Chronic Kidney Disease. *Arch. Intern. Med.* **2009**, *169*, 1156–1162. [CrossRef] [PubMed]
38. Weinberg, J.M.; Appel, L.J.; Bakris, G.L.; Gassman, J.J.; Greene, T.; Kendrick, C.A.; Wang, X.; Lash, J.P.; Lewis, J.A.; Pogue, V.; et al. Risk of Hyperkalemia in Nondiabetic Patients with Chronic Kidney Disease Receiving Antihypertensive TherapyHyperkalemia in CKD Adults Using Antihypertensives. *Arch. Intern. Med.* **2009**, *169*, 1587–1594. [CrossRef]
39. Kim, H.W.; Park, J.T.; Yoo, T.H.; Lee, J.; Chung, W.; Lee, K.B.; Chae, D.W.; Ahn, C.; Kang, S.W.; Choi, K.H.; et al. Urinary potassium excretion and progression of chronic kidney disease. *Clin. J. Am. Soc. Nephrol.* **2019**, *14*, 330–340. [CrossRef] [PubMed]

40. Kolasa, K.M. Dietary approaches to stop hypertension (DASH) in clinical practice: A primary care experience. *Clin. Cardiol.* **1999**, *22*, 16–22. [CrossRef]
41. Korgaonkar, S.; Tilea, A.; Gillespie, B.W.; Kiser, M.; Eisele, G.; Finkelstein, F.; Kotanko, P.; Pitt, B.; Saran, R. Serum potassium and outcomes in CKD: Insights from the RRI-CKD cohort study. *Clin. J. Am. Soc. Nephrol.* **2010**, *5*, 762–769. [CrossRef]
42. Miao, Y.; Dobre, D.; Heerspink, H.J.L.; Brenner, B.M.; Cooper, M.E.; Parving, H.H.; Shahinfar, S.; Grobbee, D.; Zeeuw, D.E. Increased serum potassium affects renal outcomes: A post hoc analysis of the Reduction of Endpoints in NIDDM with the Angiotesin ll Antagonist Losartan (RENAAL) trial. *Diabetologia* **2011**, *54*, 44–50. [CrossRef]
43. Smyth, A.; Dunkler, D.; Gao, P.; Teo, K.K.; Yusuf, S.; O'Donnell, M.J.; Mann, J.F.; Clase, C.M. The relationship between estimated sodium and potassium excretion and subsequent renal outcomes. *Kidney Int.* **2014**, *86*, 1205–1212. [CrossRef]
44. He, J.; Mills, K.T.; Appel, L.J.; Yang, W.; Chen, J.; Lee, B.T.; Rosas, S.E.; Porter, A.; Makos, G.; Weir, M.R.; et al. Urinary Sodium and Potassium Excretion and CKD Progression. *J. Am. Soc. Nephrol.* **2015**, *27*, 1202–1212. [CrossRef]
45. Kalantar, Z.K.; Tortorici, A.R.; Cen, J.L.T.; Kamgar, M.; Lau, W.L.; Moradi, H.; Rhee, C.M.; Streja, E.; Kovesdy, C.P. Dietary restrictions in dialysis patients: Is there anything left to eat? *Semin. Dial.* **2015**, *28*, 159–168. [CrossRef]
46. Roberts, S.B.; Fuss, P.; Heyman, M.B.; Evans, W.J.; Tsay, R.; Rasmussen, H.; Fiatarone, M.; Cortiella, J.; Dallal, G.E.; Young, V.R. Control of food intake in older men. *JAMA* **1994**, *272*, 1601–1606. [CrossRef]
47. Lynch, K.E.; Lynch, R.; Curhan, G.C.; Brunelli, S.M. Prescribed Dietary Phosphate Restriction and Survival among Hemodialysis Patients. *Clin. J. Am. Soc. Nephrol.* **2010**, *6*, 620–629. [CrossRef] [PubMed]
48. Shinaberger, C.S.; Greenland, S.; Kopple, J.D.; Wyck, D.V.; Mehrotra, R.; Kovesdy, C.P.; Kalantar-Zadeh, K. Is controlling Phosphorus by decreasing dietary protein intake beneficial or harmful in persons with chronic kidney disease? *Am. J. Clin. Nutr.* **2008**, *88*, 1511–1518. [CrossRef] [PubMed]
49. Ikizler, T.A.; Greene, J.H.; Wingard, R.L.; A Parker, R.; Hakim, R.M. Spontaneous dietary protein intake during progression of chronic renal failure. *J. Am. Soc. Nephrol.* **1995**, *6*, 1386–1391. [CrossRef] [PubMed]
50. Stenvinkel, P.; HeimbUrger, O.; Lindholm, B.; Kaysen, G.A.; Bergström, J. Are there two types of malnutrition in chronic renal failure? Evidence for relationships between malnutrition inflammation and atherosclerosis (MIA syndrome). *Nephrol. Dial. Transpl.* **2000**, *15*, 953–960. [CrossRef]
51. Fouque, D.; Kalantar-Zadeh, K.; Kopple, J.; Cano, N.; Chauveau, P.; Cuppari, L.; Franch, H.; Guarnieri, G.; Ikizler, T.; Kaysen, G.; et al. A proposed nomenclature and diagnostic criteria for protein–energy wasting in acute and chronic kidney disease. *Kidney Int.* **2008**, *73*, 391–398. [CrossRef]
52. Klahr, S.; Levey, A.S.; Beck, G.J.; Caggiula, A.W.; Hunsicker, L.; Kusek, J.W.; Striker, G. The effects of dietary protein restriction and blood pressure control on the progression of chronic renal disease. Modification of diet in renal disease study group. *N. Engl. J. Med.* **1994**, *330*, 877–884. [CrossRef]
53. Foley, R.N.; Gilbertson, D.T.; Murray, T.; Collins, A.J. Long Interdialytic Interval and Mortality among Patients Receiving Hemodialysis. *N. Engl. J. Med.* **2011**, *365*, 1099–1107. [CrossRef]
54. Zhang, H.; Schaubel, D.E.; Kalbfleisch, J.D.; Bragg-Gresham, J.L.; Robinson, B.M.; Pisoni, R.L.; Canaud, B.; Jadoul, M.; Akiba, T.; Saito, A.; et al. Dialysis outcomes and analysis of practice patterns suggests the dialysis schedule affects day-of-week mortality. *Kidney Int.* **2012**, *81*, 1108–1115. [CrossRef] [PubMed]
55. Fujita, S.; Yamaoka, Y.; Nagai, M.; Nakaya, T.; Hanba, Y.; Shigematsu, T. Analysis of factors affecting the prognosis of a hemodialysis patient-Focusing on albumin and parameters of nutrition. *Nihon Toseki Igakkai Zasshi* **2010**, *43*, 453–460. [CrossRef]
56. Johansen, K.L.; Zhang, R.; Huang, Y.; Chen, S.C.; Blagg, C.R.; Goldfarb-Rumyantzev, A.S.; Hoy, C.D.; Lockridge, R.S., Jr.; Miller, B.W.; Eggers, P.W.; et al. Survival and hospitalization among patients using nocturnal and short daily compared to conventional hemodialysis: A USRDS study. *Kindney Int.* **2009**, *76*, 984–990. [CrossRef]
57. Feriani, M.; Ronco, C.; Greca, G.L. *Replacement of Renal Function by Dialysis*, 5th ed.; Horl, W.H., Koch, K.M., Lindsay, R.M., Winchester, J.F., Eds.; Kluwer Academic Publishers: Lancaster, UK, 2004; pp. 505–537.
58. Krishnamurthy, V.M.R.; Wei, G.; Baird, B.C.; Murtaugh, M.; Chonchol, M.B.; Raphael, K.L.; Greene, T.; Beddhu, S. High dietary fiber intake is associated with decreased inflammation and all-cause mortality in patients with chronic kidney disease. *Kidney Int.* **2012**, *81*, 300–306. [CrossRef]
59. Tomemori, H.; Hamamura, K.; Tabane, K. Interactive Effects of Sodium and Potassium on the Growth and Photosynthesis of Spinach and Komatsuna. *Plant Prod. Sci.* **2002**, *5*, 281–285. [CrossRef]
60. Ogawa, A.; Eguchi, T.; Toyofuku, K. Cultivation Methods for Leafy Vegetables and Tomatoes with Low Potassium Content for Dialysis Patients. *Environ. Control. Biol.* **2012**, *50*, 407–414. [CrossRef]
61. Renna, M.; Castellino, M.; Leoni, B.; Paradiso, V.M.; Santamaria, P. Microgreens Production with Low Potassium Content for Patients with Impaired Kidney Function. *Nutrients* **2018**, *10*, 675. [CrossRef] [PubMed]
62. Asao, T.; Asaduzzaman; Mondal, F.; Tokura, M.; Adachi, F.; Ueno, M.; Kawaguchi, M.; Yano, S.; Ban, T. Impact of reduced potassium nitrate concentrations in nutrient solution on the growth, yield and fruit quality of melon in hydroponics. *Sci. Hortic.* **2013**, *164*, 221–231. [CrossRef]
63. Mondal, F.; Asaduzzaman; Ueno, M.; Kawaguchi, M.; Yano, S.; Ban, T.; Tanaka, H.; Asao, T. Reduction of Potassium (K) Content in Strawberry Fruits through KNO3 Management of Hydroponics. *Hortic. J.* **2017**, *86*, 26–36. [CrossRef]
64. Talukder, R.; Asaduzzaman; Ueno, M.; Kawaguchi, M.; Yano, S.; Ban, T.; Tanaka, H.; Asao, T. Low Potassium Content Vegetables Research for Chronic Kidney Disease Patients in Japan. *Nephrol. Open J.* **2016**, *2*, 1–8. [CrossRef]

65. Iwahori, T.; Ueshima, H.; Torii, S.; Saito, Y.; Kondo, K.; Tanaka-Mizuno, S.; Arima, H.; Miura, K. Diurnal variation of urinary sodium-to-potassium ratio in free-living Japanese individuals. *Hypertens. Res.* **2017**, *40*, 658–664. [CrossRef]
66. Ethier, J.H.; Kamel, K.S.; Magner, P.O.; Lemann, J., Jr.; Halperin, M.L. The transtubular potassium concentration in patients with hypokale-mia and hyperkalemia. *Am. J. Kidney Dis.* **1990**, *15*, 309–315. [CrossRef]
67. Choi, M.J.; Ziyadeh, F.N. The utility of the transtubular potassium gradient in the evaluation of hyperkalemia. *J. Am. Soc. Nephrol.* **2008**, *19*, 424–426. [CrossRef] [PubMed]
68. Zettle, R.M.; West, M.L.; Josse, R.G.; Richardson, R.M.; Marsden, P.A.; Halperin, M.L. Renal potassium handling during states of low al-dosterone bioactivity: A method to differentiate renal and non-renal causes. *Am. J. Nephrol.* **1987**, *7*, 360–366. [CrossRef]
69. Kamel, K.S.; Halperin, M.L. Intrarenal urea recycling leads to a higher rate of renal excretion of potassium: An hypothesis with clinical implications. *Curr. Opin. Nephrol. Hypertens.* **2011**, *20*, 547–554. [CrossRef] [PubMed]
70. Karet, F.E. Mechanisms in hyperkalelnic renal tubular acidosis. *J. Am. Soc. Nephrol.* **2009**, *20*, 251–254. [CrossRef]
71. Watson, M.; Abbott, K.; Yuan, C.M. Damned If You Do, Damned If You Don't: Potassium Binding Resins in Hyperkalemia. *Clin. J. Am. Soc. Nephrol.* **2010**, *5*, 1723–1726. [CrossRef]
72. Gardiner, G.W. Kayexalate (sodium polystyrene sulphonate) in sorbitol associated with intestinal necrosis in uremic patients. *Can. J. Gastroenterol.* **1997**, *11*, 573–577. [CrossRef]
73. Rashid, A.; Hamilton, S.R. Necrosis of the Gastrointestinal Tract in Uremic Patients as a Result of Sodium Polystyrene Sulfonate (Kayexalate) in Sorbitol. *Am. J. Surg. Pathol.* **1997**, *21*, 60–69. [CrossRef]
74. Stavros, F.; Yang, A.; Leon, A.; Nuttall, M.; Rasmussen, H.S. Characterization of structure and function of ZS-9, a K^+ selective ion trap. *PLoS ONE* **2014**, *9*, e114686. [CrossRef]
75. Greenberg, A. Hyperkalemia: Treatment options. *Semin. Nephrol.* **1998**, *18*, 46–57. [PubMed]
76. Allon, M.; Takeshian, A.; Shanklin, N. Effect of insulin plus glucose infusion with or without epirlephrine on fasting hyperkalemia. *Kidney Int.* **1993**, *43*, 212–217. [CrossRef]
77. Hsueh, W.A.; Carlson, E.J.; Luetscher, J.A.; Grislis, G. Activation and Characterization of Inactive Big Renin in Plasma of Patients with Diabetic Nephropathy and Unusual Active Renin*. *J. Clin. Endocrinol. Metab.* **1980**, *51*, 535–543. [CrossRef] [PubMed]
78. Mount, D.B. Disorders of potassium balance. In *Brenner and Rector's the Kidney*, 10th ed.; Skorecki, K., Chertow, G.M., Marsden, P.A., Taal, M.W., Wasser, W.G., Eds.; Elsevier: Philadelphia, PA, USA, 2016; pp. 559–600.
79. Palevsky, P.M.; Zhang, J.H.; O'Connor, T.Z.; Chertow, G.M.; Crowley, S.T.; Choudhury, D.; Finkel, K.W.; Kellum, J.A.; Paganini, E.P.; Schein, R.M.H.; et al. Intensity of Renal Support in Critically Ill Patients with Acute Kidney Injury. *N. Engl. J. Med.* **2008**, *359*, 7–20. [CrossRef] [PubMed]
80. Bellomo, R.; Cass, A.; Norton, R.; Gallagher, M.; Su, S.; Cole, L.; Finfer, S.; McArthur, C.; McGuinness, S.; Myburgh, J.; et al. Intensity of Continuous Renal-Replacement Therapy in Critically Ill Patients. *N. Engl. J. Med.* **2009**, *361*, 1627–1638. [CrossRef]
81. Luo, J.; Brunelli, S.M.; Jensen, D.E.; Yang, A. Association between Serum Potassium and Outcomes in Patients with Reduced Kidney Function. *Clin. J. Am. Soc. Nephrol.* **2015**, *11*, 90–100. [CrossRef]
82. Pun, P.H.; Lehrich, R.W.; Honeycutt, E.F.; Herzog, C.A.; Middleton, J.P. Modifiable risk factors associated with sudden cardiac arrest within hemodialysis clinics. *Kidney Int.* **2011**, *79*, 218–227. [CrossRef]
83. Diercks, D.B.; Shumaik, G.M.; A Harrigan, R.; Brady, W.J.; Chan, T.C. Electrocardiographic manifestations: Electrolyte abnormalities. *J. Emerg. Med.* **2004**, *27*, 153–160. [CrossRef]
84. Mujais, S.K.; Katz, A.L. Potassium deficiency. In *The Kidney: Physiology and Pathophysiology*; Seldin, D.W., Giebisch, G., Eds.; Lippincott Wiliams & Wilkins: Philadelphia, PA, USA, 2000; p. 1615.
85. Schwartz, W.B.; Relman, A.S. Effects of electrolyte disorders on renal structure and function. *N. Engl. J. Med.* **1967**, *276*, 383–389. [CrossRef]
86. Cremer, W.; Bock, K.D. Symptoms and course of chronic hypokalemic nephropathy in man. *Clin. Nephrol.* **1977**, *7*, 112–119.
87. Torres, V.E.; Young, W.F.; Offord, K.P.; Hattery, R.R. Association of Hypokalemia, Aldosteronism, and Renal Cysts. *N. Engl. J. Med.* **1990**, *322*, 345–351. [CrossRef] [PubMed]
88. Yasuhara, D.; Naruo, T.; Taguchi, S.; Umekita, Y.; Yoshida, H.; Nozoe, S. "End-stage kidney" in longstanding bulimia nervosa. *Int. J. Eat. Disord.* **2005**, *38*, 383–385. [CrossRef] [PubMed]
89. Huang, C.-L.; Kuo, E. Mechanism of Hypokalemia in Magnesium Deficiency. *J. Am. Soc. Nephrol.* **2007**, *18*, 2649–2652. [CrossRef] [PubMed]
90. Ruml, L.A.; Pak, C.Y. Effect of potassium magnesium citrate on thiazide-induced hypokalemia and magnesium loss. *Am. J. Kidney Dis.* **1999**, *34*, 107–113. [CrossRef]
91. Koeppen, B.M. The kidney and acid-base regulatio. *Adv. Physiol. Educ.* **2009**, *33*, 275–281. [CrossRef]
92. Kraut, J.A.; Kurtz, I. Metabolic Acidosis of CKD: Diagnosis, Clinical Characteristics, and Treatment. *Am. J. Kidney Dis.* **2005**, *45*, 978–993. [CrossRef]
93. Terker, A.S.; Zhang, C.; McCormick, J.A.; Lazelle, R.A.; Zhang, C.; Meermeier, N.P.; Siler, D.A.; Park, H.J.; Fu, Y.; Cohen, D.M.; et al. Potassium Modulates Electrolyte Balance and Blood Pressure through Effects on Distal Cell Voltage and Chloride. *Cell Metab.* **2015**, *21*, 39–50. [CrossRef]
94. Xu, N.; Hirohama, D.; Ishizawa, K.; Chang, W.X.; Shimosawa, T.; Fujita, T.; Uchida, S.; Shibata, S. Hypokalemia and Pendrin Induction by Aldosterone. *Hypertension* **2017**, *69*, 855–862. [CrossRef]

95. Palygin, O.; Levchenko, V.; Ilatovskaya, D.V.; Pavlov, T.S.; Pochynyuk, O.M.; Jacob, H.J.; Geurts, A.M.; Hodges, M.R.; Staruschenko, A. Essential role of Kir5.1 channels in renal salt handling and blood pressure control. *JCI Insight* **2017**, *2*, e92331. [CrossRef]
96. Kempner, W. Some effects of the rice diet treatment of kidney disease and hypertension. *Bull. N. Y. Acad. Med.* **1946**, *22*, 358–370.
97. Kawano, Y.; Omae, T. Lifestyle modifications in the management of hypertension benefits and limitations. *CVD Prev.* **1998**, *1*, 336–346.
98. Stamler, J.; Chan, Q.; Daviglus, M.L.; Dyer, A.R.; Horn, L.V.; Garside, D.B.; Miura, K.; Wu, Y.; Ueshima, H.; Zhao, L.; et al. Relation of dietary sodium (salt) to blood pressure and its possible modulation by other dietary factors: The INTERMAP study. *Hypertension* **2018**, *71*, 631–637. [CrossRef]
99. Whelton, P.K.; He, J.; Cutler, J.A.; Brancati, F.L.; Appel, L.J.; Follmann, D.; Klag, M.J. Effects of oral potassium on blood pressure meta-analysis of randomized controlled clinical trials. *JAMA* **1997**, *277*, 1624–1632. [CrossRef]
100. Akita, S.; Sacks, F.M.; Svetkey, L.P.; Conlin, P.R.; Kimura, G. DASH-sodium trial collaborative research group: Effects of the dietary approaches to stop hypertension (DASH) diet on the pressure-natriuresis relationship. *Hypertension* **2003**, *42*, 8–13. [CrossRef] [PubMed]
101. Sacks, F.M.; Svetkey, L.P.; Vollmer, W.M.; Appel, L.J.; Bray, G.A.; Harsha, D.; Obarzanek, E.; Colin, P.R.; Miller, E.R.; Simons-Morton, D.G.; et al. Effects on blood pressure of reduced dietary sodium and the Dietary Approaches to Stop Hypertension (DASH) diet. *N. Engl. J. Med.* **2001**, *344*, 3–10. [CrossRef] [PubMed]
102. Hedayati, S.S.; Minhajuddin, A.T.; Ijaz, A.; Moe, O.W.; Elsayed, E.F.; Reilly, R.F.; Huang, C.-L. Association of Urinary Sodium/Potassium Ratio with Blood Pressure: Sex and Racial Differences. *Clin. J. Am. Soc. Nephrol.* **2011**, *7*, 315–322. [CrossRef]
103. Araki, S.-I.; Haneda, M.; Koya, D.; Kondo, K.; Tanaka, S.; Arima, H.; Kume, S.; Nakazawa, J.; Chin-Kanasaki, M.; Ugi, S.; et al. Urinary Potassium Excretion and Renal and Cardiovascular Complications in Patients with Type 2 Diabetes and Normal Renal Function. *Clin. J. Am. Soc. Nephrol.* **2015**, *10*, 2152–2158. [CrossRef]
104. Macdonald, J.E.; Struthers, A.D. Optimal serum potassium level in cardiovascular patients? *J. Am. Coll Cardiol.* **2004**, *43*, 155–161. [CrossRef]
105. Wang, H.-H.; Hung, C.-C.; Kuo, M.-C.; Chiu, Y.-W.; Chang, J.-M.; Tsai, J.-C.; Seifter, J.L.; Chen, H.-C.; Hwang, D.-Y.; Hwang, S.-J. Hypokalemia, Its Contributing Factors and Renal Outcomes in Patients with Chronic Kidney Disease. *PLoS ONE* **2013**, *8*, e67140. [CrossRef] [PubMed]
106. Tyson, C.C.; Lin, P.H.; Corsino, L.; Batch, B.C.; Allen, J.; Sapp, S.; Barnhart, H.; Nwankwo, C.; Burroughs, J.; Svetkey, L.P. Short-term effects of the DASH diet in adults with moderate chronic kidney disease: A pilot feeding study. *Clin. Kidney J.* **2016**, *9*, 592–598. [CrossRef] [PubMed]
107. Iwahori, T.; Miura, K.; Ueshima, H. Time to Consider Use of the Sodium-to-Potassium Ratio for Practical Sodium Reduction and Potassium Increase. *Nutrients* **2017**, *9*, 700. [CrossRef] [PubMed]
108. Iwahori, T.; Ueshima, H.; Miyagawa, N.; Ohgami, N.; Yamashita, H.; Ohkubo, T.; Murakami, Y.; Shiga, T.; Miura, K. Six random specimens of daytime casual urine on different days are sufficient to estimate daily sodium/potassium ratio in comparison to 7-day 24-h urine collections. *Hypertens. Res.* **2014**, *37*, 765–771. [CrossRef] [PubMed]
109. Iwahori, T.; Ueshima, H.; Torii, S.; Saito, Y.; Fujiyoshi, A.; Ohkubo, T.; Miura, K. Four to seven random casual urine specimens are sufficient to estimate 24-h urinary sodium/potassium ratio in individuals with high blood pressure. *J. Hum. Hypertens.* **2016**, *30*, 328–334. [CrossRef]
110. Okuyama, Y.; Uchida, H.A.; Iwahori, T.; Segawa, H.; Kato, A.; Takeuchi, H.; Kakio, Y.; Umebayashi, R.; Kitagawa, M.; Sugiyama, H.; et al. The relationship between repeated measurement of casual and 24-h urinary sodium-to-potassium ratio in patients with chronic kidney disease. *J. Hum. Hypertens.* **2018**, *33*, 286–297. [CrossRef] [PubMed]
111. Palmer, B.F. Managing hyperkalemia caused by inhibitors of the renin angiotensin al dosterone system. *N. Engl. J. Med.* **2004**, *351*, 585–592. [CrossRef] [PubMed]
112. Chaker, B.S.; Atef, B.; Neila, F.; Raoudha, S.; Houssem, H. Drugoinduced hyperkalemia. *Drug Saf.* **2014**, *37*, 677–692.
113. Veltri, K.T.; Mason, C. Medication-Induced Hypokalemia. *Pharm. Ther.* **2015**, *40*, 185–190.

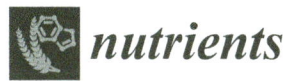

Review

Significance of Levocarnitine Treatment in Dialysis Patients

Hiroyuki Takashima, Takashi Maruyama and Masanori Abe *

Division of Nephrology, Hypertension and Endocrinology, Department of Internal Medicine, Nihon University School of Medicine, 30-1 Oyaguchi Kami-cho, Itabashi-ku, Tokyo 173-8610, Japan; takashima.hiroyuki@nihon-u.ac.jp (H.T.); maruyama.takashi@nihon-u.ac.jp (T.M.)
* Correspondence: abe.masanori@nihon-u.ac.jp; Tel.: +81-3-3972-8111; Fax: +81-3-3972-8311

Abstract: Carnitine is a naturally occurring amino acid derivative that is involved in the transport of long-chain fatty acids to the mitochondrial matrix. There, these substrates undergo β-oxidation, producing energy. The major sources of carnitine are dietary intake, although carnitine is also endogenously synthesized in the liver and kidney. However, in patients on dialysis, serum carnitine levels progressively fall due to restricted dietary intake and deprivation of endogenous synthesis in the kidney. Furthermore, serum-free carnitine is removed by hemodialysis treatment because the molecular weight of carnitine is small (161 Da) and its protein binding rates are very low. Therefore, the dialysis procedure is a major cause of carnitine deficiency in patients undergoing hemodialysis. This deficiency may contribute to several clinical disorders in such patients. Symptoms of dialysis-related carnitine deficiency include erythropoiesis-stimulating agent-resistant anemia, myopathy, muscle weakness, and intradialytic muscle cramps and hypotension. However, levocarnitine administration might replenish the free carnitine and help to increase carnitine levels in muscle. This article reviews the previous research into levocarnitine therapy in patients on maintenance dialysis for the treatment of renal anemia, cardiac dysfunction, dyslipidemia, and muscle and dialytic symptoms, and it examines the efficacy of the therapeutic approach and related issues.

Keywords: carnitine; carnitine deficiency; end-stage kidney disease; peritoneal dialysis; hemodialysis

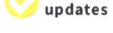

Citation: Takashima, H.; Maruyama, T.; Abe, M. Significance of Levocarnitine Treatment in Dialysis Patients. *Nutrients* **2021**, *13*, 1219. https://doi.org/10.3390/nu13041219

Academic Editor: Pramod Khosla

Received: 3 March 2021
Accepted: 4 April 2021
Published: 7 April 2021

Publisher's Note: MDPI stays neutral with regard to jurisdictional claims in published maps and institutional affiliations.

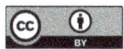

Copyright: © 2021 by the authors. Licensee MDPI, Basel, Switzerland. This article is an open access article distributed under the terms and conditions of the Creative Commons Attribution (CC BY) license (https://creativecommons.org/licenses/by/4.0/).

1. Introduction

Carnitine, with a molecular weight of 161 Da, is a water-soluble quaternary amine. It is derived from lysine and methionine, which are two essential amino acids. Its primary role is in facilitating the transport of long-chain fatty acids to the mitochondrial matrix. These substrates are delivered for β-oxidation and the subsequent production of energy. Carnitine is primarily biosynthesized in the kidney and liver and is found in virtually all tissues but predominantly in cardiac and skeletal muscle.

Patients on hemodialysis often have carnitine deficiency [1]. Carnitine deficiency is associated with several clinical disorders, such as erythropoiesis-stimulating agent (ESA)-resistant anemia, muscle weakness, myopathy, and intradialytic muscle cramps and hypotension. Additional clinical disorders of carnitine deficiency include dyslipidemia, cardiac arrhythmia, cachexia, insulin resistance, and glucose intolerance [2–4]. The characteristic features of dialysis-associated carnitine deficiency are reduced levels of free carnitine and elevated levels of acylcarnitine. Free carnitine levels are mainly decreased by its removal during hemodialysis, whereas the accumulation of acylcarnitine and an aberrantly elevated plasma acylcarnitine to free carnitine ratio are due to deficient renal clearance and β-oxidation failure [1,2]. Accordingly, carnitine supplementation in dialysis patients with carnitine insufficiency may yield clinical benefits by ameliorating several of the above-mentioned conditions.

In this review, we describe the profile of carnitine metabolism and the effects of carnitine treatment on the metabolism and function of dialysis patients. We also assess the current findings related to the carnitine treatment of patients undergoing dialysis therapy, particularly its impact on cardiac function, ESA-resistant anemia, muscle symptoms, and malnutrition.

2. Carnitine Homeostasis

The main dietary sources of carnitine are meat products, with small amounts of carnitine found in vegetables [5,6]. About 100–400 mg per day of carnitine is provided from a normal diet. Dietary carnitine is absorbed from the intestine by both active and passive transport and meets 65–75% of daily needs. The remaining 25–35% is supplied by biosynthesis in the kidney and liver from methionine and lysine. Carnitine is found both intracellularly and extracellularly and in both non-esterified and esterified forms. The former is free carnitine, while the latter is acylcarnitines. Short-, medium-, and long-chain fatty acids are found in carnitine esters and are present in biological systems. The proportion of acylcarnitine varies widely according to physical activity, disease condition, and nutritional state. Under normal conditions in humans, acylcarnitine accounts for approximately 20% of total carnitine in serum, 10–15% of that in the liver and skeletal muscle, and 50–60% of that in urine [7–9].

Under physiological conditions, the total carnitine content in the body has been estimated to be 100 mmol. More than 90% of total body carnitine is found in skeletal muscle, with 2–3% in the liver and kidney. Thus, only 0.5–1% is present in the extracellular fluid [10]. The brain has a relatively low concentration of carnitine, despite being one of the few organs with endogenous biosynthesis capability. Carnitine cannot bind to protein and is mainly filtered at the glomeruli of the kidney. However, over 90% of filtered carnitine is reabsorbed by the proximal renal tubule in individuals with normal kidney function, and the serum excretory threshold level of free carnitine in the kidney appears to be 40 μmol/L, which is near the normal serum concentration of free carnitine [5,6]. Tubular reabsorption of free carnitine predominates. Therefore, the excretion of acylcarnitine by the kidney is 4- to 8-fold higher than that of free carnitine [5]. Plasma membrane transporters and carnitine-dependent enzymes are important for maintaining carnitine homeostasis. Together, free and acylcarnitine comprise the carnitine system.

The high-affinity Na^+/carnitine cotransporter OCTN2 is the most physiologically associated plasma membrane transporter of carnitine [11]. OCTN2 is extensively found in numerous tissues, such as the heart, skeletal muscle, kidney, and placenta. OCTN2 is localized to the brush border of tubular epithelial cells in the kidney and is most active in the proximal tubules of the nephron, which is the site of approximately 65% of reabsorption and secretion [12]. The association of mutations in the OTCN2 gene with primary systemic carnitine deficiency indicates its importance [13].

Carnitine/acylcarnitine translocase (CACT) and carnitine acyltransferases are known as carnitine-dependent enzymes. CACT converts mitochondrial carnitine to cytoplasmic acylcarnitine and allows the flow of both carnitine and short-chain acyl-carnitines into and out of the mitochondria [14]. Carnitine acyltransferases exist in tissue-specific isoforms with distinct kinetic characteristics and with significant modulatory targets involved in fatty acid metabolism and coenzyme-A (CoA) release [15].

The proper function of OCTN2 and the various carnitine-dependent enzymes is needed to maintain the carnitine system. Carnitine has an important role in energy metabolism. It transports long-chain fatty acids across the inner mitochondrial membrane and modulates β-oxidation and the resulting adenosine triphosphate (ATP) production [16]. Furthermore, carnitine participates in intermediary metabolism by regulating the ratio of acyl-CoA/CoA in the cell. The main mechanisms underlying this function of carnitine are the production of short-chain acylcarnitines, which are catalyzed by carnitine acetyltransferase, and the conversion of carnitine to acylcarnitine, which is catalyzed by CACT [14,17]. Carnitine has a buffer action for accumulated acyl-CoA. The accumulation of acyl-CoA inhibits several enzymes, including acetyl CoA carboxylase, adenine nucleotide translocase, citrate synthetase, pyruvate dehydrogenase, and pyruvate carboxylase, and it induces mitochondrial dysfunction. Therefore, an accumulation of acyl groups within the mitochondria inhibits the activity of energy-producing enzymes. Acyl-CoA is restricted to the mitochondrial matrix and cannot pass the membrane. However, its acyl group is transferred from acyl-CoA to carnitine, and carnitine is metabolized into acylcarnitine. Acylcarnitine translocates from mitochondria to the extracellular fluid and is finally excreted via the urine. The detoxifying effects of carnitine are important for cell metabolism [18]. The fatty acid metabolism and functions of carnitine are shown in Figure 1.

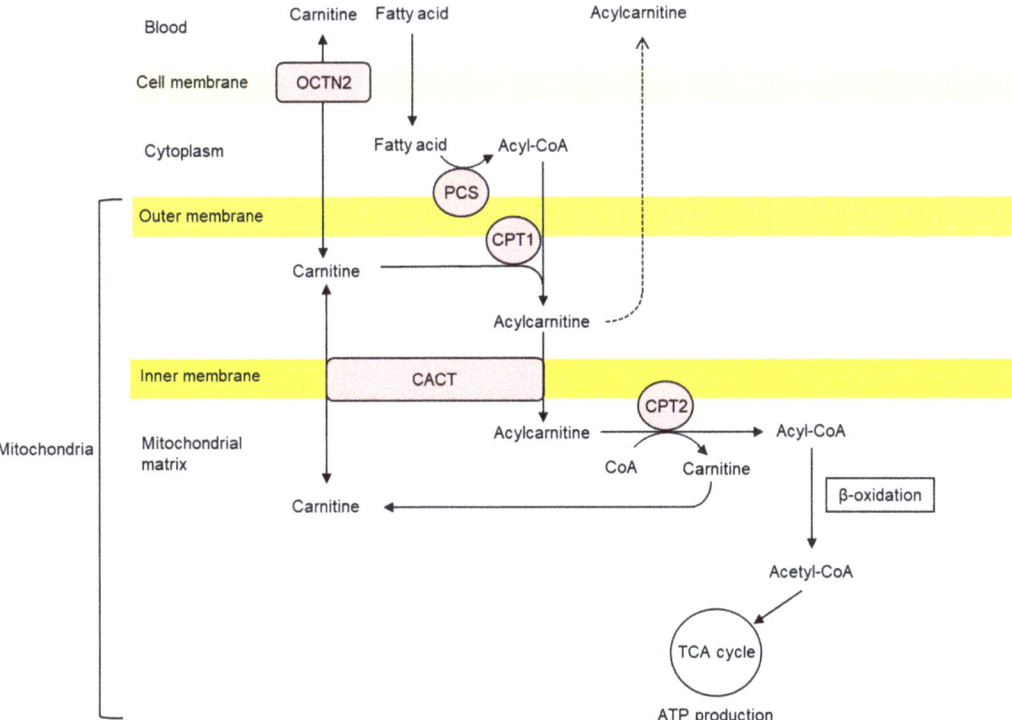

Figure 1. Fatty acid metabolism and metabolic functions of carnitine. CACT, carnitine acetyltransferase; CPT, carnitine palmitoyl transferase; OCTN2, organic cation/carnitine transporter 2, PCS, palmitoyl CoA synthetase.

Serum carnitine concentrations are 50–60 µmol/L, which is calculated as the sum of free carnitine and acylcarnitine. When serum-free carnitine drops below 20 µmol/L, the clinical symptoms of carnitine deficiency can develop. In patients with severe hereditary metabolic diseases, acylcarnitine is found in the serum and urine. In these patients, the endogenous carnitine pool falls into a deficit to manage the crucial acyl transfer, which increases the acyl/free carnitine ratio in serum. A ratio exceeding 0.4 has been used to indicate carnitine insufficiency in clinical practice [19]. Daily urinary total carnitine excretion typically consists of 50% acylcarnitine, resulting in a urinary acyl/free carnitine ratio of about 1.0 [20]. Carnitine homeostasis is shown in Figure 2.

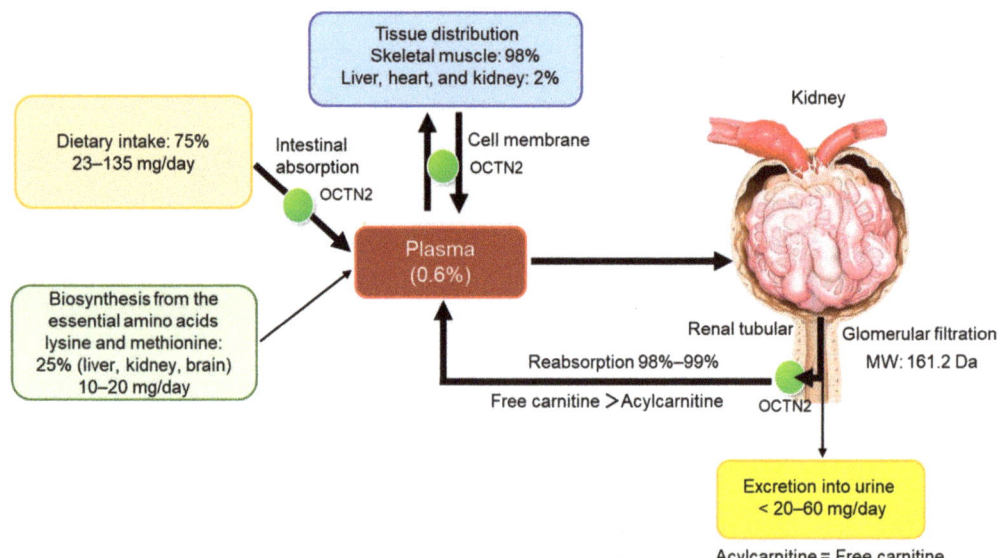

Figure 2. Carnitine homeostasis. MW, molecular weight; OCTN2, organic cation/carnitine transporter 2.

3. Carnitine Deficiency in Patients Who Are Undergoing Dialysis Therapy

Carnitine homeostasis is profoundly perturbed in patients with end-stage kidney disease, particularly patients on dialysis. Dietary intake of carnitine is decreased due to falls in appetite, total energy levels, and protein intake. In addition, accumulating evidence has linked inflammation to malnutrition, and chronic inflammation might also interrupt carnitine transfer in the intestine [21]. Protein-energy wasting (PEW) and inflammation are the most pivotal risk factors for morbidity and mortality in patients on dialysis [22–24]. Carnitine biosynthesis can also fall in patients on dialysis due to reduced biosynthesis in the kidney and limited compensation by the liver [25]. Furthermore, the kidney disease may itself modulate OCTN2 activity on the renal tubule [26]. Filtered carnitine in the glomerulus cannot be reabsorbed in anuric patients undergoing hemodialysis. Therefore, chronic hemodialysis treatment reduces serum and tissue levels of carnitine and can promote acylcarnitine accumulation. As a result of the low molecular weight of carnitine and its high hydrophilicity and absence of protein binding, carnitine is significantly removed by the dialyzer [27,28].

According to Japanese guidelines [29], a free carnitine level < 20 μmol/L is defined as carnitine deficiency, a high risk of carnitine deficiency is defined as a level in the range of 20–36 μmol/L, and carnitine insufficiency is defined as a serum acyl/free carnitine ratio > 0.4. Consequently, serum carnitine levels are significantly lower in patients receiving hemodialysis than in healthy individuals at 22.0 ± 5.4 μmol/L and 43.3 ± 8.6 μmol/L, respectively [30]. Serum endogenous carnitine levels are significantly negatively correlated with dialysis therapy duration, with most of the reduction occurring within the first few months of hemodialysis initiation [30]. Long-term hemodialysis (i.e., longer than 1 year) is also linked to a marked 38% reduction in muscle carnitine pools compared with those before hemodialysis initiation [30]. Another investigation also reported that the total carnitine and acylcarnitine levels in muscle were significantly decreased in patients on dialysis [31]. We recently reported the prevalence of carnitine deficiency in 150 patients on hemodialysis [32]. Of these, serum free carnitine levels were below the normal range (36–74 μmol/L) in 90% of the patients, and 25.3% of the participants met the definition of carnitine deficiency (<20 μmol/L). Furthermore, 64.7% were diagnosed as having high risk of carnitine deficiency (acyl/free carnitine ratio > 0.4). In addition, just 13.3% of the participants ($n = 20$) had a normal ratio of ≤ 0.4 and 86.7% of the participants ($n = 130$) were diagnosed with carnitine insufficiency. A longer duration of dialysis was significantly associated with lower serum carnitine levels in multivariate analysis [32].

Acylcarnitine levels are significantly higher in patients on maintenance hemodialysis than in healthy individuals. Acylcarnitine levels are significantly elevated in patients who have been receiving hemodialysis for at least 12 months [4,28]. Indeed, acylcarnitine levels account for about 50% of the total serum carnitine stores in these patients compared with just 15% in healthy individuals [4,28]. Hemodialysis procedures decrease free, short-chain, medium-chain, and dicarboxylic acylcarnitines but do not affect long-chain acylcarnitines [33]. The dialytic removal of acylcarnitine during a single hemodialysis session is significantly associated with the carbon chain length of the acyl groups, with no major removal of the 18-carbon chain esters [34]. The removal rate of acylcarnitine clearly decreases as the carbon chain length increases because it increases their molecular weight and alters their lipophilicity. Furthermore, longer-chain acylcarnitines can bind to protein [35]. Therefore, the acyl/free carnitine ratio is positively correlated with the number of months on hemodialysis treatment [30,36]. Acylcarnitines are classified according to carbon chain length. Tandem mass spectrometry can determine the details of acylcarnitines, such as whether they are short-chain, middle-chain, and long-chain acylcarnitines. Tandem mass spectrometry has revealed that a lower ratio of acetylcarnitine (C2)/(palmitoylcarnitine + octadecenoylcarnitine [C16+C18:1]), which indicates the ratio of short-chain/long-chain acylcarnitines, in patients on hemodialysis is associated with all-cause mortality [37].

4. Removal of Carnitine by Dialysis Therapy

In 2018, 339,841 patients underwent maintenance dialysis in Japan. Of these, 37.0% were receiving hemodiafiltration. Approximately 71% of patients who were receiving hemodiafiltration were treated with online hemodiafiltration and the pre-dilution method [38,39]. Compared with conventional high-flux hemodialysis, hemodiafiltration is a more effective technique; it relies on high-flux membranes that can remove both small solutes, such as urea, and low-molecular weight proteins, such as β2-microglobulin [40,41]. Serum carnitine is removed by hemodialysis. Previous work determined the percent reduction in serum-free carnitine in patients on hemodialysis with or without diabetes and without levocarnitine treatment. The reductions in plasma free carnitine were -64.7% and -66.6% in patients with or without diabetes, respectively [33]. However, the hemodialysis procedure was not described in detail (i.e., blood and dialysate flow rates, treatment time, and Kt/V). We previously investigated the reduction rate of the serum carnitine level after single sessions of hemodialysis and hemodiafiltration [32]. Hemodialysis using high-flux dialyzers was conducted at blood and dialysate flow rates of 200–240 mL/min and 500 mL/min, respectively. Hemodiafiltration using high-flux hemodiafilters was performed at blood flow, replacement fluid, and dialysate flow rates of 200–300, 200–250, and 250–300 mL/min, respectively. Although no significant differences were evident in the patients' baseline characteristics or in the pre-dialysis serum total, free, or acylcarnitine concentrations between the hemodialysis and hemodiafiltration groups, the Kt/V values were 1.28 ± 0.27 and 1.45 ± 0.31 in the hemodialysis and hemodiafiltration groups, respectively ($p = 0.042$). There was a significantly greater decrease in serum total, free, and acylcarnitine levels in the hemodiafiltration group. Reduction rates of serum free carnitine of $64\% \pm 4\%$ and $75\% \pm 7\%$ were obtained under hemodialysis and hemodiafiltration conditions, respectively ($p < 0.0001$). These findings indicate the greater clearance of small molecular weight solutes by hemodiafiltration.

Patients on peritoneal dialysis exhibit a decreased serum free carnitine level and increased acyl/free carnitine ratio compared with age- and sex-matched individuals with normal kidney function [42,43]. In patients on peritoneal dialysis, the mechanism of carnitine deficiency is considered to be decreased dietary intake of carnitine-containing food, decreased renal carnitine synthesis, and decreased renal excretion of acylcarnitine [27,30].

Another contributor might be the loss of free carnitine into the peritoneal dialysis fluid [44]. The prevalences of carnitine deficiency, high risk of carnitine deficiency, and carnitine insufficiency in peritoneal dialysis patients are comparable to those of age-, sex-, and dialysis vintage-matched hemodialysis patients [45]. Lower serum-free carnitine levels are associated with a longer duration of peritoneal dialysis and an older age.

5. Carnitine Supplementation in Dialysis Patients

The association between carnitine deficiency and a decreased serum-free carnitine level may result in various cellular metabolic disorders, such as reduced mitochondrial β-oxidation of fatty acids and consequent diminished energy production and storage of toxic acylcarnitines and suppression of carnitine-related enzymes involved in metabolism [46]. These carnitine-related metabolic aberrations may induce the above-mentioned clinical disorders frequently found in patients on dialysis, which include muscle weakness and cardiomyopathy, PEW, plasma lipid abnormalities, and ESA-resistant anemia, as well as hemodialysis-associated symptoms such as hypotension and muscle cramps [2–4].

Carnitine supplementation for the treatment of dialysis-related carnitine deficiency can be performed orally or intravenously. Multiple investigations have evaluated the benefits of carnitine supplementation in patients on dialysis. Intravenously administered levocarnitine has a bioavailability of 100%. When a dose of 1–2 g levocarnitine is intravenously administered to healthy individuals, the serum carnitine levels rapidly increase to 10 times that of the threshold for renal tubular reabsorption; 70–90% is consequently excreted in an unchanged form in the urine 12–24 h after administration. Therefore, a single dose of levocarnitine does not persist in the system for a sufficient length of time for any significant amount to equilibrate into the skeletal and cardiac muscle. However, for hemodialysis patients, an intravenous dose of levocarnitine remains in the blood for a long enough time for it to be taken up into the organs or tissue compartments, with up to about 90% of the administered levocarnitine possibly moved into tissues [4]. Chronic intravenous levocarnitine administration elevates muscle carnitine levels by between 60% and 200% [47–50].

In contrast, the bioavailability of oral levocarnitine administration is low, even in healthy individuals. Only 15% of a standard 2-g dose is absorbed into the blood in healthy individuals and just 5% of an oral 6-g dose [51,52]. The bioavailability of oral levocarnitine in patients on dialysis has not yet been evaluated. The metabolism of dietary carnitine and choline produces trimethylamine N-oxide (TMAO), which directly induces atherosclerosis in rodents [53,54]. Intestinal bacteria metabolize carnitine and choline to trimethylamine, which is absorbed in the intestine. Trimethylamine is itself oxidized by hepatic flavin monooxygenase to make TMAO [55]. Under normal conditions, TMAO is rapidly removed from the circulation, largely via excretion in the urine [56,57]. Accordingly, circulating TMAO levels appear to be associated with coronary artery disease and may also be associated with mortality in patients on long-term hemodialysis [58,59]. However, no study has shown whether oral levocarnitine treatment or TMAO levels would accelerate atherosclerosis in hemodialysis patients. Thus, additional work is required to evaluate the superiority, efficacy, and safety of intravenous levocarnitine administration compared with oral administration because there is no evidence of associations between the increased levels of TMAO and atherosclerosis progression in dialysis patients.

The National Kidney Foundation has stated that the detection and diagnosis of dialysis-related carnitine deficiency, as well as the decision to treat chronic dialysis patients with levocarnitine, should be determined by clinical symptoms and signs [60]. Furthermore, proof of decreased serum-free carnitine levels or an increased acyl/free carnitine ratio is dispensable for the clinical diagnosis of dialysis-related carnitine deficiency. Serum-free carnitine levels are helpful to rule out dialysis-related carnitine deficiency. However, low concentrations of serum-free carnitine cannot be used as a predictive factor of a clinical response to levocarnitine treatment.

In addition, the National Kidney Foundation has declared that the administration of levocarnitine to dialysis patients should be considered for the following four clinical conditions [60]: (1) patients with anemia who are unable to maintain optimal hemoglobin or hematocrit levels with the use of ESA, despite adequate iron status, and with no other identifiable cause of anemia or a hypo-response to ESA; (2) patients with intradialytic hypotension and no other possible causes with repeated symptomatic intradialytic hypotensive events requiring treatment; (3) patients with cardiomyopathy who have heart failure symptoms such as New York Heart Association class III–IV or symptomatic cardiomyopathy with documented impaired left ventricular ejection fraction (LVEF) and a poor response to standard medical therapy; and (4) selected patients who have symptoms that diminish their quality of life, including skeletal muscle weakness and malaise.

6. Anemia

In patients with end-stage kidney disease, anemia is induced by decreased production of erythropoietin by the kidney or fibrosis of the bone marrow. Renal anemia is commonly treated with ESA in patients with impaired kidney function. Although renal anemia strongly influences prognosis, higher-dose ESA may increase the risk of cardiovascular events in the dialysis population [61,62]. Moreover, the dosage of ESAs to maintain target hemoglobin levels varies widely among patients on dialysis [63]. A lower hematocrit level has been associated with shorter survival [64]. However, a lower hematocrit level was not a significant predictor of mortality in multivariate analysis adjusted for age, serum albumin, and the presence of diabetes. ESA resistance, which is characterized by inflammation and malnutrition, may be a significant novel predictor of mortality [64]. Patients with target hematocrit levels (i.e., 33–36%) receiving a higher ESA dose exhibit a rate of mortality double that of patients with hematocrit levels in the same range but receiving a low ESA dose. Therefore, the use of ESAs should be minimized and ESA resistance is recognized as an important marker for improving survival in the dialysis population.

Levocarnitine administration is suggested as a potential additional therapy to ESA in the management of renal anemia. The Centers for Medicare and Medicaid Services allow intravenous levocarnitine administration to patients on hemodialysis who have ESA-resistant anemia and decreased serum carnitine levels [64]. Although the most common cause of hyporesponsiveness to ESAs is iron deficiency, carnitine deficiency is proposed to be one of the causes of ESA-resistant anemia in Japanese Society for Dialysis Therapy guidelines [65]. Serum carnitine levels have been reported to be lower in patients with severe anemia needing high-dose ESA than in patients with mild-to-moderate anemia or no anemia [66]. In patients with a lower serum carnitine level and need for higher-dose ESA, erythrocyte membranes develop osmotic fragility. This shortens the survival time of erythrocytes and lowers hematocrit levels [67–70]. However, erythrocyte stability is reported to be improved by levocarnitine therapy, and this treatment would be associated with improved survival of erythrocytes through the following mechanism: levocarnitine regulates the erythrocyte membrane lipid complex, modifies the fatty acid metabolism, enhances the Na-K pump activity of erythrocytes, reduces membrane rigidity, and decreases erythrocyte calcium levels [69,71–74].

A systematic review and recent meta-analysis found that levocarnitine treatment ameliorates renal anemia and decreases ESA requirements in hemodialysis patients [75,76]. The efficacy of levocarnitine for treating renal anemia in patients on dialysis has been investigated by multiple studies. This work is summarized in Table 1 [43,69–71,77–94]. The aim of these studies was to maintain hematocrit or hemoglobin levels in carnitine and control groups by significantly decreasing the dosage of ESA in carnitine patients. ESA resistance can be determined by measuring the erythropoietin resistance index (ERI), which is calculated as the ESA dose divided by the hemoglobin level and body weight of each patient. This index is useful for assessing the response of the body to levocarnitine. Any decrease in ESA dosage or increase in the hemoglobin level during the observation period would decrease this index. The ERI was reduced by levocarnitine treatment in several studies, suggesting that levocarnitine improves erythropoietin efficiency versus control groups. However, the CARNIDIAL trial found no improvement in the ERI with levocarnitine administration in patients with a shorter duration of hemodialysis (<6 months) and no documented carnitine deficiency. In addition, levocarnitine treatment increased calcium and phosphate levels and was not associated with parathyroid hormone or fibroblast growth factor 23 [94,95].

Further studies should be conducted to determine whether levocarnitine treatment is effective in all dialysis patients with renal anemia and whether it improves long-term outcomes. Moreover, its dose–response profile in renal anemia has not yet been investigated.

Table 1. Studies of the effects of levocarnitine on renal anemia in dialysis patients.

Ref	Study Design	Subjects	Dose and Route	Treatment Duration	Findings [a]
[77]	Two-way, parallel, double-blind	29 HD patients 29 HD patients	20 mg/kg per Dx, IV Placebo, IV	6 mo	↑ RBC survival T_0: 39.1 days; T_6: 42.7 days ($p = 0.058$) → RBC survival T_0: 40.2 days; T_6: 35.4 days (NS)
[78]	One-way, open-label	14 HD patients (ESA-resistant)	500 mg/day PO	3 mo	↑ Ht T_0: 24.0% ± 2.0%; T_3: 26.1% ± 2.0% ($p = 0.003$)
[71]	One-way, open-label	15 HD patients	30 mg/kg per Dx, IV	3 mo	↑ Ht T_0: 30.8% ± 1.9%; T_3: 34.2% ± 2.4% ($p < 0.0001$), ↓ Deformability of RBCs ($p < 0.004$)
[43]	One-way, open-label	12 PD patients	2 g/day PO	3 mo	↑ Ht T_0: 35.4% ± 3.3%; T_3: 38.1% ± 3.4% ($p < 0.03$), ↑ Hb T_0: 11.0 ± 1.1 g/dL; T3: 11.9 ± 1.0 g/dL ($p < 0.01$)
[79]	Two-way, parallel, double-blind Four-way, parallel, double-blind	28 HD patients 28 HD patients 32 HD patients 30 HD patients 32 HD patients 33 HD patients	20 mg/kg per Dx, IV Placebo 10 mg/kg per Dx, IV 20 mg/kg per Dx, IV 30 mg/kg per Dx, IV Placebo	6 mo 6 mo	→ Ht T_0: 34.1% ± 3.2%; T_6: 32.8% ± 4.0% (NS) → Ht T_0: 32.9% ± 3.3%; T_6: 33.9% ± 2.9% (NS) → Ht T_0: 33.9% ± 3.2%; T_6: 35.1% ± 4.2% (NS) → Ht T_0: 33.7% ± 3.5%; T_6: 33.9% ± 3.4% (NS) → Ht T_0: 33.6% ± 3.3%; T_6: 33.5% ± 2.7% (NS) → Ht T_0: 34.2% ± 3.2%; T_6: 35.1% ± 4.2% (NS)
[80]	Two-way, parallel, double-blind	48 HD patients 65 HD patients	20 mg/kg per Dx, IV Placebo, IV	6 mo	↑ Hb T_0: 9.7 ± 1.1 g/dL; T_6: 10.8 ± 1.2 g/dL ($p < 0.0001$) → Hb T_0: 9.8 ± 1.2 g/dL; T_6: 9.9 ± 1.3 g/dL (NS)
[81]	Two-way, parallel, open label	78 HD patients 78 HD patients	1 g/Dx, IV No treatment	7 mo	↑ Hb T_0: 7.5 ± 1.5 g/dL; T_7: 11.4 ± 1.2 g/dL ($p < 0.05$) ↓ ERI T_0: 183 ± 16 U/kg; T_7: 142 ± 12 U/kg ($p < 0.05$) → Hb T_0: 7.5 ± 1.4 g/dL; T_7: 9.2 ± 1.2 g/dL (NS) → ERI T_0: 185 ± 15 U/kg; T_7: 160 ± 12 U/kg (NS)
[82]	Two-way, parallel, double-blind	18 HD patients 13 HD patients	15 mg/kg per Dx, IV Placebo, IV	6 mo	↑ Ht T_0: 24.2% ± 2.2%; T_6: 32.5% ± 3.7% ($p = 0.001$) ↑ Hb T_0: 7.9 ± 0.8 g/dL; T_6: 10.3 ± 1.1 g/dL ($p = 0.001$) → Ht T_0: 27.5% ± 4.5%; T_6: 30.2% ± 4.0% ($p = 0.1$) → Hb T_0: 8.0 ± 0.4 g/dL; T_6: 8.7 ± 2.5 g/dL ($p = 0.4$)
[83]	Two-way, parallel, single-blind	10 HD patients 10 HD patients	20 mg/kg per Dx, IV Plaxevo, IV	2 mo	↑ Hb +0.89 ± 0.56 g/dL vs. −0.47 ± 0.77 g/dL ($p = 0.001$)
[84]	Double-blind, crossover, placebo-controlled	16 HD patients	20 mg/kg per Dx, IV Placebo, IV	3 mo	→ ESA doses T_0: 8562 ± 6762 U; T_3: 8750 ± 7094 U (NS) → Hb T_0: 11.3 ± 1.9 g/dL T3: 11.5 ± 1.5 g/dL (NS)
[85]	Two-way, parallel, open-label	20 HD patients 20 HD patients	1 g per Dx, twice a week, IV No treatment	6 mo	↑ Hb T_0: 6.8 ± 1.0 g/dL; T_6: 7.7 ± 1.1 g/dL ($p < 0.001$) ↓ ERI values not reported ($p < 0.001$) → Hb T_0: 6.7 ± 1.0 g/dL; T_6: 6.9 ± 1.0 g/dL (NS), → ERI (NS)
[86]	Two-way, parallel, open-label	20 HD patients 20 HD patients	1 g/Dx, IV No treatment	3 mo	↑ Hb T_0: 7.8 ± 1.3 g/dL; T_3: 9.9 ± 1.9 g/dL ($p < 0.05$) → Hb T_0: 7.8 ± 1.1 g/dL; T_{12}: 8.5 ± 1.2 g/dL (NS)
[87]	One-way, open-label	62 HD patients 18 PD patients	600 mg/day, PO for 12 mo, then 1 g/Dx IV for 12 mo 600 mg/day, PO	24 mo 12 mo	↑ Hb T_0: 10.2 ± 1.2 g/dL; T_{12}: 10.9 ± 0.9 g/dL → Hb T_0: 10.6 ± 1.1 g/dL; T_{12}: 10.6 ± 1.3 g/dL
[88]	Two-way, parallel, double-blind	24 HD patients 27 HD patients	1 g/day, PO Placebo, PO	4 mo	→ Hb T_0: 10.5 ± 2.5 g/dL; T_4: 11.3 ± 2.1 g/dL (NS) ↓ ESA doses T_0: 7250 ± 5202 U/week; T_4: 2500 ± 4180 U/week ($p < 0.001$) → Hb T_0: 9.5 ± 2.2 g/dL; T_4: 9.9 ± 2.5 g/dL (NS) ↓ ESA doses T_0: 8000 ± 3186 U/week; T_4: 6000 ± 5083 U/week ($p = 0.033$)
[89]	Two-way, parallel, open-label	25 HD patients 35 HD patients	1 g/Dx, IV and 1 g/non-Dx, PO No treatment	36 mo	↓ ESA doses T_0: 5976 ± 1732 U/week; T_{36}: 3391 ± 659 U/week ($p < 0.001$) → ESA doses T_0: 6100 ± 1587 U/week; T_{36}: 5519 ± 1360 U/week (NS)
[90]	Two-way, parallel, double-blind	13 HD patients 13 HD patients	20 mg/kg per Dx, IV Placebo, PIV	4 mo	→ ESA doses T_4: −769 ± 1739 U/week (NS), → Hb T_4: −0.08 ± 0.90 g/dL (NS) → ESA doses T_4: +153 ± 177 U/week (NS), → Hb T_4: −0.26 ± 0.56 g/dL (NS)
[91]	Two-way, parallel, open-label	23 HD patients 22 HD patients	15 mg/kg per Dx, IV No treatment	6 mo	→ ESA doses, → Ht (NS)

Table 1. Cont.

Ref	Study Design	Subjects	Dose and Route	Treatment Duration	Findings [a]
[92]	Two-way, parallel, double-blind	13 HD patients	1 g/Dx, IV	6 mo	↓ ERI T_0: 102 ± 53 U/kg/week; T_6: 63 ± 38 U/kg/week ($p < 0.02$)
		11 HD patients	Placebo, IV		→ ERI T_0: 79 ± 32 U/kg/week; T_6: 80 ± 47 U/kg/week (NS)
[70]	Two-way, parallel, double-blind	10 HD patients	1 g/Dx, IV	6 mo	↓ ERI T_0: 135 ± 79; T_6: 118 ± 108 U/kg per week per %Ht ($p < 0.05$)
		11 HD patients	Placebo, IV		↑ ERI T_0: 136 ± 66; T_6: 217 ± 204 U/kg per week per %Ht ($p < 0.05$)
[69]	Two-way, parallel, double-blind	20 HD patients	5 mg/kg or 25 mg/kg per Dx, IV	4 mo	↓ ERI T_0: 16.0 ± 11.0; T_4: 13.6 ± 10.5 U/kg per week per gHb ($p < 0.02$)
		20 HD patients	Placebo, IV		Values not reported
[96]	Two-way, parallel, double-blind	13 HD patients	20 mg/kg per Dx, IV	6 mo	↓ ERI -1.62 ± 0.91 vs. +1.33 ± 0.79 U/kg per gHb ($p < 0.05$)
		14 HD patients	Placebo, IV		
[93]	Two-way, parallel, open-label	30 HD patients	1 g/Dx, IV	12 mo	↓ ERI T_0: 10.7 ± 7.3; T_{12}: 6.4 ± 3.8 U/kg per gHb per week ($p < 0.0001$)
		30 HD patients	No treatment		→ ERI T_0: 10.0 ± 7.9; T_{12}: 9.6 ± 6.5 U/kg per gHb per week (NS)
[94]	Two-way, parallel, double-blind	46 HD patients	1 g/Dx, IV	12 mo	→ ERI T_0: 20.6 ± 12.8; T_{12}: 15.6 ± 15.9 IU/kg per gHb ($p = 0.10$)
		46 HD patients	Placebo, IV		→ ERI T_0: 15.8 ± 11.3; T_{12}: 9.5 ± 5.8 IU/kg per gHb ($p = 0.10$)

Dx, dialysis session; HD, hemodialysis; ERI, erythropoietin resistance index; ESA, erythropoiesis-stimulating agent; Hb, hemoglobin; Ht, hematocrit; IV, intravenous injection; mo, months; NS, not significant; PO, per oral; RBC, red blood cell; Ref, reference. [a] The findings show no difference (→), a decrease (↓), or an increase (↑).

7. Cardiac Function

Cardiovascular disease is a leading cause of mortality in dialysis patients [93]. Approximately 75% of end-stage kidney disease patients commencing hemodialysis treatment experience left ventricular dysfunction, represented by reduced LVEF, which is a significant risk factor for congestive heart failure [97]. Furthermore, intradialytic hypotension has been linked to mortality and is an independent predictor of mortality in this population [97–99].

The main energy source for cardiac myocytes is β-oxidation of fatty acids. Carnitine concentrations in myocytes are some of the highest of all cell types. Furthermore, the production of intracellular acylcarnitine and lactate is induced by myocardial ischemia. Thus, levocarnitine treatment might be useful for cardiac symptoms. Numerous investigations have reported the efficacy of levocarnitine treatment in terms of cardiac function; these are summarized in Table 2 [49,50,89,100–108].

The relationship between hypotensive episodes and levocarnitine treatment has also been investigated in dialysis patients. Patients who experience hypotension during hemodialysis treatment have lower serum carnitine levels than normotensive individuals [109]. Levocarnitine treatment significantly reduces intradialytic hypotension versus placebo [49,110]. Accordingly, intravenous levocarnitine supplementation is allowed for the management of dialysis-related hypotension in hemodialysis patients who have lower serum carnitine levels by the Centers for Medicare and Medicaid Services.

A strong correlation has been found between LVEF and serum carnitine levels in patients on dialysis. In addition, 3-month administration of levocarnitine improves LVEF, significantly so in patients with repeated hypotensive events [111]. It was suggested that patients experiencing symptomatic hypotension had a significantly lower LVEF and a higher mortality risk compared with asymptomatic patients [110]. Other studies have obtained similar results [89,103,112]. Mounting evidence favors a role for levocarnitine in the management of cardiac dysfunction. On the other hand, other studies have reported the ineffectiveness of levocarnitine treatment [50,104]; however, these findings must be interpreted with caution, because these studies included patients with normal LVEF. In our previous reports, atherosclerosis assessed by brachial-ankle pulse wave velocity and cardiac function assessed by LVEF and left ventricular mass index (LVMI) were improved by levocarnitine treatment in patients on hemodialysis [107,113]. Levocarnitine administration decreased N-terminal pro-brain natriuretic peptide (NT-proBNP) levels and ameliorated the ERI. Furthermore, the responders to levocarnitine treatment were patients with left ventricular hypertrophy, as defined by the LVMI on echocardiography. These results suggest that levocarnitine treatment might be effective for patients with a larger baseline LVMI [107]. Therefore, these results indicate that levocarnitine treatment is beneficial for patients with left ventricular hypertrophy, reduced LVEF, or dialysis-related hypotension.

Table 2. Studies of the effect of levocarnitine on cardiac function and hypotension in dialysis patients.

Ref	Study Design	Population	Dose and Route	Treatment Duration	Findings [a]
[101]	Two-way, crossover, double-blind	9 HD patients 9 HD patients	990 mg/day PO then placebo for 2 mo each Placebo then 990 mg/day PO for 2 mo each	2 mo	↓ Hypotension ($p < 0.001$) → Hypotension (NS)
[50]	Two-way, parallel, double-blind	14 HD patients 14 HD patients	2 g/Dx, IV Placebo	6 weeks	No difference in cardiac function (NS)
[49]	Two-way, parallel, double-blind	38 HD patients 44 HD patients	20 mg/kg per Dx, IV Placebo	6 mo	↓ Hypotension ($p < 0.02$) → Hypotension (NS)
[102]	One-way, open-label	13 HD patients	1 g/Dx, IV	3 mo	↑ LVEF T_0: 42.4 ± 19.4%; T_3: 48.6 ± 17.6% ($p < 0.05$)
[89]	Two-way, parallel, open-label	25 HD patients 35 HD patients	1 g/Dx, IV and 1 g/non-Dx PO No treatment	36 mo	↑ LVEF ($p < 0.05$) ↓ LV end-diastolic volume ($p < 0.05$)
[103]	One-way, open-label	11 HD patients	1 g/day PO then 0.5 g/day PO for 1 mo each	2 mo	→ LVEDD, LVFS (NS) ↑ Cardiac scintigraphy ($p < 0.001$)
[104]	One-way, open-label	9 HD patients (impaired LVEF)	500 mg/day, PO	6 mo	↑ LVEF T_0: 44.9% ± 12.2%; T_6: 53.8% ± 13.8% ($p = 0.005$) ↓ CTR T_0: 56.4 ± 5.4; T_6: 53.8 ± 4.0 ($p = 0.042$)
[100]	One-way, open-label	11 HD patients (impaired LVEF)	1 g/Dx, IV	8 mo	↑ LVEF T_0: 32.0% T_8: 41.8% ($p < 0.05$)
[105]	Two-way, parallel, open-label	10 HD patients 10 HD patients	10 mg/kg/day, PO No treatment	12 mo	↓ LVMI T_0: 151.8 ± 21.2; T_{12}: 134 ± 16 g/m² ($p < 0.01$) → LVMI T_0: 153.3 ± 28.2; T_{12}: 167.1 ± 43.1 g/m² (NS)
[106]	Two-way, parallel, double-blind	20 HD patients 35 HD patients	1500 mg/day, PO No treatment	6 mo	No difference in cardiac function ($p = 0.67$) Cardiac function was not investigated.
[107]	Two-way, parallel, double-blind	10 HD patients 8 HD patients	900 mg/day, PO Placebo	3 mo	↑ LVEF T_0: 61.8% ± 16.0%; T_3: 64.4% ± 13.8% ($p < 0.05$) ↓ Hypotension T_0: 4.0 ± 1.7; T_3: 1.3 ± 0.9 times/mo ($p < 0.05$) → LVEF (NS)
[108]	Two-way, parallel, open-label	75 HD patients 73 HD patients	20 mg/kg/day, PO No treatment	12 mo	↑ LVEF T_0: 53.1% ± 5.3% T_{12}: 58.6% ± 5.5% ($p < 0.001$) ↓ LVMI T_0: 112 ± 26; T_{12}: 107 ± 24 g/m² ($p < 0.001$) → LVEF, LVMI (NS)
[109]	Two-way, parallel, double-blind	18 HD patients 15 HD patients	30 mg/kg/before Dx, IV Placebo, IV	3 mo	↓ Hypotension 9.3% vs. 33.1% ($p < 0.0001$)

CTR, cardiothoracic ratio; Dx, dialysis session; HD, hemodialysis; IV, intravenous injection; LVEDD, left ventricular end-diastolic dimension; LVFS, left ventricular fractional shortening; LVEF, left ventricular ejection fraction; LVMI, left ventricular mass index; mo, months; NS, not significant; PO, per oral; Ref, reference. [a] The findings show no difference (→), a decrease (↓), or an increase (↑).

Myocardial fatty acid metabolism, as assessed by 123-I–labeled β-methyl-p-iodophenyl-pentadecanoic acid (BMIPP), has been reported to be reduced in patients on long-term hemodialysis and recovered by levocarnitine therapy [102]. Tetradecyl glycidic acid (TDGA) impairs mitochondrial carnitine acyltransferase 1, and its administration induces left ventricular hypertrophy with enhanced lipid accumulation in the rat heart [111]. BMIPP washout from the myocardium is also decreased after TDGA administration [114]. Therefore, carnitine deficiency interrupts fatty acid metabolism in the myocardium and leads to myocardial lipid storage in patients on hemodialysis. A decreased free carnitine concentration results in disrupted fatty acid transfer into mitochondria; subsequently, the accumulation of acylcarnitine in the mitochondria disrupts carnitine-related enzymes involved in ATP production and transportation. Accordingly, levocarnitine treatment-induced amelioration of myocardial fatty acid metabolism and the acyl/free carnitine ratio might help to improve LVEF and decrease the LVMI.

Although levocarnitine treatment may be beneficial in improving LVEF, it is important to determine whether the treatment reduces cardiac events, hospitalizations, and mortality. To clarify the association between levocarnitine treatment and the hospitalization rate and number of hospital days, a large cohort study was conducted in patients on hemodialysis [115]. This study enrolled 2967 patients who were treated with levocarnitine for at least 3 months and had a 3-month or longer pre-levocarnitine period. The adjusted relative risk of hospitalization significantly decreased during the levocarnitine treatment compared with the rate before the initiation of levocarnitine treatment. Compared with the baseline hospitalization rate before levocarnitine treatment initiation, levocarnitine decreased the hospitalization rate by 34% and 58% at 6–9 months and 15–18 months, respectively. Furthermore, patients with cardiovascular disease, anemia, and hypoalbuminemia prior to levocarnitine treatment benefited most from levocarnitine treatment, in whom it was associated with fewer hospitalizations [115].

Uremia alters both carnitine and fatty acid metabolism. The combination of uremia-induced left ventricular hypertrophy and carnitine deficiency impairs myocardial metabolism and cardiac function. Levocarnitine treatment might partly improve the uremic hypertrophy, besides augmenting the metabolism. Additional large-scale clinical studies must be performed to clarify whether levocarnitine treatment ameliorates cardiovascular mortality in patients on dialysis.

8. Muscle Symptoms and Quality of Life

Sarcopenia and muscle weakness are frequent in patients with chronic kidney disease. Sarcopenia is caused by the aggravation of some physiological systems and is associated with aging. Decreased muscle strength and skeletal muscle mass are related to physical function [116,117]. In the general population, sarcopenia has been linked to adverse clinical outcomes, such as mortality, disability, hospitalization, falls, decreased quality of life, and need for long-term care [116,117]. Sarcopenia has also been associated with negative outcomes in patients with end-stage kidney disease or on dialysis [118–121]. Generally, physical activity falls with age in not only the general population, but also among patients with chronic kidney disease [122]. Patients on dialysis with decreased physical function have been found to have higher mortality than those with better physical function [123]. Although the clinical importance of sarcopenia is recognized, there are no clear intervention methods for the dialysis population. The pathophysiology of this syndrome is believed to be associated with amino acid deficiency, including that of carnitine.

In addition to sarcopenia, both inflammation and PEW are significant predictors of mortality in patients receiving dialysis therapy [22–24]. A recent meta-analysis reported a 28–50% prevalence of PEW or frailty in patients receiving dialysis [124]. Another report revealed that 30% of dialysis patients had mild or moderate malnutrition and that 6–8% of patients had severe malnutrition [125–127]. Although three pathophysiologies—sarcopenia, frailty, and PEW—are distinguished, they share some components that are associated with hospitalization and mortality. In particular, malnutrition and chronic inflammation complicated with sarcopenia are important predictors of clinical outcomes in patients on hemodialysis [128,129]. In addition, elevated proinflammatory cytokine levels stimulate protein catabolism through the ubiquitin–proteasome pathway, leading to muscle weakness or wasting [130]. The production of inflammatory cytokines, such as interleukin (IL)-1, IL-6, and tumor necrosis factor (TNF)-α, can be decreased by levocarnitine treatment [131–133].

Levocarnitine corrects insufficient energy supplies at the cellular level, alleviates long-chain fatty acid transport into mitochondria, and accelerates the removal of short- and medium-chain fatty acids stored during metabolism. Therefore, levocarnitine treatment may have beneficial effects on muscle wasting because fatty acid is the main source of energy in skeletal muscle [134]. Levocarnitine may increase the β-oxidation rate of fatty acids and maintain glycogen stores in skeletal muscle, thereby boosting ATP production [135]. Skeletal muscle function may be improved or maintained via levocarnitine-mediated augmentation of energy metabolism. Levocarnitine supplementation improves not only physical function but also mental and cognitive function in elderly individuals with normal kidney function [136,137]. Although levocarnitine supplementation fails to increase arm and leg muscle strength, it does increase the lean muscle mass of the arm and leg in elderly individuals with normal kidney function [138].

In Japan, patients receiving hemodialysis who had muscular symptoms such as cramps and asthenia have been found to have significantly lower endogenous serum carnitine levels compared with non-symptomatic patients [139]. Thirty patients on hemodialysis with muscular weakness, fatigue, or cramps were treated with levocarnitine for 12 weeks. Some muscle symptoms were improved in approximately 70% of the patients [139]. Fourteen patients on hemodialysis were treated with levocarnitine in a double-blind crossover manner to investigate carnitine levels in muscle and serum before and after 2 months of levocarnitine treatment. Although levocarnitine treatment ameliorated symptoms such as asthenia and cramps occurring during hemodialysis, these symptoms worsened during the washout period (i.e., after levocarnitine treatment was ceased) [140]. In addition, to evaluate the efficacy of levocarnitine for muscle function, a two-way parallel controlled trial was conducted for 6 months [141]. Muscle strength was significantly improved in four of the seven patients in the levocarnitine group at the study end, whereas none of the seven controls showed a significant improvement. Thereafter, all 14 patients were treated with levocarnitine for 10 months, with muscle strength increased in nine of the 14 patients. We previously conducted a randomized control trial of 91 hemodialysis patients who had lower serum carnitine levels [142]. The participants were randomly assigned to receive intravenous levocarnitine treatment (levocarnitine group) or no treatment (control group) for 12 months. Clinical dry weight, body mass index, and serum albumin levels fell significantly in the control group. However, there were no such results in the levocarnitine group. In addition, there were significant differences in the percent changes in arm muscle area, hand grip strength, and lean body mass after 12 months between the two groups [142]. Levocarnitine treatment was beneficial in patients on dialysis, particularly in elderly patients or those with diabetes, because it was able to maintain lean body mass and muscle function.

In addition to muscle and dialytic symptoms in patients on dialysis, a significant association has been reported between the acyl/free carnitine ratio and the physical component of the 36-Item Short Form Survey (SF-36) in men. Moreover, levocarnitine treatment improves SF-36 scores compared with baseline [68]. Furthermore, to evaluate health-related quality of life from the perspective of patients on dialysis, the SF-36 score was measured. Symptoms during hemodialysis were evaluated at each dialysis session using additional questionnaires. Six months of oral levocarnitine therapy boosted general health and physical function [143]. The efficacy of levocarnitine treatment for dialysis patients in terms of muscle symptoms, physical activities, and quality of life is summarized in Table 3 [49,50,83,84,87,100,139–147].

A meta-analysis failed to identify the clinical significance of levocarnitine treatment of intradialytic hypotension and muscle function [148]. However, some major limitations were noted, such as the small number of patients in many of the studies and a low associated statistical power. Furthermore, the definitions of dialysis-related hypotension and muscle cramps were not unified. To confirm the clinical efficacy of levocarnitine treatment of intradialytic hypotension and muscle cramps, additional adequately sized randomized clinical studies are required in this population.

Table 3. Studies of the effect of levocarnitine on muscle symptoms and quality of life in dialysis patients.

Ref	Study Design	Subjects	Dose and Route	Treatment Duration	Findings [a]
[101]	Double-blind, cross-over, placebo-controlled	18 HD patients	990 mg/day, PO Placebo, PO	2 mo	↓ Cramps ($p < 0.001$), ↓ Asthenia ($p < 0.001$), ↓ Dyspnea ($p < 0.001$)
[140]	Double-blind, cross-over, placebo-controlled	14 HD patients	2 g/day, PO Placebo, PO	2 mo	↑ Exercise time ($p = 0.01$), ↓ Asthenia ($p = 0.01$), ↓ Muscle cramps ($p = 0.01$)
[50]	Two-way, parallel, double-blind	14 HD patients 14 HD patients	2 g/Dx, IV Placebo, IV	1.5 mo	No difference in muscular status (NS)
[144]	One-way, open-label	6 HD patients	2 g/day, PO	1.5 mo	No difference in muscular function (NS)
[49]	Two-way, parallel, double-blind	38 HD patients 44 HD patients	20 mg/kg per Dx, IV	6 mo	↓ Cramps ($p = 0.02$), ↓ Asthenia postdialysis ($p = 0.04$), ↑ O$_2$ consumption ($p = 0.03$)
[145]	One-way, open-label	26 HD patients	2 g/dialysate ($n = 11$), 2 g/day PO ($n = 6$), 2 g/Dx IV ($n = 9$)	6 mo	↓ Cramps ($p = 0.04$), ↓ Pain ($p = 0.04$), ↑ Isometric force ($p = 0.001$)

Table 3. Cont.

Ref	Study Design	Subjects	Dose and Route	Treatment Duration	Findings [a]
[146]	One-way, open-label	6 HD patients	2 g/day, PO	2 mo	↓ Cramps ($p = 0.01$), ↓ Weakness ($p = 0.001$), ↓ Fatigue ($p = 0.05$)
[139]	Two-way, parallel, open-label	30 HD patients 21 HD patients	500 mg/day, PO No treatment	3 mo	↓ Weakness ($p < 0.005$), ↓ Fatigue ($p < 0.005$), ↓ Cramps/aches ($p < 0.05$)
[147]	Two-way, parallel, double-blind	9 HD patients 8 HD patients	10 mg/kg per Dx, IV Placebo, IV	4 mo	No difference in muscle cramps, uremic pruritus, physical strength, and general well-being
[143]	Two-way, parallel, double-blind	101 HD patients	1 g/day, PO Placebo, PO	6 mo	1.5 mo, ↑ QOL ($p = 0.02$); 3 mo, ↑ QOL ($p = 0.015$); >4.5 mo, ↓ QOL ($p = 0.013$)
[141]	Two-way, parallel, double-blind	7 HD patients	2 g/Dx, IV for 6 mo, then 1 g/Dx, IV for 10 mo	16 mo	→ Daily activity score T_0: 3.5; T_6: 2.0 (NS)
		7 HD patients	No treatment for 6 mo, then 1 g/Dx, IV for 10 mo		→ Daily activity score T_0: 3.4; T_6: 3.1 (NS)
[84]	Double-blind, cross-over, placebo-controlled	16 HD patients	20 mg/kg per Dx, IV Placebo, IV	3 mo	No changes in muscle parameters and QOL scores
[96]	Two-way, parallel, double-blind	13 HD patients 14 HD patients	20 mg/kg per Dx, IV Placebo, IV	6 mo	↑ SF-36 scores T_0: 33.9 ± 1.9; T_6: 43.2 ± 3.0 ($p < 0.05$) → SF-36 scores T_0: 40.6 ± 2.6; T_6: 40.1 ± 3.0 (NS)
[83]	Two-way, parallel, single-blind	10 HD patients 10 HD patients	20 mg/kg per Dx, IV Placebo, IV	2 mo	↑ SF-36 scores T2: +18.3 ± 12.7 vs. −6.4 ± 16.4 ($p = 0.001$)
[142]	Two-way, parallel, open-label	42 HD patients 42 HD patients	1 g/Dx, IV No treatment	12 mo	↑ AMA: +2.11% vs. −4.11% ($p < 0.01$); ↑ LBM 0.70% vs. −2.22% ($p < 0.001$); ↑ HGS: +1.58% vs. −2.69% ($p < 0.05$)
[87]	One-way, open-label	62 HD patients	600 mg/day, PO for 12 mo, then 1 g/Dx IV for 12 mo	24 mo	↓ Muscle spasms in patients who had undergone HD for >4 years (p-value not reported)
		18 PD patients	600 mg/day, PO	12 mo	

AMA, arm muscle area; Dx, dialysis session; HD, hemodialysis; HGS, hand grip strength; LBM, lean body mass; IV, intravenous injection; mo, months; NS, not significant; PD, peritoneal dialysis; PO, per oral; QOL, quality of life; Ref, reference; SF-36, 36-Item Short Form Survey.
[a] The findings showed no difference (→), or decrease (↓) or increase (↑).

9. Plasma Lipid Profiles and Inflammation-Related Parameters

Patients on dialysis exhibit a higher risk of atherosclerotic cardiovascular disease. Observational studies of dialysis patients have revealed a close relationship of dyslipidemia (e.g., elevated low-density lipoprotein (LDL) cholesterol, low high-density lipoprotein (HDL) cholesterol, elevated triglyceride, and/or elevated non-HDL cholesterol) with both atherosclerosis severity and risk of coronary artery disease [149,150]. Furthermore, dyslipidemia has a closer association with ischemic heart disease than with cerebrovascular disease. Several factors, including decreased activities of lipoprotein lipase and lecithin cholesterol acyltransferase (LCAT) and decreased hepatic lipase levels, promote dyslipidemia development in chronic kidney disease patients. The 2003 guidelines of the National Kidney Foundation's Kidney Disease Outcomes Quality Initiative recommended a triglyceride level < 500 mg/dL in a fasting blood sample, an LDL cholesterol level < 100 mg/dL, and a non-HDL cholesterol level < 130 mg/dL [151].

Levocarnitine treatment may be beneficial for dyslipidemia in dialysis patients because carnitine increases the transport of free fatty acids into mitochondria and decreases the availability of free fatty acids for triglyceride synthesis. Decreased carnitine levels may be a possible contributing factor to hyperlipidemia in the dialysis population. In addition, carnitine treatment may improve dyslipidemia because carnitine stimulates the β-oxidation of long-chain fatty acids and decreases the ester bound to glycerol, even in dialysis patients [100].

Inflammation is highly prevalent in patients on hemodialysis, and elevated C-reactive protein is a predictor of all-cause and cardiovascular mortality in this population [152–156]. Inflammation can induce hepcidin overexpression and thus cause or aggravate absolute iron deficiency by inhibiting iron enteral absorption and functional iron deficiency through decreased release of stored iron from the liver and reticuloendothelial system [157]. The antioxidant and anti-inflammatory effects of levocarnitine have been described in vitro and in vivo [158,159]. Levocarnitine has also been shown to impact insulin sensitivity and protein catabolism; it has been proposed that increased levocarnitine is likely to improve nutritional status by reducing insulin resistance [160]. In one study, when patients were divided into two groups according to albumin level (<3.5 g/dL or ≥3.5 g/dL) before levocarnitine treatment, the higher albumin group displayed a significant increase in the prealbumin level and an improved malnutrition–inflammation score (MIS) [161]. Some clinical trials have indicated that levocarnitine supplementation can improve nutritional status in hemodialysis patients. It has been reported that oral levocarnitine supplementation tended to lower graft loss within 3 months after kidney transplantation, which might be related to the antioxidant effects of carnitine [162]. Several studies have examined the effects of levocarnitine treatment on plasma lipid levels and inflammation-related parameters in patients on maintenance dialysis. These studies are listed in Table 4 [48,80,85,86,88,90,92,131–133,161,163–173].

Multiple studies have shown that levocarnitine treatment has beneficial effects on dyslipidemia. Nonetheless, conflicting results were reported in some studies. A meta-analysis failed to identify beneficial effects of levocarnitine treatment on dyslipidemia in patients on dialysis [75,174]. However, another meta-analysis reported that levocarnitine administration decreased LDL-cholesterol levels in a subgroup of patients intravenously administered levocarnitine and with a longer interventional duration, whereas it was not associated with a reduction in total cholesterol and triglycerides levels or an increase in HDL-cholesterol levels [175]. Furthermore, meta-analyses demonstrated that levocarnitine administration decreased serum C-reactive protein levels in both statistically significant and clinically relevant manners [176] and that it increased total protein, albumin, transferrin, and prealbumin levels [177]. However, there were several limitations in previous studies, including differences among studies in plasma lipid levels and serum carnitine levels, levocarnitine dosage, administration methods, and study durations. Furthermore, research is required into specific dialysis populations with dyslipidemia, such as patients with low HDL cholesterol or high triglyceride levels.

Table 4. Studies of the effect of levocarnitine on lipid profiles and inflammatory-related parameters in dialysis patients.

Ref	Study Design	Subjects	Dose and Route	Treatment Duration	Findings [a]
[163]	Two-way, parallel, open-label	8 HD patients	0.5 g/Dx IV for 2 mo, then 1.0 g/Dx IV for 1.5 mo	3.5 mo	↓ TG T_0: 336 ± 56 mg/dL; $T_{3.5}$: 244 ± 82 mg/dL ($p < 0.05$)
		8 HD patients	Placebo, IV	3.5 mo	→ TG T_0: 329 ± 72 mg/dL; $T_{3.5}$: 444 ± 82 mg/dL (NS)
[164]	Two-way, parallel, open-label	11 HD patients	1 g/Dx, IV for 1 mo then 2 g/Dx dialysate for 3 mo	4 mo	↓ TG, ↑ HDL (p-values not reported)
		11 HD patients	1 g/Dx, IV for 1 mo then 4 g/Dx dialysate for 3 mo		
[165]	Two-way, crossover, double-blind	9 HD patients	1 g t.i.d. PO then placebo for 5 wk each	5 wk	No difference in plasma lipid levels (NS)
		9 HD patients	Placebo then 1 g t.i.d. PO for 5 wk each	5 wk	
[48]	Two-way, parallel, double-blind	38 HD patients	20 mg/kg per Dx, IV	6 mo	No difference in plasma lipid levels (NS)
		44 HD patients	Placebo, IV	6 mo	
[166]	Two-way, parallel, double-blind	15 HD patients	1–1.5 g/Dx, IV	2 mo	No difference in plasma lipid levels (NS)
		15 HD patients	Placebo	2 mo	
[167]	Two-way, parallel, double-blind	11 HD patients	100 μmol/L dialysate	6 mo	No difference in plasma lipid levels (NS)
		10 HD patients	Placebo	6 mo	
[168]	Two-way, parallel, open-label	6 HD patients	900 mg t.i.d. PO	1 mo	↑ TG T_0: 180 ± 66 mg%; T_1: 219 ± 88 mg% ($p < 0.05$)
		4 HD patients	Placebo	1 mo	→ TG T_0: 222 ± 35 mg%; T_1: 222 ± 35 mg% (NS)
[131]	Two-way, parallel, open-label	21 HD patients	20 mg/kg per Dx, IV	6 mo	↓ TG T_0: 1.6 ± 0.6; T_6: 1.5 ±0.7 mmol/L ($p = 0.001$), ↑ TP T_0: 6.4 ± 0.5; T_6: 6.9 ± 0.5 g/dL ($p < 0.001$), ↑ Alb T_0: 3.6 ± 0.3; T_6: 4.1 ± 0.3 g/dL ($p < 0.001$), ↑ Tf T_0: 1.2 ± 0.2; T_6: 1.6 ± 0.4 g/L ($p < 0.001$), ↑ BMI T_0: 23.4 ± 4.0; T_6: 23.7 ± 4.0 ($p < 0.001$)
		21 HD patients	No treatment		→ TG, TP, Alb, Tf, BMI (NS)
[132]	Two-way, parallel, double-blind	20 HD patients	1 g/Dx, IV	6 mo	↓ CRP: T_0: 2.1 ± 0.6 mg/dL; T_6: 0.67 ± 0.1 mg/dL ($p = 0.02$), → TC, HDL, LDL, TG (NS)
		15 HD patients	No treatment		→ CRP, TC, HDL, LDL, TG (NS)
[88]	Two-way, parallel, double-blind	24 HD patients	1 g/day, PO	4 mo	↓ TG T_0: 166 ± 71 mg/dL; T_4: 138 ± 54 mg/dL ($p = 0.001$), ↑ HDL T_0: 30 ± 7 mg/dL; T_4: 34 ± 7 mg/dL ($p < 0.001$)
		27 HD patients	Placebo, PO		↑ TG T_0: 142 ± 58 mg/dL; T_4: 151 ± 48 mg/dL ($p = 0.029$), → HDL
[92]	Two-way, parallel, double-blind	13 HD patients	1 g/Dx, IV	6 mo	→ TC, HDL, TG (NS)
		11 HD patients	Placebo, IV		→ TC, HDL, TG (NS)

Table 4. Cont.

Ref	Study Design	Subjects	Dose and Route	Treatment Duration	Findings [a]
[90]	Two-way, parallel, double-blind	13 HD patients 13 HD patients	20 mg/kg per Dx, IV Placebo, PIV	4 mo	→ TC, TG (NS) → TC, TG (NS)
[169]	Two-way, parallel, double-blind	32 HD patients 32 HD patients	600 mg/Dx, IV Placebo, IV	12 mo	↓ MDA T_0: 2.2 ± 0.7 µmol/mL; T_3: 1.5 ± 0.7 µmol/mL ($p < 0.001$) ↑ ABI T_0: 0.71 ± 0.06; T_3: 0.78 ± 0.08 ($p < 0.001$) ↑ MDA T_0: 1.94 ± 0.5 µmol/mL; T_3: 1.9 ± 0.7 µmol/mL ($p < 0.01$) ↓ ABI T_0: 0.75 ± 0.08; T_3: 0.72 ± 0.01 ($p < 0.001$)
[85]	Two-way, parallel, open-label	20 HD patients 20 HD patients	1 g/Dx, twice a week, IV No treatment	6 mo	↓ TC ($p < 0.001$), ↑ HDL ($p < 0.001$), ↓ TG ($p < 0.001$) ↑ TC ($p < 0.001$), ↓ HDL ($p < 0.01$), → TG (NS)
[86]	Two-way, parallel, open-label	20 HD patients 20 HD patients	1 g/Dx, IV No treatment	3 mo	↓ TG T_0: 190 ± 69 mg/dL; T_3: 179 ± 51 mg/dL ($p < 0.05$) ↓ LDL 119± 21 mg/dL; T_3: 98 ± 19 mg/dL ($p < 0.05$) ↓ CRP T_0: 20.8 ± 1.7 µM; T_3: 16.5± 1.3 µM ($p < 0.05$) → TG, LDL, CRP (NS)
[161]	One-way, open-label	50 HD patients	1 g/Dx, IV	12 mo	↑ LDL ($p = 0.005$), ↓ HDL ($p = 0.001$), → TG (NS)
[133]	Two-way, parallel, open-label	18 HD patients 18 HD patients	1 g/day, PO No treatment	3 mo	↓ CRP T_3: −1.6 ± 2.3 mg/L ($p < 0.05$), ↓ IL-6 T_3: −5.5 ± 3.6 ng/L ($p < 0.001$), ↓ IL-1β T_3: −0.6 ± 0.6 ng/L ($p < 0.001$) → CRP, IL-6, IL-1β (NS)
[170]	Two-way, parallel, double-blind	18 HD patients 18 HD patients	1 g/day, PO Placebo, PO	3 mo	↓ CRP T_0: 7.5 ± 5.5 mg/L; T_3: 4.4 ± 3.3 mg/L ($p < 0.05$) → CRP T_0: 6.5 ± 5 mg/L; T_3: 6.3 ± 3.1 mg/L (NS)
[171]	Two-way, parallel, double-blind	18 HD patients 18 HD patients	1 g/day, PO Placebo, PO	3 mo	↓ SAA T_3: −32% ($p < 0.001$) → SAA (NS)
[172]	Two-way, parallel, open-label	17 HD patients 25 HD patients	1 g/day, PO No treatment	3 mo	→ BMI, Leptin, Adiponectin (NS) → BMI, Leptin, Adiponectin (NS)
[173]	Two-way, parallel, open-label	20 HD patients 20 HD patients	1 g/day, PO No treatment	2 mo	→ Alb T_0: 3.37 ± 0.40 g/dL; T_2: 3.38 ± 0.43 g/dL (NS) → Alb T_0: 3.35 ± 0.34 g/dL; T_2: 3.40 ± 0.38 g/dL (NS)
[80]	Two-way, parallel, double-blind	48 HD patients 65 HD patients	20 mg/kg per Dx, IV Placebo, IV	6 mo	↓ CRP T_0: 1.8 ± 1.2 mg/dL; T_6: 1.2 ± 0.2 ($p < 0.002$), ↑ Alb T_0: 3.6 ± 0.3 g/dL; T_6: 3.9 ± 0.4 g/dL ($p < 0.0001$), ↑ BMI T_0: 20.5 ± 0.1; T_6: 21.2 ± 0.5 ($p < 0.0001$) → CRP (NS), ↓ Alb ($p < 0.0001$), ↓ BMI ($p < 0.05$)

ABI, ankle brachial index; Alb, albumin; BMI, body mass index; CRP, C-reactive protein; Dx, dialysis session; HD, hemodialysis; HDL, high-density lipoprotein; IL, interleukin; LDL, low-density lipoprotein; MDA, malondialdehyde; IV, intravenous injection; mo, months; NS, not significant; PO, per oral; Ref, reference; SAA, serum amyloid A; TC, total cholesterol; Tf, transferrin; TG, triglyceride; TP, total protein.
[a] The findings showed no difference (→), or decrease (↓) or increase (↑).

10. Conclusions

The number of patients being treated with dialysis therapy is increasing worldwide. Patients with end-stage kidney disease who are receiving dialysis therapy frequently experience carnitine system dysfunction. Carnitine deficiency and uremic syndrome complicate the already complex pathophysiology of patients on dialysis. Furthermore, a dysfunctional fatty acid metabolism induces surplus production of free radicals and undesired apoptosis. Regarding carnitine deficiency, levocarnitine treatment positively affects pathologic processes in patients on dialysis. There are four principal indications for levocarnitine treatment in dialysis patients with carnitine deficiency according to the American National Kidney Foundation: (1) ESA-resistant anemia that has not responded to the standard ESA dosage; (2) recurrent symptomatic hypotension during hemodialysis; (3) symptomatic cardiomyopathy or confirmed cardiomyopathy with reduced LVEF; and (4) fatigability and muscle weakness that undermine quality of life. However, there were some limitations in the previous studies regarding levocarnitine treatment in the dialysis population, including sample size, adequacy of study design, and definition of target diseases. Furthermore, research has not been able to identify a dose–response relationship and the optimal administration route for levocarnitine treatment. Therefore, additional adequately sized clinical trials are required to determine whether levocarnitine treatment improves survival in patients on dialysis.

Author Contributions: Conceptualization M.A. and T.M.; methodology, H.T.; software, M.A.; validation: H.T.; investigation, T.M. and H.T.; resources: M.A.; data curation, M.A. and T.M.; writing—original draft preparation, M.A.; writing—review and editing, H.T. and T.M.; visualization, M.A.;

supervision, M.A.; project administration, T.M. All authors have read and agreed to the published version of the manuscript.

Funding: This research received no external funding.

Institutional Review Board Statement: The study was conducted according to the guidelines of the Declaration of Helsinki.

Informed Consent Statement: Not applicable.

Data Availability Statement: Not applicable.

Conflicts of Interest: M.A. and T.M. chair courses endowed by Nikkiso Co., Ltd., NIPRO Corporation, Otsuka Pharmaceutical Co., Ltd., and Terumo Corporation. The other authors declare that they have no conflict of interest.

References

1. Golper, T.A.; Ahmad, S. L-carnitine administration to hemodialysis patients: Has it times come? *Semin. Dial.* **1992**, *5*, 94–98. [CrossRef]
2. Hiatt, W.R.; Koziol, B.J.; Shapiro, J.I.; Brass, E.P. Carnitine metabolism during exercise in patients on chronic hemodialysis. *Kidney Int.* **1992**, *41*, 1613–1619. [CrossRef] [PubMed]
3. Guarnieri, G.; Situlin, R.; Biolo, G. Carnitine metabolism in uremia. *Am. J. Kidney Dis.* **2001**, *38*, S3–S7. [CrossRef] [PubMed]
4. Evans, A.M.; Faull, R.; Fornasini, G.; Lemanowicz, E.F.; Longo, A.; Pace, S.; Nation, R.L. Pharmacokinetics of L-carnitine in patients with end-stage renal disease undergoing long-term hemodialysis. *Clin. Pharmacol. Ther.* **2000**, *68*, 238–249. [CrossRef] [PubMed]
5. Borum, P.R. Carnitine. *Annu. Rev. Nutr.* **1983**, *3*, 233–259. [CrossRef]
6. Moorthy, A.V.; Rosenblum, M.; Rajaram, R.; Shug, A.L. A comparison of plasma and muscle carnitine levels in patients on peritoneal or hemodialysis for chronic renal failure. *Am. J. Nephrol.* **1983**, *3*, 205–208. [CrossRef]
7. Rebouche, C.J.; Chenard, C.A. Metabolic fate of dietary carnitine in human adults: Identification and quantification of urinary and faecal metabolism. *J. Nutr.* **1991**, *121*, 539–546. [CrossRef]
8. Lopaschuk, G.D.; Belke, D.D.; Gamble, J.; Itoi, T.; Schönekess, B.O. Regulation of fatty acid oxidation in the mammalian heart in health and disease. *Biochem. Biophys. Acta* **1994**, *1213*, 263–276. [CrossRef]
9. Marzo, A.; Martelli, E.A.; Urso, R.; Rocchetti, M.; Rizza, V.; Kelly, J.G. Metabolism and disposition of intravenously administered acetyl-L-carnitine in healthy volunteers. *Eur. J. Clin. Pharmacol.* **1989**, *37*, 59–63.
10. Matera, M.; Bellinghieri, G.; Costantino, G.; Santoro, D.; Calvani, M.; Savica, V. History of L-Carnitine: Implications for renal disease. *J. Ren. Nutr.* **2003**, *13*, 2–14. [CrossRef]
11. Tamai, I.; Ohashi, R.; Nezu, J.; Yabuuchi, H.; Oku, A.; Shimane, M.; Sai, Y.; Tsuji, A. Molecular and functional identification of sodium-dependent high affinity human carnitine trasporter OTCN2. *J. Biol. Chem.* **1998**, *273*, 20378–20382. [CrossRef]
12. Tamai, I.; China, K.; Sai, Y.; Kobayashi, D.; Nezu, J.; Kawahara, E.; Tsuji, A. Na (+)-coupled transporter of L-carnitine via high-affinity carnitine transporter OCTN2 and its subcellar localization in kidney. *Biochim. Biophys. Acta* **2001**, *1512*, 273–284.
13. Koizumi, A.; Nozaki, J.; Ohura, T.; Kayo, T.; Wada, Y.; Nezu, J.; Ohashi, R.; Tamai, I.; Shoji, Y.; Takada, G.; et al. Genetic epidemiology of the carnitine transporter OCTN2 gene in a Japanese population and phenotypic characterization in Japanese pedigrees with primary systemic carnitine deficiency. *Hum. Mol. Genet.* **1999**, *8*, 2247–2254. [CrossRef] [PubMed]
14. Pande, S.V.; Murthy, M.S.R. Carnitine-acylcarnitine translocase deficiency: Implications in human pathology. *Biochim. Biophys. Acta* **1994**, *1226*, 269–276. [CrossRef]
15. McGarry, J.D.; Brown, N.F. The mitochondrial carnitine palmitoyltransferase system: From concept to molecular analysis. *Eur. J. Biochem.* **1997**, *244*, 1–14. [CrossRef]
16. Zammit, V.A. Carnitine acyltransferase: Functional significance of subcellular distribution and membrane topology. *Prog. Lipid Res.* **1999**, *38*, 199–244. [CrossRef]
17. Bieber, L.L. Carnitine. *Annu. Rev. Biochem.* **1988**, *57*, 261–283. [CrossRef] [PubMed]
18. Shimabukuro, M.; Zhou, Y.T.; Levi, M.; Unger, R.H. Fatty acid-induced beta cell apoptosis: A link between obesity and diabetes. *Proc. Natl. Acad. Sci. USA* **1998**, *95*, 2498–2502. [CrossRef]
19. Winter, S.C.; Zorn, E.M.; Vance, W.H. Carnitine deficiency. *Lancet* **1990**, *335*, 981–982. [CrossRef]
20. Suzuki, Y.K.; Tokuyama, K.; Kinoshita, M. Urinary profile of L-Carnitine and its derivatives in starved normal persons and ACTH injected patients with myopathy. *J. Nutr. Sci. Vitaminol.* **1983**, *29*, 303–312. [CrossRef]
21. Kanda, E.; Kato, A.; Masakane, I.; Kanno, Y. A new nutritional risk index for predicting mortality in hemodialysis patients: Nationwide cohort study. *PLoS ONE* **2019**, *14*, e0214524. [CrossRef] [PubMed]
22. Kalantar-Zadeh, K.; Kopple, J.D.; Block, G.; Humphreys, M.H. A malnutrition-inflammation score is correlated with morbidity and mortality in maintenance hemodialysis patients. *Am. J. Kidney Dis.* **2001**, *38*, 1251–1263. [CrossRef] [PubMed]

23. Fouque, D.; Kalantar-Zadeh, K.; Kopple, J.; Cano, N.; Chauveau, P.; Cuppari, L.; Franch, H.; Guarnieri, G.; Ikizler, T.A.; Kaysen, G.; et al. A proposed nomenclature and diagnostic criteria for protein-energy wasting in acute and chronic kidney disease. *Kidney Int.* **2008**, *73*, 391–398. [CrossRef] [PubMed]
24. Abe, M.; Kalantar-Zadeh, K. Haemodialysis-induced hypoglycaemia and glycaemic disarrays. *Nat. Rev. Nephrol* **2015**, *11*, 302–313. [CrossRef]
25. Tein, I. Carnitine transport: Pathophysiology and metabolism of known molecular defects. *J. Inherit. Metab. Dis.* **2003**, *26*, 147–169. [CrossRef] [PubMed]
26. Kerner, J.; Hoppel, C. Genetic disorders of carnitine metabolism and their nutritional management. *Annu. Rev. Nutr.* **1998**, *18*, 179–206. [CrossRef]
27. Evans, A.M. Dialysis-related carnitine disorder and levocarnitine pharmacology. *Am. J. Kidney Dis.* **2003**, *42* (Suppl. 4), S13–S26. [CrossRef]
28. Evans, A.M.; Fornaini, G. Pharmacokinetics of L-carnitine. *Clin. Pharm.* **2003**, *42*, 941–967. [CrossRef]
29. Japan Pediatric Society. Available online: http://www.jpeds.or.jp/modules/guidelines/index.php?content_id=2 (accessed on 21 September 2018).
30. Evans, A.M.; Faull, R.J.; Nation, R.L.; Prasad, S.; Elias, T.; Reuter, S.E.; Fornasini, G. Impact of hemodialysis on endogenous plasma and muscle carnitine levels in patients with end-stage renal disease. *Kidney Int.* **2004**, *66*, 1527–1534. [CrossRef] [PubMed]
31. Spagnoli, L.G.; Palmieri, G.; Mauriello, A.; Vacha, G.M.; D'Iddio, S.; Giorcelli, G.; Corsi, M. Morphometric evidence of the trophic effect of L-carnitine on human skeletal muscle. *Nephron* **1990**, *55*, 16–23. [CrossRef]
32. Hatanaka, Y.; Higuchi, T.; Akiya, Y.; Horikami, T.; Tei, R.; Furukawa, T.; Takashima, H.; Tomita, H.; Abe, M. Prevalence of carnitine deficiency and decreased carnitine levels in patients on hemodialysis. *Blood Purif.* **2019**, *47*, 1–7. [CrossRef] [PubMed]
33. Sirolli, V.; Rossi, C.; Di Castelnuovo, A.; Felaco, P.; Amoroso, L.; Zucchelli, M.; Ciavardelli, D.; Di Ilio, C.; Sacchetta, P.; Bernardini, S.; et al. Toward personalized hemodialysis by low molecular weight aminocontaining compounds: Future perspective of patient metabolic fingerprint. *Blood Transfus.* **2012**, *10*, 78–88.
34. Reuter, S.E.; Evans, A.M.; Faull, R.J.; Chace, D.H.; Fornaini, G. Impact of haemodialysis on individual endogenous plasma acylcarnitine concentrations in end-stage renal disease. *Ann. Clin. Biochem.* **2005**, *42*, 387–393. [CrossRef]
35. Marzo, A.; Arrigoni Martelli, E.; Mancinelli, A.; Cardace, G.; Corbelletta, C.; Bassani, E.; Solbiati, M. Protein binding of L-carnitine family components. *Eur. J. Drug Metab. Pharmacokinet.* **1991**, *3*, 364–368.
36. Debska-Slizien, A.; Kawecka, A.; Wojnarowski, K.; Prajs, J.; Malgorzewicz, S.; Kunicka, D.; Zdrojewski, Z.; Walysiak, S.; Lipinski, J.; Rutkowski, B. Correlation between plasma carnitine, muscle carnitine and glycogen levels in maintenance hemodialysis patients. *Int. J. Artif. Organs* **2000**, *23*, 90–96. [CrossRef] [PubMed]
37. Kamei, Y.; Kamei, D.; Tsuchiya, K.; Mineshima, M.; Nitta, K. Association between 4-year all-cause mortality and carnitine profile in maintenance hemodialysis patients. *PLoS ONE* **2018**, *13*, e0201591. [CrossRef] [PubMed]
38. Nakai, S.; Watanabe, Y.; Masakane, I.; Wada, A.; Shoji, T.; Hasegawa, T.; Nakamoto, H.; Yamagata, K.; Kazama, J.J.; Fujii, N.; et al. Overview of regular dialysis treatment in Japan (as of 31 December 2011). *Ther. Aphel. Dial.* **2013**, *17*, 567–611. [CrossRef]
39. Masakane, I.; Kikuchi, K.; Kawanishi, H. Evidence for the clinical advantages of predilution on-line hemodiafiltration. *Contrib. Nephrol.* **2017**, *189*, 17–23.
40. Penne, E.L.; van der Weerd, N.C.; Blankestijn, P.J.; van den Dorpel, M.A.; Grooteman, M.P.; Nubé, M.J.; Ter Wee, P.M.; Lévesque, R.; Bots, M.L.; CONTRAST investigators. Role of residual kidney function and convective volume on change in beta2-microglobulin levels in hemodiafiltration patients. *Clin. J. Am. Soc. Nephrol.* **2010**, *5*, 80–86. [CrossRef]
41. Maduell, F.; Moreso, F.; Pons, M.; Ramos, R.; Mora-Macià, J.; Carreras, J.; Soler, J.; Torres, F.; Campistol, J.M.; Martinez-Castelao, A.; et al. High-efficiency postdilution online hemodiafiltration reduces all-cause mortality in hemodialysis patients. *J. Am. Soc. Nephrol.* **2013**, *24*, 487–497. [CrossRef] [PubMed]
42. Constantin-Teodosiu, D.; Kirby, D.P.; Short, A.H.; Burden, R.P.; Morgan, A.G.; Greenha, P.L. Free and esterified carnitine in continuous ambulatory peritoneal dialysis patients. *Kidney Int.* **1996**, *49*, 158–162. [CrossRef] [PubMed]
43. Sotirakopoulos, N.; Athanasiou, G.; Tsitsios, T.; Mavromatidis, K. The influence of L-carnitine supplementation on hematocrit and hemoglobin levels in patients with end stage renal failure on CAPD. *Ren. Fail.* **2002**, *24*, 505–510. [CrossRef]
44. Grzegorzewska, A.E.; Mariak, I.; Dobrowolska-Zachwieja, A. Continuous ambulatory peritoneal dialysis (CAPD) adequacy influences serum free carnitine level. *Int. Urol. Nephrol.* **1999**, *31*, 533–540. [CrossRef]
45. Shimizu, S.; Takashima, H.; Tei, R.; Furukawa, T.; Okamura, M.; Kitai, M.; Nagura, C.; Maruyama, T.; Higuchi, T.; Abe, M. Prevalence of carnitine deficiency and decreased carnitine levels in patients on peritoneal dialysis. *Nutrients* **2019**, *11*, 2645. [CrossRef]
46. Schreiber, B. Levocarnitine and dialysis: A review. *Nutr. Clin. Pract.* **2005**, *20*, 218–243. [CrossRef] [PubMed]
47. Brass, E.P. Pharmacokinetic considerations for the therapeutic use of carnitine in hemodialysis patients. *Clin. Ther.* **1995**, *17*, 176–185. [CrossRef]
48. Golper, T.A.; Wolfson, M.; Ahmad, S.; Hirschberg, R.; Kurtin, P.; Katz, L.A.; Nicora, R.; Ashbrook, D.; Kopple, J.D. Multicenter trial of L-carnitine in maintenance hemodialysis patients. I. Carnitine concentrations and lipid effects. *Kidney Int.* **1990**, *38*, 904–911. [CrossRef]

49. Ahmad, S.; Robertson, H.T.; Golper, T.A.; Wolfson, M.; Kurtin, P.; Katz, L.A.; Hirschberg, R.; Nicora, R.; Ashbrook, D.W.; Kopple, J.D. Multicenter trial of L-carnitine in maintenance hemodialysis patients. II. Clinical and biochemical effects. *Kidney Int.* **1990**, *38*, 912–918. [CrossRef]
50. Fagher, B.; Cederblad, G.; Eriksson, M.; Monti, M.; Moritz, U.; Nilsson-Ehle, P.; Thysell, H. L-carnitine and haemodialysis: Double blind study on muscle function and metabolism and peripheral nerve function. *Scand. J. Clin. Lab. Investig.* **1985**, *45*, 169–178. [CrossRef]
51. Sahajwalla, C.G.; Helton, E.D.; Purich, E.D.; Hoppel, C.L.; Cabana, B.E. Comparison of L-carnitine pharmacokinetics with and without baseline correction following administration of single 20-mg/kg intravenous dose. *J. Pharm. Sci.* **1995**, *84*, 634–639. [CrossRef]
52. Segre, G.; Bianchi, E.; Corsi, M.; D'Iddio, S.; Ghirardi, O.; Maccari, F. Plasma and urine pharmacokinetics of free and of short-chain carnitine after administration of carnitine in man. *Arzneimittelforschung* **1988**, *38*, 1830–1834.
53. Koeth, R.A.; Wang, Z.; Levison, B.S.; Buffa, J.A.; Org, E.; Sheehy, B.T.; Britt, E.B.; Fu, X.; Wu, Y.; Li, L.; et al. Intestinal microbiota metabolism of L-carnitine, a nutrient in red meat, promotes atherosclerosis. *Nat. Med.* **2013**, *19*, 576–585. [CrossRef] [PubMed]
54. Wang, Z.; Klipfell, E.; Bennett, B.J.; Koeth, R.; Levison, B.S.; Dugar, B.; Feldstein, A.E.; Britt, E.B.; Fu, X.; Chung, Y.M.; et al. Gut flora metabolism of phosphatidylcholine promotes cardiovascular disease. *Nature* **2011**, *472*, 57–63. [CrossRef]
55. Lang, D.H.; Yeung, C.K.; Peter, R.M.; Ibarra, C.; Gasser, R.; Itagaki, K.; Philpot, R.M.; Rettie, A.E. Isoform specificity of trimethylamine N-oxygenation by human flavin-containing monooxygenase (FMO) and P450 enzymes: Selective catalysis by FMO3. *Biochem. Pharmacol.* **1998**, *56*, 1005–1012. [CrossRef]
56. Al-Waiz, M.; Mitchell, S.C.; Idle, J.R.; Smith, R.L. The metabolism of 14C-labelled trimethylamine and its N-oxide in man. *Xenobiotica* **1987**, *17*, 551–558. [CrossRef] [PubMed]
57. Mitchell, S.C.; Zhang, A.Q.; Noblet, J.M.; Gillespie, S.; Jones, N.; Smith, R.L. Metabolic disposition of [14C]-trimethylamine N-oxide in rat: Variation with dose and route of administration. *Xenobiotica* **1997**, *27*, 1187–1197. [CrossRef] [PubMed]
58. Wilson, W.H.; Wang, Z.; Kennedy, D.J.; Wu, Y.; Buffa, J.A.; Agatisa-Boyle, B.; Li, X.S.; Levison, B.S.; Hazen, S.L. Gut microbiota-dependent trimethylamine N-oxide (TMAO) pathway contributes to both development of renal insufficiency and mortality risk in chronic kidney disease. *Circ. Res.* **2015**, *116*, 448–455.
59. Stubbs, J.R.; House, J.A.; Ocque, A.J.; Zhang, S.; Johnson, C.; Kimber, C.; Schmidt, K.; Gupta, A.; Wetmore, J.B.; Nolin, T.D.; et al. Serum trimethylamine-N-oxide is elevated in CKD and correlates with coronary atherosclerosis burden. *J. Am. Soc. Nephrol.* **2016**, *27*, 305–313. [CrossRef]
60. Eknoyan, G.; Latos, D.L.; Lindberg, J. Practice recommendations for the use of L-carnitine in dialysis-related carnitine disorder. National Kidney Foundation Carnitine Consensus Conference. *Am. J. Kidney Dis.* **2003**, *41*, 868–876. [CrossRef]
61. Parfrey, P.S.; Foley, R.N.; Wittreich, B.H.; Sullivan, D.J.; Zagari, M.J.; Frei, D. Double-blind comparison of full and partial anemia correction in incident hemodialysis patients without symptomatic heart disease. *J. Am. Soc. Nephrol.* **2005**, *16*, 2180–2189. [CrossRef] [PubMed]
62. Palmer, S.C.; Navaneethan, S.D.; Craig, J.C.; Johnson, D.W.; Tonelli, M.; Garg, A.X.; Pellegrini, F.; Ravani, P.; Jardine, M.; Perkovic, V.; et al. Meta-analysis: Erythropoiesis-stimulating agents in patients with chronic kidney disease. *Ann. Intern. Med.* **2010**, *153*, 23–33. [CrossRef] [PubMed]
63. Zhang, Y.; Thamer, M.; Stefanik, K.; Kaufman, J.; Cotter, D.J. Epoetin requirements predict mortality in hemodialysis patients. *Am. J. Kidney Dis.* **2004**, *44*, 866–876. [CrossRef]
64. Gunnell, J.; Yeun, J.Y.; Depner, T.A.; Kaysen, G.A. Acute-phase response predicts erythropoietin resistance in hemodialysis and peritoneal dialysis patients. *Am. J. Kidney Dis.* **1999**, *33*, 63–72. [CrossRef]
65. Yamamoto, H.; Nishi, S.; Tomo, T.; Masakane, I.; Saito, K.; Nangaku, M.; Hattori, M.; Suzuki, T.; Morita, S.; Ashida, A.; et al. 2015 Japanese Society for Dialysis Therapy: Guidelines for Renal Anemia in Chronic Kidney Disease. *Ren. Replace. Ther.* **2017**, *3*, 36. [CrossRef]
66. Kooistra, M.P.; Struyvenberg, A.; Vanes, A. The response to recombinant human erythropoietin in patients with the anemia of end-stage renal disease is correlated with serum carnitine levels. *Nephron* **1991**, *57*, 127–128. [CrossRef]
67. Matsumura, M.; Hatakeyama, S.; Koni, I.; Mabuchi, H.; Muramoto, H. Correlation between serum carnitine levels and erythrocyte osmotic fragility in hemodialysis patients. *Nephron* **1996**, *72*, 574–578. [CrossRef]
68. Steiber, A.L.; Weatherspoon, L.J.; Spry, L.; Davis, A.T. Serum carnitine concentrations correlated to clinical outcome parameters in chronic hemodialysis patients. *Clin. Nutr.* **2004**, *23*, 27–34. [CrossRef]
69. Kletzmayr, J.; Mayer, G.; Legenstein, E.; Heinz-Peer, G.; Leitha, T.; Hörl, W.H.; Kovarik, J. Anemia and carnitine supplementation in hemodialyzed patients. *Kidney Int. Suppl.* **1999**, *55*, S93–S106. [CrossRef]
70. Caruso, U.; Leone, L.; Cravotto, E.; Nava, D. Effects of L-carnitine on anemia in aged hemodialysis patients treated with recombinant human erythropoietin: A pilot study. *Dial. Transplant.* **1998**, *27*, 498–506.
71. Sotirakopoulos, N.; Athanasiou, G.; Tsitsios, T.; Stambolidou, M.; Missirlis, Y.; Mavromatidis, K. Effect of L-carnitine supplementation on red blood cells deformability in hemodialysis patients. *Ren. Fail.* **2000**, *22*, 73–80.
72. de los Reyes, B.; Perez-García, R.; Liras, A.; Arenas, J. Reduced carnitine palmitoyl transferase activity and altered acyl-trafficking in red blood cells from hemodialysis patients. *Biochim. Biophys. Acta* **1996**, *1315*, 37–39. [CrossRef]
73. Arduini, A.; Rossi, M.; Mancinelli, G.; Belfiglio, M.; Scurti, R.; Radatti, G.; Shohet, S.B. Effect of L-carnitine and acetyl-L-carnitine on the human erythrocyte membrane stability and deformability. *Life Sci.* **1990**, *47*, 2395–2400. [CrossRef]

74. Hörl, W.H. Is there a role for adjuvant therapy in patients being treated with epoetin? *Nephrol. Dial. Transplant.* **1999**, *14*, 50–60. [CrossRef]
75. Hurot, J.M.; Cucherat, M.; Haugh, M.; Fouque, D. Effects of L-carnitine supplementation in maintenance hemodialysis patients: A systematic review. *J. Am. Soc. Nephrol.* **2002**, *13*, 708–714.
76. Zhu, Y.; Xue, C.; Ou, J.; Xie, Z.; Deng, J. Effect of L-carnitine supplementation on renal anemia in patients on hemodialysis: A meta-analysis. *Int. Urol. Nephrol.* **2021**. [CrossRef] [PubMed]
77. Arduini, A.; Bonomini, M.; Clutterbuck, E.J.; Laffan, M.A.; Pusey, C.D. Effect of L-carnitine administration on erythrocyte survival in haemodialysis patients. *Nephrol. Dial. Transplant.* **2006**, *21*, 2671–2672. [CrossRef] [PubMed]
78. Matsumoto, Y.; Amano, I.; Hirose, S.; Tsuruta, Y.; Hara, S.; Murata, M.; Imai, T. Effects of L-carnitine supplementation on renal anemia in poor responders to erythropoietin. *Blood Purif.* **2001**, *19*, 24–32. [CrossRef] [PubMed]
79. Brass, E.P.; Adler, S.; Sietsema, K.E.; Hiatt, W.R.; Orlando, A.M.; Amato, A. Intravenous L-carnitine increases plasma carnitine, reduces fatigue, and may preserve exercise capacity in hemodialysis patients. *Am. J. Kidney Dis.* **2001**, *37*, 1018–1028. [CrossRef]
80. Savica, V.; Santoro, D.; Mazzaglia, G.; Ciolino, F.; Monardo, P.; Calvani, M.; Bellinghieri, G.; Kopple, J.D. L-carnitine infusions may suppress serum C-reactive protein and improve nutritional status in maintenance hemodialysis patients. *J. Ren. Nutr.* **2005**, *15*, 225–230. [CrossRef] [PubMed]
81. Cui, H.X.; Wu, E.L. Effect of levocarnitine/iron saccharate combination on renal anaemia and oxidative stress in patients undergoing haemodialysis. *Trop. J. Pharm. Res.* **2016**, *15*, 2269–2274. [CrossRef]
82. Mitwalli, A.H.; Al-Wakeel, J.S.; Alam, A.; Tarif, N.; Abu-Aisha, H.; Rashed, M.; Al Nahed, N. L-carnitine supplementation in hemodialysis patients. *Saudi J. Kidney Dis. Transplant.* **2005**, *16*, 17–22.
83. Rathod, R.; Baig, M.S.; Khandelwal, P.N.; Kulkarni, S.G.; Gade, P.R.; Siddiqui, S. Results of a single blind, randomized, placebo-controlled clinical trial to study the effect of intravenous L-carnitine supplementation on health-related quality of life in Indian patients on maintenance hemodialysis. *Indian J. Med. Sci.* **2006**, *60*, 143–153.
84. Semeniuk, J.; Shalansky, K.F.; Taylor, N.; Jastrzebski, J.; Cameron, E.C. Evaluation of the effect of intravenous l-carnitine on quality of life in chronic hemodialysis patients. *Clin. Nephrol.* **2000**, *54*, 470–477.
85. Singh, H.; Jain, D.; Bhaduri, G.; Gupta, N.; Sangwan, R. Study on effects of L-carnitine supplementation on anaemia with erythropoietin hyporesponsiveness and lipid profile in chronic kidney disease patients on maintenance haemodialysis. *Indian J. Basic Appl. Med. Res.* **2020**, *9*, 224–232.
86. Fu, R.G.; Wang, L.; Zhou, J.P.; Ma, F.; Liu, X.D.; Ge, H.; Zhang, J. The effect of levocarnitine on nutritional status and lipid metabolism during long-term maintenance hemodialysis. *Acad. J. Xi'an Jiaotong Univ.* **2010**, *22*, 203–207.
87. Kuwasawa-Iwasaki, M.; Io, H.; Muto, M.; Ichikawa, S.; Wakabayashi, K.; Kanda, R.; Nakata, J.; Nohara, N.; Tomino, Y.; Suzuki Y. Effects of L-carnitine supplementation in patients receiving hemodialysis or peritoneal dialysis. *Nutrients* **2020**, *12*, 3371. [CrossRef] [PubMed]
88. Emami Naini, A.; Moradi, M.; Mortazavi, M.; Amini Harandi, A.; Hadizadeh, M.; Shirani, F.; Basir Ghafoori, H.; Emami Naini, P. Effects of oral L-carnitine supplementation on lipid profile, anemia, and quality of life in chronic renal disease patients under hemodialysis: A randomized, double-blinded, placebo-controlled trial. *J. Nutr. Metab.* **2012**, *2012*, 510483. [CrossRef]
89. Trovato, G.M.; Iannetti, E.; Murgo, A.M.; Carpinteri, G.; Catalano, D. Body composition and long-term levo-carnitine supplementation. *Clin. Ter.* **1998**, *149*, 209–214. [PubMed]
90. Vaux, E.C.; Taylor, D.J.; Altmann, P.; Rajagopalan, B.; Graham, K.; Cooper, R.; Bonomo, Y.; Styles, P. Effects of carnitine supplementation on muscle metabolism by the use of magnetic resonance spectroscopy and near-infrared spectroscopy in end-stage renal disease. *Nephron. Clin. Pract.* **2004**, *97*, 41–48. [CrossRef]
91. Chazot, C.; Blanc, C.; Hurot, J.M.; Charra, B.; Jean, G.; Laurent, G. Nutritional effects of carnitine supplementation in hemodialysis patients. *Clin. Nephrol.* **2003**, *59*, 24–30. [CrossRef] [PubMed]
92. Labonia, W.D. L-carnitine effects on anemia in hemodialyzed patients treated with erythropoietin. *Am. J. Kidney Dis.* **1995**, *26*, 757–764. [CrossRef]
93. Maruyama, T.; Higuchi, T.; Yamazaki, T.; Okawa, E.; Ando, H.; Oikawa, O.; Inoshita, A.; Okada, K.; Abe, M. Levocarnitine injections decrease the need for erythropoiesis-stimulating agents in hemodialysis patients with renal anemia. *Cardiorenl. Med.* **2017**, *7*, 188–197. [CrossRef] [PubMed]
94. Mercadal, L.; Coudert, M.; Vassault, A.; Pieroni, L.; Debure, A.; Ouziala, M.; Depreneuf, H.; Fumeron, C.; Servais, A.; Bassilios, N.; et al. L-carnitine treatment in incident hemodialysis patients: The multicenter, randomized, doubleblinded, placebo-controlled CARNIDIAL trial. *Clin. J. Am. Soc. Nephrol.* **2012**, *7*, 1836–1842. [CrossRef]
95. Mercadal, L.; Tezenas du Montcel, S.; Chonchol, M.B.; Debure, A.; Depreneuf, H.; Servais, A.; Bassilios, N.; Assogba, U.; Allouache, M.; Prié, D. Effects of L-carnitine on mineral metabolism in the multicentre, randomized, double blind, placebo-controlled CARNIDIAL trial. *Am. J. Nephrol.* **2018**, *48*, 349–356. [CrossRef] [PubMed]
96. Steiber, A.L.; Davis, A.T.; Spry, L.; Strong, J.; Buss, M.L.; Ratkiewicz, M.M.; Weatherspoon, L.J. Carnitine treatment improved quality-of-life measure in a sample of Midwestern hemodialysis patients. *JPEN J. Parenter. Enteral. Nutr.* **2006**, *30*, 10–15. [CrossRef] [PubMed]
97. Reuter, S.E.; Faull, R.J.; Evans, A.M. L-carnitine supplementation in the dialysis population: Are Australian patients missing out? *Nephrology* **2008**, *13*, 3–16. [CrossRef]

98. Fotiadou, E.; Georgianos, P.I.; Chourdakis, M.; Zebekakis, P.E.; Liakopoulos, V. Eating during the Hemodialysis Session: A Practice Improving Nutritional Status or a Risk Factor for Intradialytic Hypotension and Reduced Dialysis Adequacy? *Nutrients* **2020**, *12*, 1703. [CrossRef]
99. Shoji, T.; Tsubakihara, Y.; Fujii, M.; Imai, E. Hemodialysis-associated hypotension as an independent risk factor for two-year mortality in hemodialysis patients. *Kidney Int.* **2004**, *66*, 1212–1220. [CrossRef]
100. Casciani, C.U.; Caruso, U.; Cravotto, E.; Corsi, M.; Maccari, F. Benefitial effects of L-carnitine in post-dialysis syndrome. *Curr. Ther. Res.* **1982**, *32*, 116–127.
101. van Es, A.; Henny, F.C.; Kooistra, M.P.; Lobatto, S.; Scholte, H.R. Amelioration of cardiac function by L-carnitine administration in patients on haemodialysis. *Contrib. Nephrol.* **1992**, *98*, 28–35. [PubMed]
102. Sakurabayashi, T.; Takaesu, Y.; Haginoshita, S.; Takeda, T.; Aoike, I.; Miyazaki, S.; Koda, Y.; Yuasa, Y.; Sakai, S.; Suzuki, M.; et al. Improvement of myocardial fatty acid metabolism through L-carnitine administration to chronic hemodialysis patients. *Am. J. Nephrol.* **1999**, *19*, 480–484. [CrossRef]
103. Matsumoto, Y.; Sato, M.; Ohashi, H.; Araki, H.; Tadokoro, M.; Osumi, Y.; Ito, H.; Morita, H.; Amano, I. Effects of L-carnitine supplementation on cardiac morbidity in hemodialyzed patients. *Am. J. Nephrol.* **2000**, *20*, 201–207. [CrossRef] [PubMed]
104. Sakurabayashi, T.; Miyazaki, S.; Yuasa, Y.; Sakai, S.; Suzuki, M.; Takahashi, S.; Hirasawa, Y. L-carnitine supplementation decreases the left ventricular mass in patients undergoing hemodialysis. *Circ. J.* **2008**, *72*, 926–931. [CrossRef]
105. Sabry, A.A. The role of oral L-carnitine therapy in chronic hemodialysis patients. *Saudi J. Kidney Dis. Transplant.* **2010**, *21*, 454–459.
106. Kudoh, Y.; Aoyama, S.; Torii, T.; Chen, Q.; Nagahara, D.; Sakata, H.; Nozawa, A. Hemodynamic stabilizing effects of L-carnitine in chronic hemodialysis patients. *Cardiorenal Med.* **2013**, *3*, 200–207. [CrossRef]
107. Higuchi, T.; Abe, M.; Yamazaki, T.; Okawa, E.; Ando, H.; Hotta, S.; Oikawa, O.; Kikuchi, F.; Okada, K.; Soma, M. Levocarnitine Improves Cardiac Function in Hemodialysis Patients with Left Ventricular Hypertrophy: A Randomized Controlled Trial. *Am. J. Kidney Dis.* **2016**, *67*, 260–270. [CrossRef] [PubMed]
108. Ibarra-Sifuentes, H.R.; Del Cueto-Aguilera, Á.; Gallegos-Arguijo, D.A.; Castillo-Torres, S.A.; Vera-Pineda, R.; Martínez-Granados, R.J.; Atilano-Díaz, A.; Cuellar-Monterrubio, J.E.; Pezina-Cantú, C.O.; Martínez-Guevara, E.J.; et al. Levocarnitine decreases intradialytic hypotension episodes: A randomized controlled trial. *Ther. Apher. Dial.* **2017**, *21*, 459–464. [CrossRef] [PubMed]
109. Riley, S.; Rutherford, S.; Rutherford, P.A. Low carnitine levels in hemodialysis patients: Relationship with functional activity status and intra-dialytic hypotension. *Clin. Nephrol.* **1997**, *48*, 392–393. [CrossRef] [PubMed]
110. Poldermans, D.; Man in't Veld, A.J.; Rambaldi, R.; Van Den Meiracker, A.H.; Van Den Dorpel, M.A.; Rocchi, G.; Boersma, E.; Bax, J.J.; Weimar, W.; Roelandt, J.R.; et al. Cardiac evaluation in hypotension-prone and hypotension-resistant hemodialysis patients. *Kidney Int.* **1999**, *56*, 1905–1911. [CrossRef]
111. Litwin, S.E.; Raya, T.E.; Gay, R.G.; Bedotto, J.B.; Bahl, J.J.; Anderson, P.G.; Goldman, S.; Bressler, R. Chronic inhibition of fatty acid oxidation: New model of diastolic dysfunction. *Am. J. Physiol.* **1990**, *258*, 51–56. [CrossRef] [PubMed]
112. Romagnoli, G.F.; Naso, A.; Carraro, G.; Lidestri, V. Beneficial effects of L-carnitine in dialysis patients with impaired left ventricular function: An observational study. *Curr. Med. Res. Opin.* **2002**, *18*, 172–175. [CrossRef]
113. Higuchi, T.; Abe, M.; Yamazaki, T.; Mizuno, M.; Okawa, E.; Ando, H.; Oikawa, O.; Okada, K.; Kikuchi, F.; Soma, M. Effects of levocarnitine on brachial-ankle pulse wave velocity in hemodialysis patients: A randomized controlled trial. *Nutrients* **2014**, *6*, 5992–6004. [CrossRef] [PubMed]
114. Fujibayashi, Y.; Som, P.; Yonekura, Y.; Knapp, F.F., Jr.; Tamaki, N.; Yamamoto, K.; Konishi, J.; Yokoyama, A. Myocardial accumulation of iodinated beta-methyl-branched fatty acid analog, [125I] (p-iodophenyl)-3-(R, S)-methylpentadecanoic acid (BMIPP), and correlation to ATP concentration–II. Studies in salt-induced hypertensive rats. *Nucl. Med. Biol.* **1993**, *20*, 163–166. [CrossRef]
115. Kazmi, W.H.; Obrador, G.T.; Sternberg, M.; Lindberg, J.; Schreiber, B.; Lewis, V.; Pereira, B.J. Carnitine therapy is associated with decreased hospital utilization among hemodialysis patients. *Am. J. Nephrol.* **2005**, *25*, 106–115.
116. Cruz-Jentoft, A.J.; Landi, F.; Topinková, E.; Michel, J.P. Understanding sarcopenia as a geriatric syndrome. *Curr. Opin. Clin. Nutr. Metab. Care* **2010**, *13*, 1–7. [CrossRef] [PubMed]
117. Muscaritoli, M.; Anker, S.D.; Argilés, J.; Aversa, Z.; Bauer, J.M.; Biolo, G.; Boirie, Y.; Bosaeus, I.; Cederholm, T.; Costelli, P.; et al. Consensus definition of sarcopenia, cachexia and precachexia: Joint document elaborated by Special Interest Groups (SIG) "cachexia-anorexia in chronic wasting diseases" and "nutrition in geriatrics". *Clin. Nutr.* **2010**, *29*, 154–159. [CrossRef]
118. Fielding, R.A.; Vellas, B.; Evans, W.J.; Bhasin, S.; Morley, J.E.; Newman, A.B.; Abellan van Kan, G.; Andrieu, S.; Bauer, J.; Breuille, D.; et al. Sarcopenia: An undiagnosed condition in older adults. Current consensus definition: Prevalence, etiology, and consequences. International Working Group on Sarcopenia. *J. Am. Med. Dir. Assoc.* **2011**, *12*, 249–256. [CrossRef]
119. Ikizler, T.A.; Cano, N.J.; Franch, H.; Fouque, D.; Himmelfarb, J.; Kalantar-Zadeh, K.; Kuhlmann, M.K.; Stenvinkel, P.; TerWee, P.; Teta, D.; et al. International Society of Renal Nutrition and Metabolism. Prevention and treatment of protein energy wasting in chronic kidney disease patients: A consensus statement by the International Society of Renal Nutrition and Metabolism. *Kidney Int.* **2013**, *84*, 1096–1107. [CrossRef] [PubMed]
120. Kim, J.C.; Kalantar-Zadeh, K.; Kopple, J.D. Frailty and protein-energy wasting in elderly patients with end stage kidney disease. *J. Am. Soc. Nephrol.* **2013**, *24*, 337–351. [CrossRef]

121. Carrero, J.J.; Stenvinkel, P.; Cuppari, L.; Ikizler, T.A.; Kalantar-Zadeh, K.; Kaysen, G.; Mitch, W.E.; Price, S.R.; Wanner, C.; Wang, A.Y.; et al. Etiology of the protein-energy wasting syndrome in chronic kidney disease: A consensus statement from the International Society of Renal Nutrition and Metabolism (ISRNM). *J. Ren. Nutr.* **2013**, *23*, 77–90. [CrossRef]
122. Johansen, K.L.; Chertow, G.M.; Ng, A.V.; Mulligan, K.; Carey, S.; Schoenfeld, P.Y.; Kent-Braun, J.A. Physical activity levels in patients on hemodialysis and healthy sedentary controls. *Kidney Int.* **2000**, *57*, 2564–2570. [CrossRef] [PubMed]
123. Stack, A.G.; Martin, D.R. Association of patient autonomy with increased transplantation and survival among new dialysis patients in the United States. *Am. J. Kidney Dis.* **2005**, *45*, 730–742. [CrossRef] [PubMed]
124. Carrero, J.J.; Thomas, F.; Nagy, K.; Arogundade, F.; Avesani, C.M.; Chan, M.; Chmielewski, M.; Cordeiro, A.C.; Espinosa-Cuevas, A.; Fiaccadori, E.; et al. Global Prevalence of Protein-Energy Wasting in Kidney Disease: A Meta-analysis of Contemporary Observational Studies From the International Society of Renal Nutrition and Metabolism. *J. Ren. Nutr.* **2018**, *28*, 380–392. [CrossRef] [PubMed]
125. Johansen, K.L. The frail dialysis population: A growing burden for the dialysis community. *Blood Purif.* **2015**, *40*, 288–292. [CrossRef] [PubMed]
126. Johansen, K.L.; Chertow, G.M.; Jin, C.; Kutner, N.G. Significance of frailty among dialysis patients. *J. Am. Soc. Nephrol.* **2007**, *18*, 2960–2967. [CrossRef]
127. Bellinghieri, G.; Santoro, D.; Calvani, M.; Savica, V. Role of carnitine in modulating acute-phase protein synthesis in hemodialysis patients. *J. Ren. Nutr.* **2005**, *15*, 13–17. [CrossRef]
128. Stenvinkel, P.; Heimbürger, O.; Lindholm, B.; Kaysen, G.A.; Bergström, J. Are there two types of malnutrition in chronic renal failure? Evidence for relationship between malnutrition, inflammation and atherosclerosis (MIA syndrome). *Nephrol. Dial. Transplant.* **2000**, *15*, 953–960. [CrossRef]
129. Kalantar-Zadeh, K.; Block, G.; McAllister, C.J.; Humphreys, M.H.; Kopple, J.D. Appetite and inflammation, nutrition, anemia, and clinical outcome in hemodialysis patients. *Am. J. Clin. Nutr.* **2004**, *80*, 299–307. [CrossRef] [PubMed]
130. Bistrian, B.R.; Schwartz, J.; Istfan, N.W. Cytokines, muscle proteolysis, and the catabolic response to infection and inflammation. *Proc. Soc. Exp. Biol. Med.* **1992**, *200*, 220–223. [CrossRef]
131. Duranay, M.; Akay, H.; Yilmaz, F.M.; Senes, M.; Tekeli, N.; Yücel, D. Effects of L-carnitine infusions on inflammatory and nutritional markers in haemodialysis patients. *Nephrol. Dial. Transplant.* **2006**, *21*, 3211–3214. [CrossRef] [PubMed]
132. Suchitra, M.M.; Ashalatha, V.L.; Sailaja, E.; Rao, A.M.; Reddy, V.S.; Bitla, A.R.; Sivakumar, V.; Rao, P.V. The effect of L-carnitine supplementation on lipid parameters, inflammatory and nutritional markers in maintenance hemodialysis patients. *Saudi J. Kidney Dis. Transpl.* **2011**, *22*, 1155–1159. [PubMed]
133. Shakeri, A.; Tabibi, H.; Hedayati, M. Effects of L-carnitine supplement on serum inflammatory cytokines, C-reactive protein, lipoprotein (a), and oxidative stress in hemodialysis patients with Lp (a) hyperlipoproteinemia. *Hemodial Int.* **2010**, *14*, 498–504. [CrossRef] [PubMed]
134. Hoppel, C. The role of carnitine in normal and altered fatty acid metabolism. *Am. J. Kidney Dis.* **2003**, *41*, 4–12. [CrossRef]
135. Malaguarnera, M.; Cammalleri, L.; Gargante, M.P.; Vacante, M.; Colonna, V.; Motta, M. L-Carnitine treatment reduces severity of physical and mental fatigue and increases cognitive functions in centenarians: A randomized and controlled clinical trial. *Am. J. Clin. Nutr.* **2007**, *86*, 1738–1744. [CrossRef] [PubMed]
136. Badrasawi, M.; Shahar, S.; Zahara, A.M.; Nor Fadilah, R.; Singh, D.K. Efficacy of L-carnitine supplementation on frailty status and its biomarkers, nutritional status, and physical and cognitive function among prefrail older adults: A double-blind, randomized, placebocontrolled clinical trial. *Clin. Interv. Aging* **2016**, *11*, 1675–1686. [CrossRef] [PubMed]
137. Evans, M.; Guthrie, N.; Pezzullo, J.; Sanli, T.; Fielding, R.A.; Bellamine, A. Efficacy of a novel formulation of L-Carnitine, creatine, and leucine on lean body mass and functional muscle strength in healthy older adults: A randomized, double-blind placebo-controlled study. *Nutr. Metab.* **2017**, *14*, 7. [CrossRef] [PubMed]
138. Malaguarnera, M.; Gargante, M.P.; Cristaldi, E.; Colonna, V.; Messano, M.; Koverech, A.; Neri, S.; Vacante, M. Acetyl L-carnitine (ALC) treatment in elderly patients with fatigue. *Arch. Gerontol. Geriatr.* **2008**, *46*, 181–190. [CrossRef] [PubMed]
139. Sakurauchi, Y.; Matsumoto, Y.; Shinzato, T.; Takai, I.; Nakamura, Y.; Sato, M.; Nakai, S.; Miwa, M.; Morita, H.; Miwa, T.; et al. Effects of L-carnitine supplementation on muscular symptoms in hemodialyzed patients. *Am. J. Kidney Dis.* **1998**, *32*, 258–264. [CrossRef] [PubMed]
140. Bellinghieri, G.; Savica, V.; Mallamace, A.; Di Stefano, C.; Consolo, F.; Spagnoli, L.G.; Villaschi, S.; Palmieri, G.; Corsi, M.; Maccari, F. Correlation between increased serum and tissue L-carnitine levels and improved muscle symptoms in hemodialyzed patients. *Am. J. Clin. Nutr.* **1983**, *38*, 523–531. [CrossRef]
141. Siami, G.; Clinton, M.E.; Mrak, R.; Griffis, J.; Stone, W. Evaluation of the effect of intravenous L-carnitine therapy on function, structure and fatty acid metabolism of skeletal muscle in patients receiving chronic hemodialysis. *Nephron* **1991**, *57*, 306–313. [CrossRef] [PubMed]
142. Maruyama, T.; Maruyama, N.; Higuchi, T.; Nagura, C.; Takashima, H.; Kitai, M.; Utsunomiya, K.; Tei, R.; Furukawa, T.; Yamazaki, T.; et al. Efficacy of L-carnitine supplementation for improving lean body mass and physical function in patients on hemodialysis: A randomized controlled trial. *Eur. J. Clin. Nutr.* **2019**, *73*, 293–301. [CrossRef] [PubMed]
143. Sloan, R.S.; Kastan, B.; Rice, S.I.; Sallee, C.W.; Yuenger, N.J.; Smith, B.; Ward, R.A.; Brier, M.E.; Golper, T.A. Quality of life during and between hemodialysis treatments: Role of L-carnitine supplementation. *Am. J. Kidney Dis.* **1998**, *32*, 265–272. [CrossRef] [PubMed]

144. Rogerson, M.E.; Rylance, P.B.; Wilson, R.; De Sousa, C.; Lanigan, C.; Rose, P.E.; Howard, J.; Parsons, V. Carnitine and weakness in haemodialysis patients. *Nephrol. Dial. Transplant.* **1989**, *4*, 366–371. [CrossRef] [PubMed]
145. Giovenali, P.; Fenocchio, D.; Montanari, G.; Cancellotti, C.; D'Iddio, S.; Buoncristiani, U.; Pelagaggia, M.; Ribacchi, R. Selective trophic effect of L-carnitine in type I and IIa skeletal muscle fibers. *Kidney Int.* **1994**, *46*, 1616–1619. [CrossRef] [PubMed]
146. Feinfeld, D.A.; Kurian, P.; Cheng, J.T.; Dilimetin, G.; Arriola, M.R.; Ward, L.; Manis, T.; Carvounis, C.P. Effect of oral L-carnitine on serum myoglobin in hemodialysis patients. *Ren. Fail.* **1996**, *18*, 91–96. [CrossRef] [PubMed]
147. Thomas, S.; Fischer, F.P.; Mettang, T.; Pauli-Magnus, C.; Weber, J.; Kuhlmann, U. Effects of L-carnitine on leukocyte function and viability in hemodialysis patients: A double-blind randomized trial. *Am. J. Kidney Dis.* **1999**, *34*, 678–687. [CrossRef]
148. Lynch, K.E.; Feldman, H.I.; Berlin, J.A.; Flory, J.; Rowan, C.G.; Brunelli, S.M. Effects of L-carnitine on dialysis-related hypotension and muscle cramps: A meta-analysis. *Am. J. Kidney Dis.* **2008**, *52*, 962–971. [CrossRef]
149. Shoji, T.; Emoto, M.; Tabata, T.; Kimoto, E.; Shinohara, K.; Maekawa, K.; Kawagishi, T.; Tahara, H.; Ishimura, E.; Nishizawa, Y. Advanced atherosclerosis in predialysis patients with chronic renal failure. *Kidney Int.* **2002**, *61*, 2187–2192. [CrossRef]
150. Shoji, T.; Masakane, I.; Watanabe, Y.; Iseki, K.; Tsubakihara, Y. Elevated non-high-density lipoprotein cholesterol (non-HDL-C) predicts atherosclerotic cardiovascular events in hemodialysis patients. *Clin. J. Am. Soc. Nephrol.* **2011**, *6*, 1112–1120. [CrossRef]
151. Kidney Disease Outcomes Quality Initiative (K/DOQI) Group. K/DOQI clinical practice guidelines for management of dyslipidemias in patients with kidney disease. *Am. J. Kidney Dis.* **2003**, *41*, 1–91.
152. Yeun, J.Y.; Levine, R.A.; Mantadilok, V.; Kaysen, G.A. C-Reactive protein predicts all-cause and cardiovascular mortality in hemodialysis patients. *Am. J. Kidney Dis.* **2000**, *35*, 469–476. [CrossRef]
153. Krane, V.; Wanner, C. Statins, inflammation and kidney disease. *Nat. Rev. Nephrol.* **2011**, *7*, 385–397. [CrossRef]
154. Abe, M.; Hamano, T.; Hoshino, J.; Wada, A.; Nakai, S.; Hanafusa, N.; Masakane, I.; Nitta, K.; Nakamoto, H. Predictors of outcomes in patients on peritoneal dialysis: A 2-year nationwide cohort study. *Sci. Rep.* **2019**, *9*, 3967. [CrossRef]
155. Abe, M.; Hamano, T.; Wada, A.; Nakai, S.; Masakane, I.; Renal Data Registry Committee, Japanese Society for Dialysis Therapy. Effect of dialyzer membrane materials on survival in chronic hemodialysis patients: Results from the annual survey of the Japanese Nationwide Dialysis Registry. *PLoS ONE* **2017**, *12*, e0184424. [CrossRef] [PubMed]
156. Abe, M.; Hamano, T.; Wada, A.; Nakai, S.; Masakane, I. High-performance membrane dialyzers and mortality in hemodialysis patients: A 2-year cohort study from the Annual Survey of the Japanese Renal Data Registry. *Am. J. Nephrol.* **2017**, *46*, 82–92. [CrossRef] [PubMed]
157. Eleftheriadis, T.; Liakopoulos, V.; Antoniadi, G.; Kartsios, C.; Stefanidis, I. The role of hepcidin in iron homeostasis and anemia in hemodialysis patients. *Semin. Dial.* **2009**, *22*, 70–77. [CrossRef]
158. Yu, J.; Ye, J.; Liu, X.; Han, Y.; Wang, C. Protective effect of L-carnitine against H(2)O(2)-induced neurotoxicity in neuroblastoma (SH-SY5Y) cells. *Neurol. Res.* **2011**, *33*, 708–716. [CrossRef] [PubMed]
159. Ribas, G.S.; Biancini, G.B.; Mescka, C.; Wayhs, C.Y.; Sitta, A.; Wajner, M.; Vargas, C.R. Oxidative stress parameters in urine from patients with disorders of propionate metabolism: A beneficial effect of L-carnitine supplementation. *Cell. Mol. Neurobiol.* **2012**, *32*, 77–82. [CrossRef] [PubMed]
160. Biolo, G.; Stulle, M.; Bianco, F.; Mengozzi, G.; Barazzoni, R.; Vasile, A.; Panzetta, G.; Guarnieri, G. Insulin action on glucose and protein metabolism during L-carnitine supplementation in maintenance haemodialysis patients. *Nephrol. Dial. Transplant.* **2008**, *23*, 991–997. [CrossRef]
161. Katalinic, L.; Krtalic, B.; Jelakovic, B.; Basic-Jukic, N. The unexpected effects of L-carnitine supplementation on lipid metabolism in hemodialysis patients. *Kidney Blood Press. Res.* **2018**, *43*, 1113–1120. [CrossRef] [PubMed]
162. Jafari, A.; Khatami, M.R.; Dashti-Khavidaki, S.; Lessan-Pezeshki, M.; Abdollahi, A.; Moghaddas, A. Protective effects of L-carnitine against delayed graft function in kidney transplant recipients: A pilot, randomized, double-blinded, placebo-controlled clinical trial. *J. Ren. Nutr.* **2017**, *27*, 113–126. [CrossRef] [PubMed]
163. Guarnieri, G.F.; Ranieri, F.; Toigo, G.; Vasile, A.; Ciman, M.; Rizzoli, V.; Moracchiello, M.; Campanacci, L. Lipid-lowering effect of carnitine in chronically uremic patients treated with maintenance hemodialysis. *Am. J. Clin. Nutr.* **1980**, *33*, 1489–1492. [CrossRef] [PubMed]
164. Vacha, G.M.; Giorcelli, G.; D'Iddio, S.; Valentini, G.; Bagiella, E.; Procopio, A.; di Donato, S.; Ashbrook, D.; Corsi, M. L-carnitine addition to dialysis fluid. A therapeutic alternative for hemodialysis patients. *Nephron* **1989**, *51*, 237–242. [CrossRef]
165. Bellinghieri, G.; Savica, V.; Barbera, C.M.; Ricciardi, B.; Egitto, M.; Torre, F.; Valentini, G.; D'Iddio, S.; Bagiella, E.; Mallamace, A.; et al. L-carnitine and platelet aggregation in uremic patients subjected to hemodialysis. *Nephron* **1990**, *55*, 28–32. [CrossRef] [PubMed]
166. Sohn, H.J.; Choi, G.B.; Yoon, K.I. L-Carnitine in maintenance hemodialysis clinical lipid and biochemical effects. *Korean J. Nephrol.* **1992**, *2*, 260–268.
167. Yderstraede, K.B.; Pedersen, F.B.; Dragsholt, C.; Trostmann, A.; Laier, E.; Larsen, H.F. The effect of L-carnitine on lipid metabolism in patients on chronic haemodialysis. *Nephrol. Dial. Transplant.* **1987**, *1*, 238–241. [PubMed]
168. Weschler, A.; Aviram, M.; Levin, M.; Better, O.S.; Brook, J.G. High dose of L-carnitine increases platelet aggregation and plasma triglyceride levels in uremic patients on hemodialysis. *Nephron* **1984**, *38*, 120–124. [CrossRef] [PubMed]
169. Signorelli, S.S.; Fatuzzo, P.; Rapisarda, F.; Neri, S.; Ferrante, M.; Oliveri Conti, G.; Fallico, R.; Di Pino, L.; Pennisi, G.; Celotta, G.; et al. A randomised, controlled clinical trial evaluating changes in therapeutic efficacy and oxidative parameters after treatment with propionyl L-carnitine in patients with peripheral arterial disease requiring haemodialysis. *Drugs Aging* **2006**, *23*, 263–270. [CrossRef]

170. Hakeshzadeh, F.; Tabibi, H.; Ahmadinejad, M.; Malakoutian, T.; Hedayati, M. Effects of L-Carnitine supplement on plasma coagulation and anticoagulation factors in hemodialysis patients. *Ren. Fail.* **2010**, *32*, 1109–1114. [CrossRef]
171. Tabibi, H.; Hakeshzadeh, F.; Hedayati, M.; Malakoutian, T. Effects of l-carnitine supplement on serum amyloid A and vascular inflammation markers in hemodialysis patients: A randomized controlled trial. *J. Ren. Nutr.* **2011**, *21*, 485–491. [CrossRef]
172. Ahmadi, S.; Banadaki, S.D.; Mozaffari-Khosravi, H. Effects of oral L-carnitine supplementation on leptin and adiponectin levels and body weight of hemodialysis patients: A randomized clinical trial. *Iran. J. Kidney. Dis.* **2016**, *10*, 144–150. [PubMed]
173. Alattiya, T.N.; Jaleel, N.A.; Al-Sabbag, M.S.; Jamil, N.S.; Mohammed, M.M. Effect of oral L-carnitine supplementation on the mortality markers in hemodialysis patients. *Int. J. Pharm. Sci. Rev. Res.* **2016**, *14*, 64–69.
174. Yang, S.K.; Xiao, L.; Song, P.A.; Xu, X.; Liu, F.Y.; Sun, L. Effect of L-carnitine therapy on patients in maintenance hemodialysis: A systematic review and meta-analysis. *J. Nephrol.* **2014**, *27*, 317–329. [CrossRef]
175. Huang, H.; Song, L.; Zhang, H.; Zhang, H.; Zhang, J.; Zhao, W. Influence of L-carnitine supplementation on serum lipid profile in hemodialysis patients: A systematic review and meta-analysis. *Kidney Blood Press Res.* **2013**, *38*, 31–41. [CrossRef]
176. Chen, Y.; Abbate, M.; Tang, L.; Cai, G.; Gong, Z.; Wei, R.; Zhou, J.; Chen, X. L-Carnitine supplementation for adults with end-stage kidney disease requiring maintenance hemodialysis: A systematic review and meta-analysis. *Am. J. Clin. Nutr.* **2014**, *99*, 408–422. [CrossRef]
177. Zhou, J.; Yang, T. The efficacy of L-carnitine in improving malnutrition in patients on maintenance hemodialysis: A meta-analysis. *Biosci. Rep.* **2020**, *40*, BSR20201639. [CrossRef] [PubMed]

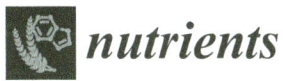

Review

Association of Zinc Deficiency with Development of CVD Events in Patients with CKD

Shinya Nakatani [1], Katsuhito Mori [2,*], Tetsuo Shoji [3,4] and Masanori Emoto [1,2,4]

1. Department of Metabolism, Endocrinology and Molecular Medicine, Osaka City University Graduate School of Medicine, 1-4-3 Asahi-machi, Abeno-ku, Osaka 545-8585, Japan; m2026719@med.osaka-cu.ac.jp (S.N.); memoto@med.osaka-cu.ac.jp (M.E.)
2. Department of Nephrology, Osaka City University Graduate School of Medicine, 1-4-3 Asahi-machi, Abeno-ku, Osaka 545-8585, Japan
3. Department of Vascular Medicine, Osaka City University Graduate School of Medicine, 1-4-3 Asahi-machi, Abeno-ku, Osaka 545-8585, Japan; t-shoji@med.osaka-cu.ac.jp
4. Vascular Science Center for Translational Research, Osaka City University Graduate School of Medicine, 1-4-3 Asahi-machi, Abeno-ku, Osaka 545-8585, Japan
* Correspondence: ktmori@med.osaka-cu.ac.jp; Tel.: +81-666-045-3806; Fax: +81-666-453-808

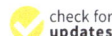

Citation: Nakatani, S.; Mori, K.; Shoji, T.; Emoto, M. Association of Zinc Deficiency with Development of CVD Events in Patients with CKD. Nutrients 2021, 13, 1680. https://doi.org/10.3390/nu13051680

Academic Editor: Pietro Manuel Ferraro

Received: 25 March 2021
Accepted: 11 May 2021
Published: 15 May 2021

Publisher's Note: MDPI stays neutral with regard to jurisdictional claims in published maps and institutional affiliations.

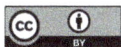

Copyright: © 2021 by the authors. Licensee MDPI, Basel, Switzerland. This article is an open access article distributed under the terms and conditions of the Creative Commons Attribution (CC BY) license (https://creativecommons.org/licenses/by/4.0/).

Abstract: Deficiency of the micronutrient zinc is common in patients with chronic kidney disease (CKD). The aim of this review is to summarize evidence presented in literature for consolidation of current knowledge regarding zinc status in CKD patients, including those undergoing hemodialysis. Zinc deficiency is known to be associated with various risk factors for cardiovascular disease (CVD), such as increased blood pressure, dyslipidemia, type 2 diabetes mellitus, inflammation, and oxidative stress. Zinc may protect against phosphate-induced arterial calcification by suppressing activation of nuclear factor kappa light chain enhancer of activated B. Serum zinc levels have been shown to be positively correlated with T_{50} (shorter T_{50} indicates higher calcification propensity) in patients with type 2 diabetes mellitus as well as those with CKD. Additionally, higher intake of dietary zinc was associated with a lower risk of severe abdominal aortic calcification. In hemodialysis patients, the beneficial effects of zinc supplementation in relation to serum zinc and oxidative stress levels was demonstrated in a meta-analysis of 15 randomized controlled trials. Thus, evidence presented supports important roles of zinc regarding antioxidative stress and suppression of calcification and indicates that zinc intake/supplementation may help to ameliorate CVD risk factors in CKD patients.

Keywords: zinc; hemodialysis; chronic kidney disease; cardiovascular disease

1. Introduction

The micronutrient zinc is an essential trace element and the second most abundant divalent cation in the body (2–4 g), with approximately 57% existing in skeletal muscle and 29% in bone [1]. Inadequate intake, decreased absorption, and/or increased loss of zinc can result in a deficiency. Zinc deficiency is common throughout the world and affects over two billion people [2]. In patients with chronic kidney disease (CKD), several previous studies have demonstrated lower blood zinc levels, with the prevalence of zinc deficiency ranging from 40% to 78% in those undergoing hemodialysis [3,4].

Zinc plays important roles in various biochemical pathways, including as a cofactor with >300 enzymes. Additionally, zinc is involved in structural integrity maintenance, basic cellular functions such as proliferation, DNA and RNA synthesis, control of the expression of several genes, and regulation of the immune functions of many types of cells [5,6]. In previous reports, zinc deficiency has been shown to be associated with growth disturbance [7,8], taste impairment [9], anorexia and loss of appetite [10], dermatitis [11], delayed wound healing [12], and infection [13]. Zinc is also essential in an active site of superoxide dismutase (SOD), an important antioxidant enzyme that catalyzes the dismutation of superoxide [14]. Furthermore, treatment with zinc has been found to attenuate reactive oxygen species (ROS) production [15].

In a recent in vitro study, zinc attenuated phosphate-induced osteochondrogenic phenotypic switch of vasculature smooth muscle cells (VSMCs) leading to development of vascular calcification [16]. Additionally, an in vivo study demonstrated that zinc can protect against phosphate-induced arterial calcification by inducing production of a zinc-finger protein, tumor necrosis factor (TNF)-a-induced protein 3 (TNFAIP3), and suppressing activation of nuclear factor kappa-light-chain-enhancer of activated B (NF-k B) [17].

Cardiovascular disease (CVD) is the leading cause of morbidity and mortality throughout the world [18–20]. Furthermore, vascular calcification is a striking feature of chronic inflammatory diseases including CKD and has been shown to be associated with increased risk of CVD events [18,20]. An in vitro test (T_{50}-test) for determination of serum calcification propensity has been developed [21], as that has been shown to be a novel surrogate marker of CVD events [22]. A shorter T_{50} means a higher calcification propensity [21]. In other studies, serum zinc levels were found to be positively correlated with T_{50} in patients with type 2 diabetes mellitus [23] and CKD [17], and higher intake of dietary zinc was independently associated with lower risk of severe abdominal aortic calcification (AAC) in noninstitutionalized adults in the United States [24]. Indeed, several cohort studies have shown that low zinc intake is associated with cardiovascular mortality [25,26].

Given the importance of zinc regarding both attenuating antioxidative stress and suppressing calcification, it is not surprising that accumulated evidence suggests an association of zinc deficiency with the development of CVD events in patients with CKD, especially those undergoing hemodialysis. The aim of this review is to summarize results presented in literature so as to consolidate current knowledge regarding zinc status, including zinc status in patients affected by CKD and receiving hemodialysis treatments.

2. Zinc and Nutrition

The daily requirement of zinc for adults throughout the world ranges from 7 to 11 mg [27]. In Japan, the recommended dietary intake (RDI) of zinc for adults is 9–10 mg/day for males and 7–8 mg/day for females [28], although intake is insufficient in 60–70% of both genders aged over 20 years [29]. Additionally, zinc intake was found to be lower in patients with advanced stage CKD as compared with those without advanced stage CKD who participated in the National Health and Nutrition Examination Survey conducted in the United States [24].

Meats as well as oysters and scallops contain abundant zinc [30], while some cereals and Japanese foods, including tofu, rice, and fermented soybeans (*natto*), also have large amounts [29]. Generally, red meat contains more zinc than white meat and fish [30]. It is also known that leaf vegetables and fruits have low zinc concentrations, along with high water and potassium content [31]; thus, patients undergoing hemodialysis must be careful regarding their overconsumption so as to avoid hyperkalemia and volume overload.

It is important to recognize that the content of zinc in food (nutrients) is not necessarily identical with its availability [30,32]. For example, the availability of zinc present in peas, lentils, and beans is limited because it is released during milling [30]. In addition, food components, such as phytate [27], casein [27,31], and fiber, as well as higher calcium concentrations are known to impair zinc absorption [33]. Phytate forms insoluble complexes with zinc in the intestines [27,34], which then hinder its absorption and bioavailability; consequently, zinc absorption is reduced in intestinal cells [35]. It is very likely that the absorption-inhibiting effects of fiber and higher calcium concentrations are also due to the phytate they contain [33]. Methods used for processing, such as grinding, soaking, germination, malting, and/or fermentation, can reduce the phytate content of foods and thus its protective effect in regard to absorption of zinc [31]. Furthermore, various organic acids including citric acid (citrus fruits) and lactic acid (sour milk) as well as fruit acid bind to zinc and increase its absorption [31].

3. Zinc Deficiency in CKD

Reduced levels of zinc in serum or plasma of patients with CKD have been demonstrated (Table 1). Several factors may contribute to and explain zinc deficiency seen in association with CKD. Some studies have demonstrated a negative zinc balance in CKD patients [36,37]. This may be due to decreased intestinal absorption, decreased food intake, uremic toxicity, bioavailability, and/or increased loss, such as through the face, urine, or hemodialysis. It is also important to note that many CKD patients are elderly and using multiple medications that can affect taste sensation and increase zinc deficiency [38]. In a recent study by Chen et al., 5/6 nephrectomized rats as well as phenylhydrazine-induced anemic mice were found to have zinc redistributed to bone marrow from bone and plasma, causing the zinc level in plasma to decrease, which produced reticulocytes [39]. Their novel findings of pools of zinc in plasma and bone redistributed to bone marrow in the majority of those nephrectomized rats indicate the mechanism of zinc deficiency in CKD.

Table 1. Summary of observational studies regarding zinc deficiency in patients with CKD.

Author, Year [30]	Country	Number of CKD/HD Patients	Number of Healthy Subjects	Sample	Zinc level, CKD vs. Control †
CKD					
Tavares et al. 2020 [40]	Brazil	21	22	Plasma	70.1 ± 19.2 vs. 123.2 ± 24.6 (µg/dL)
Shen et al. 2020 [41]	China	193	173	Plasma	188 vs. 229 (µg/dL)
Damianaki et al. 2020 [42]	Switzerland	108	42	Plasma	60.6 ± 10.6 vs. 66.4 ± 10.1 (µg/dL)
Pan et al. 2019 [43]	Taiwan	204	2853	Serum	76.9 ± 1.29 vs. 82.8 ± 0.67 (µg/dL)
Aziz et al. 2016 [44]	Iraq	49	42	Plasma	83 ± 10 vs. 112 ± 19 (µg/dL)
Mafra et al. 2002 [45]	Brazil	29	19	Plasma	74 ± 17.7 vs. 82.1 ± 15.5 (µg/dL)
HD					
Hasanato 2014 [46]	Saudi Arabia	42	18	Plasma	9.5 vs. 13.2 (nmol/L)
Lobo et al. 2013 [47]	Brazil	45	20	Plasma	54.9 ± 16.1 vs. 78.8 ± 9.4 (µg/dL)
Guo et al. 2011 [48]	Taiwan	20	20	Plasma	68 ± 3 vs. 76 ± 8 (µg/L)
Dashti-Khavidaki et al. 2010 [49]	Iran	94	47	Serum	69.2 ± 17.3 vs. 82.9 ± 14.8 (µg/dL)
Kiziltas et al. 2008 [50]	Turkey	30	30	Serum	15.7 ± 1.25 vs. 21.2 ± 1.44 (µmol/L)
Batista et al. 2006 [51]	Brazil	30	20	Plasma	81.2 ± 19.8 vs. 93.3 ± 12.1 (µg/dL)

† Zinc level values are shown as the mean ± standard deviation. Abbreviations: CKD, chronic kidney disease; HD, hemodialysis.

3.1. Urinary Zinc Excretion in CKD

Due to the fact that zinc is bound to proteins in plasma [52], it is generally believed that glomerular filtration of zinc and consecutive urinary zinc excretion are limited [1]. However, Damianaki et al. recently found that urinary zinc excretion was significantly higher in CKD patients (612.4 ± 425.9 µg/24 h) (n = 108) as compared with non-CKD patients with preserved kidney function (479.2 ± 293.0 µg/24 h) (n = 81) (p = 0.02) [42]. That study also noted that zinc fractional excretion was stable in the early stage of CKD, then a sudden and strong increase was seen in stage 3 patients, while that was correlated negatively and linearly with estimated glomerular filtration rate (eGFR). Although the mechanism related to increased fractional excretion of zinc in CKD patients remains unclear, increased urinary zinc excretion has been shown to be linked to tubular dysfunction in patients with cancer [53], type 1 diabetes mellitus [54], and type 2 diabetes mellitus [55], possibly due to impaired tubular activity. In the study presented by Damianaki et al., zinc fractional excretion was correlated negatively with 24 h urinary uromodulin excretion (r = 0.29; p < 0.01) [42]. Uromodulin, a protein produced by tubular cells of the ascending loops of Henle, was recently identified as a marker of tubular mass and function in the general population [56]. The negative correlation between urinary uromodulin excretion and fractional excretion of zinc suggests that urinary zinc loss may be linked to the low number of functional tubules associated with CKD.

3.2. Taste Change Associated with CKD

Many CKD patients are elderly and using multiple medications that can affect taste sensations and increase zinc deficiency [38]. Taste change has been reported by 40–60% of pre-dialysis CKD [57] and hemodialysis [58,59] patients, with taste changes of "bland" and "bitter" found to be associated with upper gastrointestinal symptoms, including nausea, vomiting, anorexia, and malnutrition [59].

In addition, taste change is one of the major symptoms of zinc deficiency [29]. There are roughly 7000 taste buds, peripheral receptors of taste, present in the oral cavity, pharynx, and larynx, with a particularly high concentration in lingual papillae on the tongue surface [29]. In findings obtained with an in vivo zinc-deficient model, microstructural abnormalities including microvilli rupture and vacuolation were shown in taste cells [60]. Taste cell differentiation from basal cells is also impaired when zinc deficiency is present [61], and an in vitro study demonstrated that reduced expression of bitter taste receptors was the result of that deficiency [62]. Furthermore, several reports have noted recovery of taste change by treatment with various forms of zinc, such as zinc gluconate [63,64], zinc picolinate [65], and polaprezinc [66]. Additional studies are needed to investigate whether recovery of taste change by use of these medications has effects on clinical hard endpoints such as CVD events or mortality.

3.3. Albumin and Zinc in CKD

Zinc is actively absorbed throughout the small intestine, and in circulation, zinc is present predominantly as being bound to proteins such as albumin, α-macroglobulin, and transferrin, with approximately 60–80% of zinc in serum bound to albumin [67,68]. Patients undergoing hemodialysis often show low serum albumin along with chronic malnutrition. Because albumin is the primary carrier protein for circulating zinc [69], hypoalbuminemia should be considered as another confounding factor in interpreting plasma zinc concentration.

3.4. Other Factors of Zinc Deficiency in CKD

Several hypotheses related to low zinc levels in CKD patients have been proposed, such as low dietary intake due to protein restriction and decreased gastrointestinal absorption of dietary zinc due to impairment of formation of 1.25-dihydroxycholecalciferol or drug interactions [70,71]. Indeed, zinc intake has been shown to be lower in patients with advanced stage CKD [24]. In addition, phosphate binding decreases zinc absorption [72]. Physicians should pay careful attention to possible effects on plasma zinc levels when they start protein restriction and use phosphate binder medication in the management of patients with CKD.

4. Vascular Calcification and CVD in CKD

One of the most characteristic features of vascular change seen in dialysis patients is vascular calcification, which is associated with several types of target organ damage, including stroke, ischemic heart disease, and peripheral arterial disease. Gorriz et al. demonstrated that vascular calcification is a predictor of cardiovascular death in patients with varying CKD stages before starting dialysis [19].

CVD events are well known to increase as kidney function declines. The largest population-based study, conducted by Go et al. with 1,120,295 adult subjects, revealed that the adjusted hazard ratio (HR) for CVD events was inversely associated with eGFR, with an HR of 1.4 for subjects with an eGFR of 45–59 mL/min/1.73 m^2, 2.0 for those with an eGFR of 30–44 mL/min/1.73 m^2, 2.8 for those with an eGFR of 15–29 mL/min/per1.73 m^2, and 3.4 for those with an eGFR <15 mL/min/1.73 m^2 [73]. Additionally, adjusted risk of hospitalization and mortality followed a similar pattern. A collaborative meta-analysis of 10 cohorts with a total of 266,975 patients performed by van der Velde et al. revealed a similar trend showing a relationship of CVD mortality with eGFR [74].

5. Vascular Calcification and Vascular Smooth Muscle Cells

The pathophysiology of vascular calcification in CKD patients involves several factors, including changes related to oxidative stress, inflammation, imbalance between calcification promoters and inhibitors, and extracellular matrix metabolism, as well as calcium and phosphate metabolism imbalances [75,76].

5.1. Vascular Smooth Muscle Cells

Excess CVD morbidity and mortality in CKD patients might be explained by redistribution and/or overload of calcium and phosphorus. The primary mechanism of vascular calcification is considered to be related to ectopic deposition of hydroxyapatite [77] induced by an increase in calcium–phosphorus product (Ca $\times$ P) in serum [78]. VSMCs play a pivotal tool for investigation of vascular calcification [79]. Previous studies have reported transdifferentiation of VSMCs into osteoblast-like cells [80,81]. Bone morphogenetic protein-2 (BMP-2), oxidized lipids, and inflammation are known to accelerate vascular calcification [82], whereas matrix Gla protein (MGP), osteoprotegerin, and osteopontin act on the vascular wall as calcification inhibitors [83]. A recent work focused on runt-related transcription factor 2 (Runx2), an essential transcriptional factor for osteogenesis, and reported that Runx2 appears to be involved in repression of the primary VSMC phenotype, in addition to acceleration of the osteogenic phenotype [84]. Phenotypical transdifferentiation of VSMCs is regulated by complex signaling pathways [85] that are linked to generalized inflammation and dependent, at least in part, on the transcription factor NF-kB, which has emerged as a key regulator of vascular calcification [86].

5.2. Zinc Inhibits Phosphate-Induced VSMC Calcification

Some recently presented studies reported that zinc plays an important role in inhibition of calcification using VSMCs. Zinc sulfate blunted phosphate-induced calcification and decreased messenger RNA expression by osteogenic markers including TNFAIP3 expression, which subsequently was shown to inhibit NF-kB activation and osteo-/chondrogenic reprograming, resulting in suppression of phosphate-induced calcification of VSMCs [17] (Figure 1).

Hypoxia-inducible factor (HIF) stabilizers, also known as HIF prolyl hydroxylase inhibitors (PHI), are promising candidates for treatment of CKD-associated anemia as they increase erythropoietin synthesis [87,88]. Moreover, recent findings suggest that HIFs also play a pivotal role in vascular calcification [89,90]. Indeed, FG4592, an orally bioavailable PHI, promoted phosphate-induced loss of smooth muscle cell markers (ACTA-2, MYH11, SM22a) and enhanced osteochondrogenic gene expression (Msx-2, BMP-2, Sp7), thus triggering an osteochondrogenic phenotypic switch by VSMCs [16]. These effects of PHI occurred in parallel with increased pyruvate dehydrogenase kinase 4 (PDK4) expression. Additionally, zinc was shown to inhibit an osteochondrogenic phenotypic switch of VSMCs, reflected by lowered phosphate uptake, which resulted in decreased expressions of Msx-2, BMP-2, and Sp7, as well as loss of smooth muscle cell specific markers. That previous study [16] also found that zinc preserved the phosphorylation state of Runx2, decreased PDK4 level, and restored cell viability, suggesting that it inhibits PHI aggravated by VSMC calcification induced by a high phosphate level (Figure 1). Clinical trials are needed to examine whether zinc supplementation attenuates aortic calcification and CVD events in CKD patients with high phosphate overload or treated with PHI.

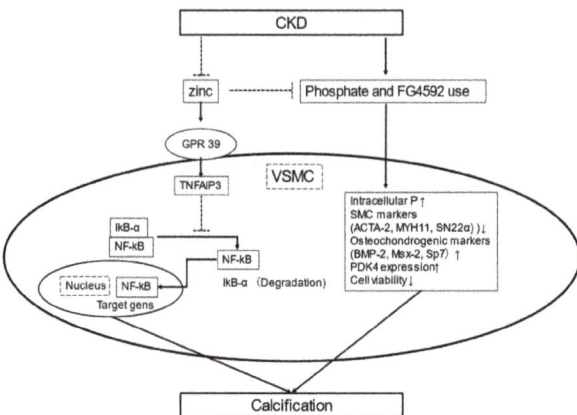

Figure 1. Schematic illustration of zinc and calcification. CKD induces hypozincemia and hyperphosphatemia. Zinc supplementation may increase zinc finger protein TNFAIP3 levels by upregulating zinc-sensing receptor ZnR/GPR39-dependent TNFAIP3 gene expression. Increased TNFAIP3 inhibits NF-kB activation and osteo-/chondrogenic reprograming, resulting in suppression of phosphate-induced VSMC calcification [17]. FG4592, an orally bioavailable PHI, promotes phosphate uptake in VSMCs and phosphate-induced loss of smooth muscle cell markers (ACTA-2, MYH11, SM22a) and also enhances osteochondrogenic gene expression (Msx-2, BMP-2, Sp7). Zinc inhibits FG4592-aggravated calcification caused by high phosphate by maintaining the VSMC phenotype, decreasing phosphate uptake, and lowering osteochondrogenic gene expression and levels of PDK4, as well as preserving Runx2 phosphorylation and cell variability [16]. Abbreviations: ACTA-2, smooth muscle a-2 actin; BMP-2, bone morphogenic protein-2; CKD, chronic kidney disease; NF-kB, nuclear factor kappa light chain enhancer of activated B; Msx-2, Msh Homeobox 2; MYH11, smooth muscle myosin heavy chain 11; PDK4, pyruvate dehydrogenase kinase 4; PHI, prolyl hydroxylase inhibitors; Runx2, runt-related transcription factor 2; TNFAIP3, TNFa-induced protein 3; VSMCs; vasculature smooth muscle cells.

6. Zinc and Calcification Propensity in Serum

6.1. Serum Calcification Propensity (T_{50})

In serum, precipitation of supersaturated calcium and phosphate is prevented by formation of amorphous primary calciprotein particles [91,92]. Primary calciprotein particles spontaneously convert into secondary calciprotein particles that contain crystalline hydroxyapatite [91,92]. The propensity for transformation to secondary calciprotein particles can be assessed by determining the time required to transform into secondary calciprotein particles, termed serum calcification propensity or T_{50}, and an in vitro test (T_{50}-test) has been developed for determination of serum calcification propensity [21]. This assay determines the time required for primary calciprotein particles to transform into secondary calciprotein particles in the presence of supersaturating doses of calcium and phosphate, resulting in increased turbidity of the samples. Serum T_{50} can be examined by laser light scatter in turbid samples using nephelometry and a shorter T_{50} time means a higher calcification propensity. Studies have shown that lower T_{50} predicts vascular stiffness progression and all-cause mortality in patients with stage 3 or 4 CKD [22], as well as all-cause mortality and cardiovascular composite endpoint in hemodialysis patients [93]. A lower T_{50} level was also shown to predict cardiovascular and all-cause mortality in renal transplant recipients [94,95]. While it remains unclear how well in vitro T_{50} assay results represent the mineralization process in vivo, the mineralization process has been shown to be associated with arterial calcification, arterial stiffness, cardiovascular outcomes, and mortality in at least 18 observational and 11 interventional studies [96]. Thus, T_{50} may be useful as a surrogate marker of calcification stress which is closely associated with CVD risk in CKD.

6.2. Association of Zinc and Serum Calcification Propensity

A cross-sectional study of 132 type 2 diabetes mellitus patients with various levels of kidney function showed a weak but positive correlation of serum zinc with T_{50} [23], while another study that included healthy subjects and patients with CKD also reported a positive correlation [17]. Furthermore, in vitro experiments demonstrated that addition of a physiological concentration of exogenous zinc chloride significantly increased serum T_{50}. Together, these findings indicate that serum zinc is an independent factor with a potential role in suppression of calcification propensity in serum [23].

7. Zinc and Vascular Change

7.1. Zinc and Abdominal Aortic Calcification

AAC is common in CKD cases and is known to be an independent predictor of cardiovascular mortality in both the general population and CKD patients [97,98]. Recently, Chen et al. showed that high dietary zinc intake was independently associated with lower risk of severe AAC in non-institutionalized adults in the United States (n = 2535) [24]. In that study, 18.1% of the subjects were CKD patients, and higher zinc intake in those was associated with reduced risk of severe AAC after adjustment for age, gender, and ethnicity, while no association between zinc intake and AAC was found in the fully adjusted model. However, that lack of association might have been due to the low statistical power due to the small sample size.

7.2. Zinc and Carotid Intima-Media Thickness

Carotid intima-media thickness (CIMT) is a valuable marker of subclinical atherosclerosis [99]. In a study that included middle-aged and elderly subjects, the low zinc intake group showed a greater CIMT than the high zinc intake group [100]. A reduced serum zinc level is also associated with increased CIMT in patients receiving hemodialysis [101]. To clarify the effects of zinc intake and/or supplementation for AAC and/or CIMT, further studies focused on advanced CKD stage are necessary.

8. Zinc Deficiency and Risk Factors for CVD

Zinc deficiency is also associated with various risk factors related to CVD events, such as high blood pressure, dyslipidemia, type 2 diabetes mellitus, inflammation, and oxidative stress (Figure 2).

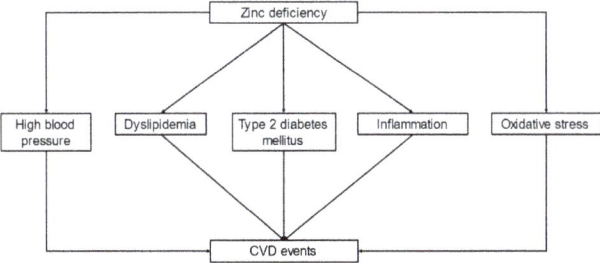

Figure 2. Association of zinc deficiency. Zinc deficiency is associated with major risk factors for CVD, including higher blood pressure, dyslipidemia, type 2 diabetes mellitus, inflammation, and oxidative stress. Zinc deficiency is associated with CVD events in CKD patients, including those undergoing hemodialysis. Abbreviations: CKD, chronic kidney disease; CVD, cardio vascular disease.

8.1. Zinc Deficiency and Blood Pressure

Zinc is also known to be involved in arterial pressure regulation. In salt-sensitive hypertensive model rats, plasma zinc levels were found to be reduced [102]. Additionally, in spontaneous hypertension-prone rats, dietary zinc restriction exacerbated systolic blood pressure [102], whereas zinc supplementation attenuated blood pressure response [103].

Of interest, Williams et al. revealed a possible mechanism of zinc related to blood pressure regulation, as an Na^+-Cl^- cotransporter (NCC) was found to be a zinc-regulated transporter upregulated in mice with zinc deficiency, and NCC upregulation contributed to increased blood pressure by stimulating renal sodium reabsorption [104]. In human studies, it has been reported that populations with low dietary zinc intake have a high prevalence of hypertension, and a possible inverse correlation between zinc levels and blood pressure has also been noted [105,106].

8.2. Zinc Deficiency and Dyslipidemia

Animal studies have demonstrated profound effects of zinc deficiency on the cell structure of the aorta, as well as fatty acids and carbohydrate metabolism, which are disadvantageous for maintaining vascular health [107]. In low-density lipoprotein (LDL) receptor knock-out mice, acute zinc deficiency elicited changes in key transcription factors and adhesion molecules found to be pro-atherogenic [108]. In addition, zinc is a cofactor for desaturases and elongases involved in endogenous fatty acid synthesis [109,110]; thus, an alteration in its plasma level may influence the activities of these enzymes and consequently regulation of fatty acid metabolism.

A systematic review and meta-analysis of 24 studies that included 14,515 subjects showed favorable effects of zinc supplementation on lipid parameters [111]. It was found that zinc supplementation (average 39.3 mg/day) achieved a significant reduction in LDL cholesterol (-4.78 mg/dL) and total cholesterol (-10.72 mg/dL), as well as triglycerides (-8.73 mg/dL). Hypercholesterolemia and hypertriglyceridemia have been reported in previous studies that used a zinc-deficient diet, which might induce CVD events and insulin resistance in CKD patients [112,113], while others have suggested that zinc supplementation improves blood lipid metabolism in hemodialysis patients [114,115]. More evidence is needed to better understand the effects of zinc supplementation on the lipid profile of patients undergoing hemodialysis.

8.3. Zinc Deficiency and Type 2 Diabetes

Zinc deficiency is also an important risk factor in regard to type 2 diabetes mellitus [116,117]. Although the mechanism by which zinc may have an impact on risk of type 2 diabetes mellitus development has not been completely elucidated, zinc is known to participate in adequate insulin synthesis, storage, crystallization, and secretion in pancreatic β-cells, as well as be involved in the action and translocation of insulin into cells [118,119]. In addition, zinc apparently has a role in insulin sensitivity via activation of the phosphoinositol-3-kinase/protein kinase B cascade [119]. Due to its insulin–mimetic action, zinc also stimulates glucose uptake in insulin-dependent tissues [120].

Regarding zinc intake, a systematic review and meta-analysis of prior cohort showed that a moderately high dietary zinc intake in relation to the dietary recommended intake values was associated with a lower risk of type 2 diabetes mellitus by 13%, and it was associated with 41% lower risk in subjects living in rural areas [121]. A randomized controlled trial (RCT) also showed that zinc supplementation improved glucose metabolism and insulin sensitivity in diabetic patients [122]. Nevertheless, additional evidence is needed to clarify the effects of zinc intake and/or supplementation on glucose metabolism, as well as the association between blood zinc status and glycemic status in patients undergoing hemodialysis.

8.4. Zinc Deficiency and Inflammation

Inflammation is another major risk factor that contributes to the pathological process of CVD. Zinc is well known to be essential for normal functions of the immune system in both innate and adaptive immunity responses to pathogens or tissue damage [123]. NF-κB, a transcription factor and key modulator in inflammatory response pathways [124], has an ability to enter the nucleus and induce expression of targeted genes. NF-κB-regulated genes include a variety of inflammatory cytokines, such as interleukin-1 (IL-1), IL-6, TNF-α, lymphotoxin, and interferon-γ (IFN-γ) [123]. Dietary zinc deficiency and intracellular zinc deprivation have been shown to result in increased activation of NF-κB, as well as inflammatory cytokine expression in cultured cells and animal models regulated by NF-κB [125,126]. Supplementation with zinc might also suppress NF-κB activation and NF-κB-regulated inflammatory cytokine release [127].

Furthermore, in a calcification model with klotho-hypomorphic, subtotal nephrectomy, and cholecalciferol overload mice, zinc sulfate supplementation was found to increase aortic expression of the zinc finger proteinTNFAIP3, which is a suppressor of the NF-kB transcription factor pathway and which is reused when NF-κB is suppressed [17]. Supplementation with zinc may suppress NF-κB activation and NF-κB-regulated inflammatory cytokine release, as well as aortic calcification, likely by inhibiting phosphorylation and degradation of IκB and increasing TNFAIP3.

Mousavi et al. (2018) showed a significant reduction in circulating C-reactive protein (CRP) level after zinc supplementation and concluded that such supplementation might have a beneficial effect on serum CRP, especially at a dose of 50 mg/day, in adult kidney failure patients [128].

8.5. Zinc Deficiency and Oxidative Stress

Oxidative stress is also a key risk factor that contributes to the development and progression of CVD [129]. Nuclear factor erythroid 2-related factor 2 (Nrf2) is a master transcriptional regulator of genes related to redox status and antioxidant effects [130]. Zinc has been shown to be involved in modulation of Nrf2 [14]. In endothelial cells, zinc positively regulates glutamate cysteine ligase expression by activating and promoting translocation of the transcription factor Nrf2 to the nucleus [131], while it also activates the antioxidant responsive element–Nrf2 pathway in epithelial cells [132]. In human renal tubular cells under diabetic conditions, treatment with zinc significantly increased nuclear expression of Nrf2 [133]. Human studies also showed that CKD patients have downregulation of Nrf2 mRNA expression [134]. In addition, bardoxolone methyl, a potent activator of Nrf2 was shown to increase eGFR in patients with type 2 diabetes mellitus and CKD stage 3 when administered over a 52-week period [135]. Thus, additional RCTs are needed to investigate whether zinc supplementation, such as with bardoxolone methyl, has protective effects on kidney function in CKD patients.

ROS production is increased by zinc deficiency in various cells, such as in mouse 3T3 cells, in human fibroblasts, and in neuronal and epithelial cells [136]. Zinc is also essential in the active site of SOD, an important antioxidant enzyme that catalyzes the dismutation of superoxide. In addition, zinc treatment of human peritoneal mesothelial cells was found to inhibit activation of the nucleotide-binding domain and leucine-rich repeat-containing family, pyrin domain-containing-3 (NLRP3) inflammasome, by attenuating ROS production [15]. Thus, zinc has an important role as an antioxidant agent [14,137]. Together, these results indicate that zinc supplementation may contribute to an increase in Nrf2 expression and SOD synthesis, as well as to an improvement in antioxidant defense, resulting in reduced CVD risk in CKD patients. Further studies are anticipated.

9. Zinc Levels and CVD Events

In a systematic review of prospective cohort studies regarding zinc status and CVD events, Chu et al. found that higher serum zinc level was associated with lower risk of a CVD event [138], especially in vulnerable populations, including individuals with type 2 diabetes mellitus [139] and patients referred for coronary angiography [140]. Only a few studies of hemodialysis patients have been conducted. Recently, Toda et al. prospectively investigated the association of zinc status and CVD events in 142 incident hemodialysis patients [141]. Although all patients undergoing hemodialysis are at risk for a CVD event, this longitudinal study (mean follow-up 2.5 years, 20 cases with CVD events) showed an insignificant association of a lower zinc level with a higher risk of CVD. The relatively small sample size is a limitation of that investigation. To clarify the relationship between serum zinc levels and cardiovascular events in patients with CKD and hemodialysis, studies with a greater number of cases will be necessary.

10. Zinc and CVD Mortality

10.1. Blood Zinc Level and CVD Mortality

We identified and summarized four cohort studies [25,129,131,132] that investigated the association between the level of zinc in blood and CVD mortality (Table 2). Results obtained in two of those showed increased risk in association with lower zinc level [25,140], while the other studies found no such association [142,143]. The subjects examined in the studies that showed increased risk with lower zinc level had increased CVD risk factors at the baseline, such as having been referred for coronary angiography. Thus, future studies that investigate blood zinc levels and CVD-related mortality in populations with increased risk for CVD, including CKD, hemodialysis, and type 2 diabetes mellitus, may provide additional important information. These four studies were conducted in Europe; thus, it will also be necessary to examine other subjects in other regions, as the sources of dietary zinc differ throughout the world.

Table 2. Summary of cohort studies regarding blood zinc levels and CVD mortality.

Author, Year, (Reference)	Country	Number of Subjects	Age (Years) †	Follow-Up Period (years) ‡	Number of CVD Deaths	Association of Lower Blood Zinc Levels with Higher CVD Mortality
Bates et al. 2011 [25]	UK	1054 (general population)	≥65 years old Male: 75.8 ± 6.9 Female: 77.3 ± 7.9	n/a	189	Yes (HR 0.79; 95% CI 0.72–0.87)
Pilz et al. 2009 [140]	Germany	3316 (patients referred for coronary angiopathy)	Male: 62 ± 11 Female: 65 ± 10	7.75	484	Yes (HR 1.10; 95% CI 1.01–1.21) (Reference: high serum zinc group)
Leone et al. 2006 [142]	France	4035 males (general population)	30–60 years old 43 ± 5 (alive) 44 ± 4 (dead)	18 ± 2.9	56	No (RR 0.7; 95% CI 0.3–1.5)
Marniemi et al. 1998 [143]	Finland	344 (general population)	≥65 years old 65–69 (n = 99), 70–74 (n = 98) 75–80 (n = 84), ≥80–(n = 63)	13	142	No (HR 0.77; 95% CI 0.42–1.41)

† Age shown as mean ± standard deviation or range (lower limit, upper limit). ‡ Follow-up period shown as mean or mean ± standard deviation. Abbreviations: CVD, cardiovascular disease; HR, hazard ratio; NA, not available; RR, relatively risk.

10.2. Dietary Zinc Intake and CVD Mortality

General population studies have found that zinc intake is correlated with serum zinc level [144,145]. We investigated and summarized five cohort studies [25,26,146–148] that investigated the association between dietary zinc intake and CVD mortality (Table 3). Four studies showed a decreased risk of mortality in association with greater dietary zinc intake [25,26,135,137]. However, findings in the study showing no such association [147] could be explained, at least in part, by the relatively lower incidence of CVD mortality and adequate dietary zinc intake in those subjects. Higher dietary zinc intake likely has positive effects on CVD mortality. Nevertheless, results showing dietary zinc intake by CKD patients are few; thus, further observational and interventional studies that include those patients are needed.

Table 3. Summary of observational studies regarding zinc intake and CVD mortality.

Author, Year (Reference)	Country	Number of Subjects	Age (Years) †	Follow-Up Period (years) ‡	Number of CVD Deaths	Outcomes
Chen et al. 2019 [146]	USA	30,899	46.9	6.1	945	Adequate nutrient intake of zinc associated with lower CVD mortality (RR = 0.50; 95% CI 0.36–0.71).
Shi et al. 2018 [147]	China	2832	47.1	9.8	70	Dietary zinc intake not related to CVD mortality.
Eshak et al. 2018 [26]	Japan	58,646	40–79	19.3	3388	Higher intake of zinc inversely associated with mortality from coronary heart disease (n = 702) in males; 0.68 (0.58–1.03; p-trend = 0.05) but not females; 1.13 (0.71–1.49; p-trend = 0.61).
Bates et al. 2011 [25]	UK	1054	75.8 ± 6.9 (males) 77.3 ± 7.9 (females)	n/a	189	Plasma zinc associated with vascular disease mortality (HR 0.73; 95% CI 0.61–0.88).
Lee et al. 2005 [148]	USA	34,492	(55–69)	>15	1767	Inverse association of dietary zinc with CVD mortality.

† Age shown as mean ± standard deviation or range (lower limit, upper limit). ‡ Follow-up period shown as mean. Abbreviations: CVD: cardiovascular disease; NA, not available; RR: relatively risk.

To properly interpret previous studies of zinc intake, the various sources must be considered. In Japan, the main dietary source of zinc is rice [149], and higher dietary zinc intake was shown to be associated with lower mortality due to lower incidence of coronary heart disease [26]. In contrast, red meat is the main source of zinc in the United States [24], and a high level of consumption has been reported to be associated with vascular mortality [150], while increased iron load due to meat-derived heme iron intake has been discussed as a potential underlying mechanism [151,152].

11. Zinc and Progression of CKD

Damimanaki et al. assessed the relationship between baseline plasma zinc level and yearly kidney function decline in a cohort with 3-year follow-up data and found a significant association of a lower baseline zinc level with a large decline of kidney function [42]. Furthermore, the association remained statistically significant in multivariable models adjusted for age, gender, diabetes, and arterial hypertension, while it was no longer significant when baseline eGFR or proteinuria were introduced into the model [42]. Unfortunately, the number of subjects was relatively small (n = 108); thus, additional large scale longitudinal observational studies are necessary to clarify the association between blood zinc level and progression of CKD. Additionally, RCTs are needed to determine the effect of zinc supplementation on kidney function in pre-dialysis CKD patients.

12. Zinc Supplementation in Patients with CKD

Table 4 summarizes 17 RCTs [153–155] among which 15 trials were included in a previous systematic review and meta-analysis by Wang et al. [155]. Although the median intervention period was 60 days and the daily dose ~45 mg, zinc supplementation resulted in higher serum zinc, SOD, and dietary protein intake levels and lower levels of CRP and malondialdehyde [155]. In consideration of previously presented RCTs, zinc supplementation greater than 45 mg/day may be necessary to increase the serum zinc level in hemodialysis patients.

Table 4. Summary of RCTs of zinc supplementation in patients with hemodialysis.

Author, Year (Reference)	Country	Number of Subjects	Age (Years) †	Elemental Zinc Dose (mg/day)	Administration Duration (Days)	Outcomes
Escobedo-Monge et al. 2019 [153]	Peru	48 (children)	12.8 ± 4	15/30	365	Increase: BMI (30 mg/day group only)
Kobayashi et al. 2015 [156]	Japan	70	69 ± 10	34	90/180/270/360	Increase: serum zinc Decrease: serum copper, ferritin
El-Shazly et al. 2015 [157]	Egypt	30	13.2 ± 2.1	16.5	90	Increase: serum zinc, BMI Decrease: serum leptin
Tonelli et al. 2015 [154]	Canada	150	62	25 and 50	90 and 180	None
Argani et al. 2014 [114]	Iran	60	(50,60)	90	60	Increase: serum zinc, albumin, hemoglobin, BMI Decrease: serum leptin
Pakfetrat et al. 2013 [158]	Iran	97	51.6 ± 16.8	50	43	Increase: serum zinc Decrease: homocysteine
Mazani et al. 2013 [159]	Iran	65	52.7 ± 12.6	100	60	Increase: serum zinc, GSH, MDA, SOD, TAC
Guo and Wang. 2013 [160]	Taiwan	65	59.7 ± 9.2	11	56	Increase: plasma zinc, albumin, hemoglobin, hematocrit, nPNA, SOD, vitamin C, vitamin E, CD4, D19 Decrease: plasma copper, CRP, MDA INF-b, TNF-α,
Rahimi-Ardabili et al. 2012 [161]	Iran	60	52.7 ± 12.7	100	60	Increase: Apo-AI, HDL-C, PON
Roozbeh et al. 2009 [115]	Iran	53	55.7	45	42	Increase: serum zinc, TC, HDL-C, LDL-C, TG
Rashidi et al. 2009 [162]	Iran	55	57.6	45	42	Increase: serum zinc
Nava-Hernandez and Amato 2005 [163]	Mexico	25	16.6	100	90	n/a
Matson et al. 2003 [164]	UK	15	60 (31–76)	45	42	Not significant
Chevalier et al. 2002 [165]	USA	27	51.9	50	40/90/90	Increase: serum zinc, LDL-C
Candan et al. 2002 [166]	Turkey	34	45.6 (28,64)	20	90	Increase: serum zinc Decrease: lipid peroxidation osmotic fragility
Jern et al. 2000 [167]	USA	14	56.5 (23,80)	45	40/90	Increase: serum zinc, nPNA
Brodersen et al. 1995 [168]	Germany	40	60	60	112	Increase: serum zinc

Note. † Age is shown as mean, mean ± standard deviation, or mean (lower limit, upper limit). Abbreviations: Apo-AI, apolipoprotein AI; BMI, body mass index; Ccr, creatinine clearance rate; CRP, C-reactive protein; ESA, erythropoiesis-stimulating agent; ERI, ESA resistance index; GFR, glomerular filtration rate; GSH, whole blood glutathione peroxidase; HDL-C, high-density lipoprotein cholesterol; IL, interleukin; LDL-C, low-density lipoprotein cholesterol; MDA, malondialdehyde; NA, not available; nPNA, normalized protein equivalent of nitrogen appearance; PON, paraoxonase; SOD, superoxide dismutase; TAC, total antioxidant capacity; TC, total cholesterol; TG, triglyceride; TNF, tumor necrosis factor.

In children with CKD, adequate nutritional status is important for normal growth and development; thus, careful monitoring is essential [169]. The Chronic Kidney Disease in Children study revealed that 7–20% of pediatric CKD patients showed protein-energy wasting [170]. Recently, an RCT was conducted with 48 CKD patients including 33 undergoing hemodialysis to compare the effects of two different doses of zinc supplementation (15 and 30 mg/day) given for 12 months [153]. There was no significant change in mean serum zinc level in children in either group. On the other hand, a small but positive and significant change in body mass as well as normalization of body mass index (BMI) Z-score, hypoalbuminemia, hypozincemia, and high CRP was noted, especially with a dose of 30 mg/day, which suggested that zinc supplementation could be beneficial for nutritional status in children with CKD. Another interventional study of 40 hemodialysis patients aged between 5 and 18 years old and given daily zinc supplementation of 50–100 mg for 90 days found that serum zinc was significantly increased from 53.2 ± 8.15 to 90.75 ± 12.2 μg/dL ($p = 0.001$) [157].

13. Optimal Serum Zinc Level

The optimal level of zinc in serum remains controversial. The American Society for Parenteral and Enteral Nutrition guidelines suggests that trace minerals, including zinc, should be provided to critically ill patients [171]. Additionally, according to the European Society for Clinical Nutrition and Metabolism guidelines, zinc levels should be measured as a part of nutrition screening [172]. The Japanese Practical Guidelines have generally proposed a level > 80 μg/dL as normal zinc status in all individuals [29]. However, a recent nationally representative cross-sectional study that enrolled subjects from participants in the National Health and Nutrition Examination Survey [173] showed that a higher zinc level per every 10 μg/dL was associated with a 1.12-times higher risk for diabetes mellitus and a 1.23-times higher risk for CVD in those with a serum zinc level $\geq$ 100 μg/dL. Furthermore, each 10 μg/dL increase was also associated with a 1.40-fold increase in stroke in participants with a serum zinc level $\geq$120 μg/dL [173]. The mechanisms underlying these relationships are unclear, though it may be important to avoid hyperzincemia in regard to CVD events in the general population. Regarding hemodialysis patients, a recent study recommended a lower level of serum zinc (78.3 μg/dL) because of the potential for copper deficiency [174]. Additional studies are needed to determine the optimal zinc blood level in the general population, as well as in pre-dialysis CKD patients and those receiving hemodialysis treatments.

14. Conclusions

In patients with CKD, zinc deficiency is common and shown by taste change, decreased food intake, and/or increased urinary excretion. Zinc deficiency is also known to be associated with various risk factors for CVD, including increased blood pressure, dyslipidemia, type 2 diabetes mellitus, inflammation, and oxidative stress. Various clinical studies have revealed that zinc intake/supplementation can increase blood zinc levels in patients with CKD. In addition, zinc may prevent phosphate-induced arterial calcification by inducing the production of TNFIAP3 as well as suppressing activation of NF-kB. High-quality prospective cohort studies and RCTs are needed to provide evidence for zinc intake/supplementation as an effective therapeutic tool for preventing CVD events in patients with CKD, including those undergoing hemodialysis.

Author Contributions: S.N. wrote the manuscript. K.M., T.S., and M.E. critically reviewed and corrected all versions of the manuscript. All authors have read and agreed to the published version of the manuscript.

Funding: This research received no external funding.

Institutional Review Board Statement: The study was conducted according to the guidelines of the Declaration of Helsinki.

Informed Consent Statement: Not applicable.

Data Availability Statement: Not applicable.

Acknowledgments: The authors would like to thank Ai Yamada for the secretarial assistance.

Conflicts of Interest: The authors have no conflicts of interest to declare.

Abbreviations

AAC	abdominal aortic calcification
ACTA-2	smooth muscle a-2 actin
BMI	body mass index
BMP2	bone morphogenetic protein-2
CIMT	carotid intima-media thickness
CKD	chronic kidney disease
CRP	C-reactive protein
CVD	cardiovascular disease
eGFR	estimated glomerular rate
HIF	hypoxia-inducible factor
LDL	low-density lipoprotein
MGP	matrix Gla protein
Msx-2	Msh homeobox 2
MYH11	smooth muscle myosin heavy chain 11;
NCC	Na^+-Cl^- cotransporter
NF-k B	nuclear factor kappa light chain enhancer of activated B
NLRP3	nucleotide-binding domain and leucine-rich repeat-containing family, pyrin domain-containing-3
Nrf2	nuclear factor erythroid 2-related factor 2
PDK4	pyruvate dehydrogenase kinase 4
PHI	prolyl hydroxylase inhibitors
RCT	randomized controlled trial
RDI	recommended dietary intake
ROS	reactive oxygen species
Runx2	runt-related transcription factor 2
SOD	chronic kidney disease
T_{50}	serum calcification propensity
TNF	tumor necrosis factor
TNFAIP3	TNFa-induced protein 3
VSMC	vasculature smooth muscle cell

References

1. King, J.C.; Shames, D.M.; Woodhouse, L.R. Zinc homeostasis in humans. *J. Nutr.* **2000**, *130*, 1360S–1366S. [CrossRef] [PubMed]
2. Prasad, A.S. Discovery of human zinc deficiency: 50 years later. *J. Trace Elem. Med. Biol.* **2012**, *26*, 66–69. [CrossRef]
3. Dvornik, S.; Cuk, M.; Racki, S.; Zaputovic, L. Serum zinc concentrations in the maintenance hemodialysis patients. *Coll. Antropol.* **2006**, *30*, 125–129.
4. Lee, S.H.; Huang, J.W.; Hung, K.Y.; Leu, L.J.; Kan, Y.T.; Yang, C.S.; Chung Wu, D.; Huang, C.L.; Chen, P.Y.; Chen, J.S.; et al. Trace Metals' abnormalities in hemodialysis patients: Relationship with medications. *Artif. Organs.* **2000**, *24*, 841–844. [CrossRef]
5. Prasad, A.S. Zinc: Role in immunity, oxidative stress and chronic inflammation. *Curr. Opin. Clin. Nutr. Metab. Care* **2009**, *12*, 646–652. [CrossRef] [PubMed]
6. MacDonald, R.S. The role of zinc in growth and cell proliferation. *J. Nutr.* **2000**, *130*, 1500S–1508S. [CrossRef]
7. Golden, M.H.; Golden, B.E. Effect of zinc supplementation on the dietary intake, rate of weight gain, and energy cost of tissue deposition in children recovering from severe malnutrition. *Am. J. Clin. Nutr.* **1981**, *34*, 900–908. [CrossRef] [PubMed]
8. Walravens, P.A.; Hambidge, K.M.; Koepfer, D.M. Zinc supplementation in infants with a nutritional pattern of failure to thrive: A double-blind, controlled study. *Pediatrics* **1989**, *83*, 532–538.
9. Henkin, R.I. Zinc in taste function: A critical review. *Biol. Trace Elem. Res.* **1984**, *6*, 263–280. [CrossRef]
10. Lask, B.; Fosson, A.; Rolfe, U.; Thomas, S. Zinc deficiency and childhood-onset anorexia nervosa. *J. Clin. Psychiatry* **1993**, *54*, 63–66.
11. Gray, N.A.; Dhana, A.; Stein, D.J.; Khumalo, N.P. Zinc and atopic dermatitis: A systematic review and meta-analysis. *J. Eur. Acad. Dermatol. Venereol.* **2019**, *33*, 1042–1050. [CrossRef]
12. Prasad, A.S. Clinical manifestations of zinc deficiency. *Annu. Rev. Nutr.* **1985**, *5*, 341–363. [CrossRef]
13. Yang, C.Y.; Wu, M.L.; Chou, Y.Y.; Li, S.Y.; Deng, J.F.; Yang, W.C.; Ng, Y.Y. Essential trace element status and clinical outcomes in long-term dialysis patients: A two-year prospective observational cohort study. *Clin. Nutr.* **2012**, *31*, 630–636. [CrossRef]
14. Prasad, A.S.; Bao, B. Molecular Mechanisms of Zinc as a Pro-Antioxidant Mediator: Clinical Therapeutic Implications. *Antioxidants (Basel)* **2019**, *8*, 164. [CrossRef] [PubMed]

15. Fan, Y.; Zhang, X.; Yang, L.; Wang, J.; Hu, Y.; Bian, A.; Liu, J.; Ma, J. Zinc inhibits high glucose-induced NLRP3 inflammasome activation in human peritoneal mesothelial cells. *Mol. Med. Rep.* **2017**, *16*, 5195–5202. [CrossRef] [PubMed]
16. Nagy, A.; Petho, D.; Gall, T.; Zavaczki, E.; Nyitrai, M.; Posta, J.; Zarjou, A.; Agarwal, A.; Balla, G.; Balla, J. Zinc Inhibits HIF-Prolyl Hydroxylase Inhibitor-Aggravated VSMC Calcification Induced by High Phosphate. *Front. Physiol.* **2019**, *10*, 1584. [CrossRef] [PubMed]
17. Voelkl, J.; Tuffaha, R.; Luong, T.T.D.; Zickler, D.; Masyout, J.; Feger, M.; Verheyen, N.; Blaschke, F.; Kuro, O.M.; Tomaschitz, A.; et al. Zinc Inhibits Phosphate-Induced Vascular Calcification through TNFAIP3-Mediated Suppression of NF-kappaB. *J. Am. Soc. Nephrol.* **2018**, *29*, 1636–1648. [CrossRef]
18. Chen, J.; Budoff, M.J.; Reilly, M.P.; Yang, W.; Rosas, S.E.; Rahman, M.; Zhang, X.; Roy, J.A.; Lustigova, E.; Nessel, L.; et al. Coronary Artery Calcification and Risk of Cardiovascular Disease and Death Among Patients With Chronic Kidney Disease. *JAMA Cardiol.* **2017**, *2*, 635–643. [CrossRef]
19. Gorriz, J.L.; Molina, P.; Cerveron, M.J.; Vila, R.; Bover, J.; Nieto, J.; Barril, G.; Martinez-Castelao, A.; Fernandez, E.; Escudero, V.; et al. Vascular calcification in patients with nondialysis CKD over 3 years. *Clin. J. Am. Soc. Nephrol.* **2015**, *10*, 654–666. [CrossRef]
20. Levin, A. Clinical epidemiology of cardiovascular disease in chronic kidney disease prior to dialysis. *Semin. Dial.* **2003**, *16*, 101–105. [CrossRef]
21. Pasch, A.; Farese, S.; Graber, S.; Wald, J.; Richtering, W.; Floege, J.; Jahnen-Dechent, W. Nanoparticle-based test measures overall propensity for calcification in serum. *J. Am. Soc. Nephrol.* **2012**, *23*, 1744–1752. [CrossRef]
22. Smith, E.R.; Ford, M.L.; Tomlinson, L.A.; Bodenham, E.; McMahon, L.P.; Farese, S.; Rajkumar, C.; Holt, S.G.; Pasch, A. Serum calcification propensity predicts all-cause mortality in predialysis CKD. *J. Am. Soc. Nephrol.* **2014**, *25*, 339–348. [CrossRef]
23. Nakatani, S.; Mori, K.; Sonoda, M.; Nishide, K.; Uedono, H.; Tsuda, A.; Emoto, M.; Shoji, T. Association between Serum Zinc and Calcification Propensity (T50) in Patients with Type 2 Diabetes Mellitus and In Vitro Effect of Exogenous Zinc on T50. *Biomedicines* **2020**, *8*, 337. [CrossRef]
24. Chen, W.; Eisenberg, R.; Mowrey, W.B.; Wylie-Rosett, J.; Abramowitz, M.K.; Bushinsky, D.A.; Melamed, M.L. Association between dietary zinc intake and abdominal aortic calcification in US adults. *Nephrol Dial. Transplant.* **2020**, *35*, 1171–1178. [CrossRef] [PubMed]
25. Bates, C.J.; Hamer, M.; Mishra, G.D. Redox-modulatory vitamins and minerals that prospectively predict mortality in older British people: The National Diet and Nutrition Survey of people aged 65 years and over. *Br. J. Nutr.* **2011**, *105*, 123–132. [CrossRef]
26. Eshak, E.S.; Iso, H.; Yamagishi, K.; Maruyama, K.; Umesawa, M.; Tamakoshi, A. Associations between copper and zinc intakes from diet and mortality from cardiovascular disease in a large population-based prospective cohort study. *J. Nutr. Biochem.* **2018**, *56*, 126–132. [CrossRef]
27. Lonnerdal, B. Dietary factors influencing zinc absorption. *J. Nutr.* **2000**, *130*, 1378S–1383S. [CrossRef] [PubMed]
28. Inoue, Y. [Dietary reference intakes of trace elements for Japanese and problems in clinical fields]. *Nihon Rinsho* **2016**, *74*, 1066–1073.
29. Kodama, H.; Tanaka, M.; Naito, Y.; Katayama, K.; Moriyama, M. Japan's Practical Guidelines for Zinc Deficiency with a Particular Focus on Taste Disorders, Inflammatory Bowel Disease, and Liver Cirrhosis. *Int. J. Mol. Sci.* **2020**, *21*, 2941. [CrossRef]
30. Maret, W.; Sandstead, H.H. Zinc requirements and the risks and benefits of zinc supplementation. *J. Trace Elem. Med. Biol.* **2006**, *20*, 3–18. [CrossRef] [PubMed]
31. Saunders, A.V.; Craig, W.J.; Baines, S.K. Zinc and vegetarian diets. *Med. J. Aust.* **2013**, *199*, S17–S21. [CrossRef] [PubMed]
32. Grungreiff, K.; Gottstein, T.; Reinhold, D. Zinc Deficiency-An Independent Risk Factor in the Pathogenesis of Haemorrhagic Stroke? *Nutrients* **2020**, *12*, 3548. [CrossRef] [PubMed]
33. Hunt, J.R. Bioavailability of iron, zinc, and other trace minerals from vegetarian diets. *Am. J. Clin. Nutr* **2003**, *78*, 633S–639S. [CrossRef]
34. Hambidge, K.M.; Miller, L.V.; Westcott, J.E.; Sheng, X.; Krebs, N.F. Zinc bioavailability and homeostasis. *Am. J. Clin. Nutr.* **2010**, *91*, 1478S–1483S. [CrossRef]
35. Wessels, I.; Rink, L. Micronutrients in autoimmune diseases: Possible therapeutic benefits of zinc and vitamin D. *J. Nutr. Biochem.* **2020**, *77*, 108240. [CrossRef] [PubMed]
36. Mahajan, S.K.; Bowersox, E.M.; Rye, D.L.; Abu-Hamdan, D.K.; Prasad, A.S.; McDonald, F.D.; Biersack, K.L. Factors underlying abnormal zinc metabolism in uremia. *Kidney Int. Suppl.* **1989**, *27*, S269–S273. [PubMed]
37. Cardozo, L.; Mafra, D. Don't forget the zinc. *Nephrol. Dial. Transplant.* **2020**, *35*, 1094–1098. [CrossRef]
38. Pisano, M.; Hilas, O. Zinc and Taste Disturbances in Older Adults: A Review of the Literature. *Consult. Pharm.* **2016**, *31*, 267–270. [CrossRef]
39. Chen, Y.H.; Jeng, S.S.; Hsu, Y.C.; Liao, Y.M.; Wang, Y.X.; Cao, X.; Huang, L.J. In anemia zinc is recruited from bone and plasma to produce new red blood cells. *J. Inorg. Biochem.* **2020**, *210*, 111172. [CrossRef]
40. Tavares, A.; Mafra, D.; Leal, V.O.; Gama, M.D.S.; Vieira, R.; Brum, I.; Borges, N.A.; Silva, A.A. Zinc Plasma Status and Sensory Perception in Nondialysis Chronic Kidney Disease Patients. *J. Ren. Nutr.* **2020**. [CrossRef]
41. Shen, Y.; Yin, Z.; Lv, Y.; Luo, J.; Shi, W.; Fang, J.; Shi, X. Plasma element levels and risk of chronic kidney disease in elderly populations (>/= 90 Years old). *Chemosphere* **2020**, *254*, 126809. [CrossRef]

42. Damianaki, K.; Lourenco, J.M.; Braconnier, P.; Ghobril, J.P.; Devuyst, O.; Burnier, M.; Lenglet, S.; Augsburger, M.; Thomas, A.; Pruijm, M. Renal handling of zinc in chronic kidney disease patients and the role of circulating zinc levels in renal function decline. *Nephrol. Dial. Transplant.* **2020**, *35*, 1163–1170. [CrossRef] [PubMed]
43. Pan, C.F.; Lin, C.J.; Chen, S.H.; Huang, C.F.; Lee, C.C. Association between trace element concentrations and anemia in patients with chronic kidney disease: A cross-sectional population-based study. *J. Investig. Med.* **2019**, *67*, 995–1001. [CrossRef]
44. Aziz, M.A.; Majeed, G.H.; Diab, K.S.; Al-Tamimi, R.J. The association of oxidant-antioxidant status in patients with chronic renal failure. *Ren. Fail.* **2016**, *38*, 20–26. [CrossRef] [PubMed]
45. Mafra, D.; Cuppari, L.; Cozzolino, S.M. Iron and zinc status of patients with chronic renal failure who are not on dialysis. *J. Ren. Nutr.* **2002**, *12*, 38–41. [CrossRef] [PubMed]
46. Hasanato, R.M. Assessment of trace elements in sera of patients undergoing renal dialysis. *Saudi Med. J.* **2014**, *35*, 365–370. [PubMed]
47. Lobo, J.C.; Stockler-Pinto, M.B.; Farage, N.E.; Faulin Tdo, E.; Abdalla, D.S.; Torres, J.P.; Velarde, L.G.; Mafra, D. Reduced plasma zinc levels, lipid peroxidation, and inflammation biomarkers levels in hemodialysis patients: Implications to cardiovascular mortality. *Ren. Fail.* **2013**, *35*, 680–685. [CrossRef]
48. Guo, C.H.; Wang, C.L.; Chen, P.C.; Yang, T.C. Linkage of some trace elements, peripheral blood lymphocytes, inflammation, and oxidative stress in patients undergoing either hemodialysis or peritoneal dialysis. *Perit. Dial. Int.* **2011**, *31*, 583–591. [CrossRef]
49. Dashti-Khavidaki, S.; Khalili, H.; Vahedi, S.M.; Lessan-Pezeshki, M. Serum zinc concentrations in patients on maintenance hemodialysis and its relationship with anemia, parathyroid hormone concentrations and pruritus severity. *Saudi. J. Kidney Dis. Transpl.* **2010**, *21*, 641–645.
50. Kiziltas, H.; Ekin, S.; Erkoc, R. Trace element status of chronic renal patients undergoing hemodialysis. *Biol. Trace Elem. Res.* **2008**, *124*, 103–109. [CrossRef]
51. Batista, M.N.; Cuppari, L.; de Fatima Campos Pedrosa, L.; Almeida, M.; de Almeida, J.B.; de Medeiros, A.C.; Canziani, M.E. Effect of end-stage renal disease and diabetes on zinc and copper status. *Biol. Trace Elem. Res.* **2006**, *112*, 1–12. [CrossRef]
52. Barnett, J.P.; Blindauer, C.A.; Kassaar, O.; Khazaipoul, S.; Martin, E.M.; Sadler, P.J.; Stewart, A.J. Allosteric modulation of zinc speciation by fatty acids. *Biochim. Biophys. Acta.* **2013**, *1830*, 5456–5464. [CrossRef]
53. Melichar, B.; Malir, F.; Jandik, P.; Malirova, E.; Vavrova, J.; Mergancova, J.; Voboril, Z. Increased urinary zinc excretion in cancer patients is linked to immune activation and renal tubular cell dysfunction. *Biometals* **1995**, *8*, 205–208. [CrossRef] [PubMed]
54. Brun, J.F.; Fons, C.; Fussellier, M.; Bardet, L.; Orsetti, A. Urinary zinc and its relationships with microalbuminuria in type I diabetics. *Biol. Trace Elem. Res.* **1992**, *32*, 317–323. [CrossRef]
55. Marreiro, D.N.; do Perpetuo Socorro, C.M.M.; de Sousa, S.S.; Ibiapina, V.; Torres, S.; Pires, L.V.; do Nascimento Nogueira, N.; Lima, J.M.; do Monte, S.J. Urinary excretion of zinc and metabolic control of patients with diabetes type 2. *Biol. Trace Elem. Res.* **2007**, *120*, 42–50. [CrossRef] [PubMed]
56. Pruijm, M.; Ponte, B.; Ackermann, D.; Paccaud, F.; Guessous, I.; Ehret, G.; Pechere-Bertschi, A.; Vogt, B.; Mohaupt, M.G.; Martin, P.Y.; et al. Associations of Urinary Uromodulin with Clinical Characteristics and Markers of Tubular Function in the General Population. *Clin. J. Am. Soc. Nephrol* **2016**, *11*, 70–80. [CrossRef]
57. Manley, K.J. Saliva composition and upper gastrointestinal symptoms in chronic kidney disease. *J. Ren. Care.* **2014**, *40*, 172–179. [CrossRef]
58. Fitzgerald, C.; Wiese, G.; Moorthi, R.N.; Moe, S.M.; Hill Gallant, K.; Running, C.A. Characterizing Dysgeusia in Hemodialysis Patients. *Chem. Senses* **2019**, *44*, 165–171. [CrossRef]
59. Dawson, J.; Brennan, F.P.; Hoffman, A.; Josland, E.; Li, K.C.; Smyth, A.; Brown, M.A. Prevalence of Taste Changes and Association with Other Nutrition-Related Symptoms in End-Stage Kidney Disease Patients. *J. Ren. Nutr.* **2021**, *31*, 80–84. [CrossRef]
60. Naganuma, M.; Ikeda, M.; Tomita, H. Changes in soft palate taste buds of rats due to aging and zinc deficiency–scanning electron microscopic observation. *Auris. Nasus. Larynx.* **1988**, *15*, 117–127. [CrossRef]
61. Kobayashi, T.; Tomita, H. Electron microscopic observation of vallate taste buds of zinc-deficient rats with taste disturbance. *Auris. Nasus. Larynx.* **1986**, *13 Suppl 1*, S25–31. [CrossRef]
62. Sekine, H.; Takao, K.; Yoshinaga, K.; Kokubun, S.; Ikeda, M. Effects of zinc deficiency and supplementation on gene expression of bitter taste receptors (TAS2Rs) on the tongue in rats. *Laryngoscope* **2012**, *122*, 2411–2417. [CrossRef]
63. Yoshida, S.; Endo, S.; Tomita, H. A double-blind study of the therapeutic efficacy of zinc gluconate on taste disorder. *Auris. Nasus. Larynx.* **1991**, *18*, 153–161. [CrossRef]
64. Heckmann, S.M.; Hujoel, P.; Habiger, S.; Friess, W.; Wichmann, M.; Heckmann, J.G.; Hummel, T. Zinc gluconate in the treatment of dysgeusia–a randomized clinical trial. *J. Dent. Res.* **2005**, *84*, 35–38. [CrossRef]
65. Sakai, F.; Yoshida, S.; Endo, S.; Tomita, H. Double-blind, placebo-controlled trial of zinc picolinate for taste disorders. *Acta Otolaryngol.* **2002**. [CrossRef]
66. Sakagami, M.; Ikeda, M.; Tomita, H.; Ikui, A.; Aiba, T.; Takeda, N.; Inokuchi, A.; Kurono, Y.; Nakashima, M.; Shibasaki, Y.; et al. A zinc-containing compound, Polaprezinc, is effective for patients with taste disorders: Randomized, double-blind, placebo-controlled, multi-center study. *Acta Otolaryngol.* **2009**, *129*, 1115–1120. [CrossRef]
67. Scott, B.J.; Bradwell, A.R. Identification of the serum binding proteins for iron, zinc, cadmium, nickel, and calcium. *Clin. Chem.* **1983**, *29*, 629–633. [CrossRef]

68. Kambe, T.; Hashimoto, A.; Fujimoto, S. Current understanding of ZIP and ZnT zinc transporters in human health and diseases. *Cell Mol. Life Sci.* **2014**, *71*, 3281–3295. [CrossRef]
69. King, J.C.; Brown, K.H.; Gibson, R.S.; Krebs, N.F.; Lowe, N.M.; Siekmann, J.H.; Raiten, D.J. Biomarkers of Nutrition for Development (BOND)-Zinc Review. *J. Nutr.* **2015**, *146*, 858S–885S. [CrossRef] [PubMed]
70. Mahajan, S.K.; Prasad, A.S.; Rabbani, P.; Briggs, W.A.; McDonald, F.D. Zinc metabolism in uremia. *J. Lab. Clin. Med.* **1979**, *94*, 693–698. [CrossRef] [PubMed]
71. Kambe, T.; Tsuji, T.; Hashimoto, A.; Itsumura, N. The Physiological, Biochemical, and Molecular Roles of Zinc Transporters in Zinc Homeostasis and Metabolism. *Physiol. Rev.* **2015**, *95*, 749–784. [CrossRef]
72. Takagi, K.; Masuda, K.; Yamazaki, M.; Kiyohara, C.; Itoh, S.; Wasaki, M.; Inoue, H. Metal ion and vitamin adsorption profiles of phosphate binder ion-exchange resins. *Clin. Nephrol.* **2010**, *73*, 30–35. [CrossRef]
73. Go, A.S.; Chertow, G.M.; Fan, D.; McCulloch, C.E.; Hsu, C.Y. Chronic kidney disease and the risks of death, cardiovascular events, and hospitalization. *N. Engl. J. Med.* **2004**, *351*, 1296–1305. [CrossRef]
74. van der Velde, M.; Matsushita, K.; Coresh, J.; Astor, B.C.; Woodward, M.; Levey, A.; de Jong, P.; Gansevoort, R.T.; Chronic Kidney Disease Prognosis, C.; van der Velde, M.; et al. Lower estimated glomerular filtration rate and higher albuminuria are associated with all-cause and cardiovascular mortality. A collaborative meta-analysis of high-risk population cohorts. *Kidney Int.* **2011**, *79*, 1341–1352. [CrossRef]
75. Paloian, N.J.; Giachelli, C.M. A current understanding of vascular calcification in CKD. *Am. J. Physiol. Ren. Physiol.* **2014**, *307*, F891–S900. [CrossRef] [PubMed]
76. Ruderman, I.; Holt, S.G.; Hewitson, T.D.; Smith, E.R.; Toussaint, N.D. Current and potential therapeutic strategies for the management of vascular calcification in patients with chronic kidney disease including those on dialysis. *Semin Dial.* **2018**, *31*, 487–499. [CrossRef]
77. Lanzer, P.; Boehm, M.; Sorribas, V.; Thiriet, M.; Janzen, J.; Zeller, T.; St Hilaire, C.; Shanahan, C. Medial vascular calcification revisited: Review and perspectives. *Eur. Heart J.* **2014**, *35*, 1515–1525. [CrossRef] [PubMed]
78. Houben, E.; Neradova, A.; Schurgers, L.J.; Vervloet, M. The influence of phosphate, calcium and magnesium on matrix Gla-protein and vascular calcification: A systematic review. *G. Ital. Nefrol.* **2016**, *33*.
79. Lang, F.; Ritz, E.; Voelkl, J.; Alesutan, I. Vascular calcification–is aldosterone a culprit? *Nephrol. Dial. Transplant.* **2013**, *28*, 1080–1084. [CrossRef] [PubMed]
80. Cozzolino, M.; Gallieni, M.; Brancaccio, D. Vascular calcification in uremic conditions: New insights into pathogenesis. *Semin. Nephrol.* **2006**, *26*, 33–37. [CrossRef]
81. Jablonski, K.L.; Chonchol, M. Vascular calcification in end-stage renal disease. *Hemodial Int.* **2013**, *17 Suppl 1*, S17–21. [CrossRef]
82. Demer, L.L.; Tintut, Y. Mineral exploration: Search for the mechanism of vascular calcification and beyond: The 2003 Jeffrey M. Hoeg Award lecture. *Arterioscler Thromb Vasc. Biol.* **2003**, *23*, 1739–1743. [CrossRef]
83. Wallin, R.; Wajih, N.; Greenwood, G.T.; Sane, D.C. Arterial calcification: A review of mechanisms, animal models, and the prospects for therapy. *Med. Res. Rev.* **2001**, *21*, 274–301. [CrossRef]
84. Tanaka, T.; Sato, H.; Doi, H.; Yoshida, C.A.; Shimizu, T.; Matsui, H.; Yamazaki, M.; Akiyama, H.; Kawai-Kowase, K.; Iso, T.; et al. Runx2 represses myocardin-mediated differentiation and facilitates osteogenic conversion of vascular smooth muscle cells. *Mol. Cell Biol.* **2008**, *28*, 1147–1160. [CrossRef] [PubMed]
85. Lin, M.E.; Chen, T.M.; Wallingford, M.C.; Nguyen, N.B.; Yamada, S.; Sawangmake, C.; Zhang, J.; Speer, M.Y.; Giachelli, C.M. Runx2 deletion in smooth muscle cells inhibits vascular osteochondrogenesis and calcification but not atherosclerotic lesion formation. *Cardiovasc. Res.* **2016**, *112*, 606–616. [CrossRef] [PubMed]
86. Zhao, G.; Xu, M.J.; Zhao, M.M.; Dai, X.Y.; Kong, W.; Wilson, G.M.; Guan, Y.; Wang, C.Y.; Wang, X. Activation of nuclear factor-kappa B accelerates vascular calcification by inhibiting ankylosis protein homolog expression. *Kidney Int.* **2012**, *82*, 34–44. [CrossRef] [PubMed]
87. Besarab, A.; Chernyavskaya, E.; Motylev, I.; Shutov, E.; Kumbar, L.M.; Gurevich, K.; Chan, D.T.; Leong, R.; Poole, L.; Zhong, M.; et al. Roxadustat (FG-4592): Correction of Anemia in Incident Dialysis Patients. *J. Am. Soc. Nephrol.* **2016**, *27*, 1225–1233. [CrossRef]
88. Besarab, A.; Provenzano, R.; Hertel, J.; Zabaneh, R.; Klaus, S.J.; Lee, T.; Leong, R.; Hemmerich, S.; Yu, K.H.; Neff, T.B. Randomized placebo-controlled dose-ranging and pharmacodynamics study of roxadustat (FG-4592) to treat anemia in nondialysis-dependent chronic kidney disease (NDD-CKD) patients. *Nephrol Dial. Transplant.* **2015**, *30*, 1665–1673. [CrossRef]
89. Mokas, S.; Lariviere, R.; Lamalice, L.; Gobeil, S.; Cornfield, D.N.; Agharazii, M.; Richard, D.E. Hypoxia-inducible factor-1 plays a role in phosphate-induced vascular smooth muscle cell calcification. *Kidney Int.* **2016**, *90*, 598–609. [CrossRef]
90. Zhu, Y.; Ma, W.Q.; Han, X.Q.; Wang, Y.; Wang, X.; Liu, N.F. Advanced glycation end products accelerate calcification in VSMCs through HIF-1alpha/PDK4 activation and suppress glucose metabolism. *Sci. Rep.* **2018**, *8*, 13730. [CrossRef]
91. Heiss, A.; Jahnen-Dechent, W.; Endo, H.; Schwahn, D. Structural dynamics of a colloidal protein-mineral complex bestowing on calcium phosphate a high solubility in biological fluids. *Biointerphases* **2007**, *2*, 16–20. [CrossRef]
92. Heiss, A.; DuChesne, A.; Denecke, B.; Grotzinger, J.; Yamamoto, K.; Renne, T.; Jahnen-Dechent, W. Structural basis of calcification inhibition by alpha 2-HS glycoprotein/fetuin-A. Formation of colloidal calciprotein particles. *J. Biol. Chem.* **2003**, *278*, 13333–13341. [CrossRef]

93. Pasch, A.; Block, G.A.; Bachtler, M.; Smith, E.R.; Jahnen-Dechent, W.; Arampatzis, S.; Chertow, G.M.; Parfrey, P.; Ma, X.; Floege, J. Blood Calcification Propensity, Cardiovascular Events, and Survival in Patients Receiving Hemodialysis in the EVOLVE Trial. *Clin. J. Am. Soc. Nephrol.* **2017**, *12*, 315–322. [CrossRef] [PubMed]
94. Keyzer, C.A.; de Borst, M.H.; van den Berg, E.; Jahnen-Dechent, W.; Arampatzis, S.; Farese, S.; Bergmann, I.P.; Floege, J.; Navis, G.; Bakker, S.J.; et al. Calcification Propensity and Survival among Renal Transplant Recipients. *J. Am. Soc. Nephrol.* **2016**, *27*, 239–248. [CrossRef]
95. Dahle, D.O.; Asberg, A.; Hartmann, A.; Holdaas, H.; Bachtler, M.; Jenssen, T.G.; Dionisi, M.; Pasch, A. Serum Calcification Propensity Is a Strong and Independent Determinant of Cardiac and All-Cause Mortality in Kidney Transplant Recipients. *Am. J. Transplant.* **2016**, *16*, 204–212. [CrossRef]
96. Silaghi, C.N.; Ilyes, T.; Van Ballegooijen, A.J.; Craciun, A.M. Calciprotein Particles and Serum Calcification Propensity: Hallmarks of Vascular Calcifications in Patients with Chronic Kidney Disease. *J. Clin. Med.* **2020**, *9*, 1287. [CrossRef]
97. Wilson, P.W.; Kauppila, L.I.; O'Donnell, C.J.; Kiel, D.P.; Hannan, M.; Polak, J.M.; Cupples, L.A. Abdominal aortic calcific deposits are an important predictor of vascular morbidity and mortality. *Circulation* **2001**, *103*, 1529–1534. [CrossRef] [PubMed]
98. Peeters, M.J.; van den Brand, J.A.; van Zuilen, A.D.; Koster, Y.; Bots, M.L.; Vervloet, M.G.; Blankestijn, P.J.; Wetzels, J.F.; Group, M.S. Abdominal aortic calcification in patients with CKD. *J. Nephrol.* **2017**, *30*, 109–118. [CrossRef]
99. Yang, C.W.; Guo, Y.C.; Li, C.I.; Liu, C.S.; Lin, C.H.; Liu, C.H.; Wang, M.C.; Yang, S.Y.; Li, T.C.; Lin, C.C. Subclinical Atherosclerosis Markers of Carotid Intima-Media Thickness, Carotid Plaques, Carotid Stenosis, and Mortality in Community-Dwelling Adults. *Int. J. Environ. Res. Public Health* **2020**, *17*, 4745. [CrossRef]
100. Yang, Y.J.; Choi, B.Y.; Chun, B.Y.; Kweon, S.S.; Lee, Y.H.; Park, P.S.; Kim, M.K. Dietary zinc intake is inversely related to subclinical atherosclerosis measured by carotid intima-media thickness. *Br. J. Nutr.* **2010**, *104*, 1202–1211. [CrossRef] [PubMed]
101. Ari, E.; Kaya, Y.; Demir, H.; Asicioglu, E.; Keskin, S. The correlation of serum trace elements and heavy metals with carotid artery atherosclerosis in maintenance hemodialysis patients. *Biol. Trace Elem. Res.* **2011**, *144*, 351–359. [CrossRef]
102. Sato, M.; Yanagisawa, H.; Nojima, Y.; Tamura, J.; Wada, O. Zn deficiency aggravates hypertension in spontaneously hypertensive rats: Possible role of Cu/Zn-superoxide dismutase. *Clin. Exp. Hypertens* **2002**, *24*, 355–370. [CrossRef]
103. Dimitrova, A.A.; Strashimirov, D.; Betova, T.; Russeva, A.; Alexandrova, M. Zinc content in the diet affects the activity of Cu/ZnSOD, lipid peroxidation and lipid profile of spontaneously hypertensive rats. *Acta Biol. Hung.* **2008**, *59*, 305–314. [CrossRef] [PubMed]
104. Williams, C.R.; Mistry, M.; Cheriyan, A.M.; Williams, J.M.; Naraine, M.K.; Ellis, C.L.; Mallick, R.; Mistry, A.C.; Gooch, J.L.; Ko, B.; et al. Zinc deficiency induces hypertension by promoting renal Na(+) reabsorption. *Am. J. Physiol. Renal Physiol.* **2019**, *316*, F646–F653. [CrossRef] [PubMed]
105. Kunutsor, S.K.; Laukkanen, J.A. Serum zinc concentrations and incident hypertension: New findings from a population-based cohort study. *J. Hypertens* **2016**, *34*, 1055–1061. [CrossRef] [PubMed]
106. Bergomi, M.; Rovesti, S.; Vinceti, M.; Vivoli, R.; Caselgrandi, E.; Vivoli, G. Zinc and copper status and blood pressure. *J. Trace Elem. Med. Biol.* **1997**, *11*, 166–169. [CrossRef]
107. Beattie, J.H.; Gordon, M.J.; Rucklidge, G.J.; Reid, M.D.; Duncan, G.J.; Horgan, G.W.; Cho, Y.E.; Kwun, I.S. Aorta protein networks in marginal and acute zinc deficiency. *Proteomics* **2008**, *8*, 2126–2135. [CrossRef]
108. Reiterer, G.; MacDonald, R.; Browning, J.D.; Morrow, J.; Matveev, S.V.; Daugherty, A.; Smart, E.; Toborek, M.; Hennig, B. Zinc deficiency increases plasma lipids and atherosclerotic markers in LDL-receptor-deficient mice. *J. Nutr.* **2005**, *135*, 2114–2118. [CrossRef]
109. Reed, S.; Qin, X.; Ran-Ressler, R.; Brenna, J.T.; Glahn, R.P.; Tako, E. Dietary zinc deficiency affects blood linoleic acid: Dihomo-gamma-linolenic acid (LA:DGLA) ratio; a sensitive physiological marker of zinc status in vivo (Gallus gallus). *Nutrients* **2014**, *6*, 1164–1180. [CrossRef]
110. Knez, M.; Stangoulis, J.C.R.; Glibetic, M.; Tako, E. The Linoleic Acid: Dihomo-gamma-Linolenic Acid Ratio (LA:DGLA)-An Emerging Biomarker of Zn Status. *Nutrients* **2017**, *9*, 825. [CrossRef]
111. Ranasinghe, P.; Wathurapatha, W.S.; Ishara, M.H.; Jayawardana, R.; Galappatthy, P.; Katulanda, P.; Constantine, G.R. Effects of Zinc supplementation on serum lipids: A systematic review and meta-analysis. *Nutr. Metab. (Lond)* **2015**, *12*, 26. [CrossRef] [PubMed]
112. Lobo, J.C.; Torres, J.P.; Fouque, D.; Mafra, D. Zinc deficiency in chronic kidney disease: Is there a relationship with adipose tissue and atherosclerosis? *Biol. Trace Elem. Res.* **2010**, *135*, 16–21. [CrossRef]
113. Kalkan Ucar, S.; Coker, M.; Sozmen, E.; Goksen Simsek, D.; Darcan, S. An association among iron, copper, zinc, and selenium, and antioxidative status in dyslipidemic pediatric patients with glycogen storage disease types IA and III. *J. Trace Elem. Med. Biol* **2010**, *24*, 42–45. [CrossRef] [PubMed]
114. Argani, H.; Mahdavi, R.; Ghorbani-haghjo, A.; Razzaghi, R.; Nikniaz, L.; Gaemmaghami, S.J. Effects of zinc supplementation on serum zinc and leptin levels, BMI, and body composition in hemodialysis patients. *J. Trace Elem. Med. Biol* **2014**, *28*, 35–38. [CrossRef]
115. Roozbeh, J.; Hedayati, P.; Sagheb, M.M.; Sharifian, M.; Hamidian Jahromi, A.; Shaabani, S.; Jalaeian, H.; Raeisjalali, G.A.; Behzadi, S. Effect of zinc supplementation on triglyceride, cholesterol, LDL, and HDL levels in zinc-deficient hemodialysis patients. *Ren. Fail.* **2009**, *31*, 798–801. [CrossRef]
116. Chausmer, A.B. Zinc, insulin and diabetes. *J. Am. Coll. Nutr.* **1998**, *17*, 109–115. [CrossRef] [PubMed]

117. Farooq, D.M.; Alamri, A.F.; Alwhahabi, B.K.; Metwally, A.M.; Kareem, K.A. The status of zinc in type 2 diabetic patients and its association with glycemic control. *J. Family Community Med.* **2020**, *27*, 29–36. [CrossRef]
118. Keller, S.R. Role of the insulin-regulated aminopeptidase IRAP in insulin action and diabetes. *Biol. Pharm. Bull.* **2004**, *27*, 761–764. [CrossRef]
119. Tang, X.; Shay, N.F. Zinc has an insulin-like effect on glucose transport mediated by phosphoinositol-3-kinase and Akt in 3T3-L1 fibroblasts and adipocytes. *J. Nutr.* **2001**, *131*, 1414–1420. [CrossRef]
120. Chabosseau, P.; Rutter, G.A. Zinc and diabetes. *Arch. Biochem. Biophys.* **2016**, *611*, 79–85. [CrossRef]
121. Fernandez-Cao, J.C.; Warthon-Medina, M.; Horan, V.H.; Arija, V.; Doepking, C.; Serra-Majem, L.; Lowe, N.M. Zinc Intake and Status and Risk of Type 2 Diabetes Mellitus: A Systematic Review and Meta-Analysis. *Nutrients* **2019**, *11*, 1027. [CrossRef] [PubMed]
122. Islam, M.R.; Attia, J.; Ali, L.; McEvoy, M.; Selim, S.; Sibbritt, D.; Akhter, A.; Akter, S.; Peel, R.; Faruque, O.; et al. Zinc supplementation for improving glucose handling in pre-diabetes: A double blind randomized placebo controlled pilot study. *Diabetes Res. Clin. Pract.* **2016**, *115*, 39–46. [CrossRef] [PubMed]
123. Choi, S.; Liu, X.; Pan, Z. Zinc deficiency and cellular oxidative stress: Prognostic implications in cardiovascular diseases. *Acta Pharmacol. Sin.* **2018**, *39*, 1120–1132. [CrossRef] [PubMed]
124. Lawrence, T. The nuclear factor NF-kappaB pathway in inflammation. *Cold Spring Harb. Perspect. Biol.* **2009**, *1*, a001651. [CrossRef] [PubMed]
125. Wong, C.P.; Ho, E. Zinc and its role in age-related inflammation and immune dysfunction. *Mol. Nutr. Food Res.* **2012**, *56*, 77–87. [CrossRef]
126. Beattie, J.H.; Gordon, M.J.; Duthie, S.J.; McNeil, C.J.; Horgan, G.W.; Nixon, G.F.; Feldmann, J.; Kwun, I.S. Suboptimal dietary zinc intake promotes vascular inflammation and atherogenesis in a mouse model of atherosclerosis. *Mol. Nutr. Food Res.* **2012**, *56*, 1097–1105. [CrossRef]
127. Jarosz, M.; Olbert, M.; Wyszogrodzka, G.; Mlyniec, K.; Librowski, T. Antioxidant and anti-inflammatory effects of zinc. Zinc-dependent NF-kappaB signaling. *Inflammopharmacology* **2017**, *25*, 11–24. [CrossRef] [PubMed]
128. Mousavi, S.M.; Djafarian, K.; Mojtahed, A.; Varkaneh, H.K.; Shab-Bidar, S. The effect of zinc supplementation on plasma C-reactive protein concentrations: A systematic review and meta-analysis of randomized controlled trials. *Eur. J. Pharmacol.* **2018**, *834*, 10–16. [CrossRef]
129. Senoner, T.; Dichtl, W. Oxidative Stress in Cardiovascular Diseases: Still a Therapeutic Target? *Nutrients* **2019**, *11*, 2090. [CrossRef]
130. Suzuki, T.; Yamamoto, M. Molecular basis of the Keap1-Nrf2 system. *Free Radic. Biol. Med.* **2015**, *88*, 93–100. [CrossRef]
131. Cortese, M.M.; Suschek, C.V.; Wetzel, W.; Kroncke, K.D.; Kolb-Bachofen, V. Zinc protects endothelial cells from hydrogen peroxide via Nrf2-dependent stimulation of glutathione biosynthesis. *Free Radic. Biol. Med.* **2008**, *44*, 2002–2012. [CrossRef]
132. Ha, K.N.; Chen, Y.; Cai, J.; Sternberg, P., Jr. Increased glutathione synthesis through an ARE-Nrf2-dependent pathway by zinc in the RPE: Implication for protection against oxidative stress. *Invest. Ophthalmol Vis. Sci* **2006**, *47*, 2709–2715. [CrossRef]
133. Li, B.; Cui, W.; Tan, Y.; Luo, P.; Chen, Q.; Zhang, C.; Qu, W.; Miao, L.; Cai, L. Zinc is essential for the transcription function of Nrf2 in human renal tubule cells in vitro and mouse kidney in vivo under the diabetic condition. *J. Cell Mol. Med.* **2014**, *18*, 895–906. [CrossRef]
134. Pedruzzi, L.M.; Cardozo, L.F.; Daleprane, J.B.; Stockler-Pinto, M.B.; Monteiro, E.B.; Leite, M., Jr.; Vaziri, N.D.; Mafra, D. Systemic inflammation and oxidative stress in hemodialysis patients are associated with down-regulation of Nrf2. *J. Nephrol.* **2015**, *28*, 495–501. [CrossRef]
135. Pergola, P.E.; Raskin, P.; Toto, R.D.; Meyer, C.J.; Huff, J.W.; Grossman, E.B.; Krauth, M.; Ruiz, S.; Audhya, P.; Christ-Schmidt, H.; et al. Bardoxolone methyl and kidney function in CKD with type 2 diabetes. *N. Engl. J. Med.* **2011**, *365*, 327–336. [CrossRef]
136. Eide, D.J. The oxidative stress of zinc deficiency. *Metallomics* **2011**, *3*, 1124–1129. [CrossRef] [PubMed]
137. Rink, L.; Gabriel, P. Zinc and the immune system. *Proc. Nutr. Soc.* **2000**, *59*, 541–552. [CrossRef]
138. Chu, A.; Foster, M.; Samman, S. Zinc Status and Risk of Cardiovascular Diseases and Type 2 Diabetes Mellitus-A Systematic Review of Prospective Cohort Studies. *Nutrients* **2016**, *8*, 707. [CrossRef] [PubMed]
139. Soinio, M.; Marniemi, J.; Laakso, M.; Pyorala, K.; Lehto, S.; Ronnemaa, T. Serum zinc level and coronary heart disease events in patients with type 2 diabetes. *Diabetes Care* **2007**, *30*, 523–528. [CrossRef]
140. Pilz, S.; Dobnig, H.; Winklhofer-Roob, B.M.; Renner, W.; Seelhorst, U.; Wellnitz, B.; Boehm, B.O.; Marz, W. Low serum zinc concentrations predict mortality in patients referred to coronary angiography. *Br. J. Nutr.* **2009**, *101*, 1534–1540. [CrossRef] [PubMed]
141. Toida, T.; Toida, R.; Ebihara, S.; Takahashi, R.; Komatsu, H.; Uezono, S.; Sato, Y.; Fujimoto, S. Association between Serum Zinc Levels and Clinical Index or the Body Composition in Incident Hemodialysis Patients. *Nutrients* **2020**, *12*, 3187. [CrossRef]
142. Leone, N.; Courbon, D.; Ducimetiere, P.; Zureik, M. Zinc, copper, and magnesium and risks for all-cause, cancer, and cardiovascular mortality. *Epidemiology* **2006**, *17*, 308–314. [CrossRef] [PubMed]
143. Marniemi, J.; Jarvisalo, J.; Toikka, T.; Raiha, I.; Ahotupa, M.; Sourander, L. Blood vitamins, mineral elements and inflammation markers as risk factors of vascular and non-vascular disease mortality in an elderly population. *Int. J. Epidemiol.* **1998**, *27*, 799–807. [CrossRef] [PubMed]
144. Kogirima, M.; Kurasawa, R.; Kubori, S.; Sarukura, N.; Nakamori, M.; Okada, S.; Kamioka, H.; Yamamoto, S. Ratio of low serum zinc levels in elderly Japanese people living in the central part of Japan. *Eur. J. Clin. Nutr.* **2007**, *61*, 375–381. [CrossRef]

145. Whittaker, P. Iron and zinc interactions in humans. *Am. J. Clin. Nutr.* **1998**, *68*, 442S–446S. [CrossRef]
146. Chen, F.; Du, M.; Blumberg, J.B.; Ho Chui, K.K.; Ruan, M.; Rogers, G.; Shan, Z.; Zeng, L.; Zhang, F.F. Association Among Dietary Supplement Use, Nutrient Intake, and Mortality Among U.S. Adults: A Cohort Study. *Ann. Intern. Med.* **2019**, *170*, 604–613. [CrossRef] [PubMed]
147. Shi, Z.; Chu, A.; Zhen, S.; Taylor, A.W.; Dai, Y.; Riley, M.; Samman, S. Association between dietary zinc intake and mortality among Chinese adults: Findings from 10-year follow-up in the Jiangsu Nutrition Study. *Eur. J. Nutr.* **2018**, *57*, 2839–2846. [CrossRef]
148. Lee, D.H.; Folsom, A.R.; Jacobs, D.R., Jr. Iron, zinc, and alcohol consumption and mortality from cardiovascular diseases: The Iowa Women's Health Study. *Am. J. Clin. Nutr.* **2005**, *81*, 787–791. [CrossRef]
149. Sarukura, N.; Kogirima, M.; Takai, S.; Kitamura, Y.; Kalubi, B.; Yamamoto, S.; Takeda, N. Dietary zinc intake and its effects on zinc nutrition in healthy Japanese living in the central area of Japan. *J. Med. Investig.* **2011**, *58*, 203–209. [CrossRef]
150. Quintana Pacheco, D.A.; Sookthai, D.; Wittenbecher, C.; Graf, M.E.; Schubel, R.; Johnson, T.; Katzke, V.; Jakszyn, P.; Kaaks, R.; Kuhn, T. Red meat consumption and risk of cardiovascular diseases-is increased iron load a possible link? *Am. J. Clin. Nutr.* **2018**, *107*, 113–119. [CrossRef]
151. Ascherio, A.; Willett, W.C.; Rimm, E.B.; Giovannucci, E.L.; Stampfer, M.J. Dietary iron intake and risk of coronary disease among men. *Circulation* **1994**, *89*, 969–974. [CrossRef] [PubMed]
152. Wolk, A. Potential health hazards of eating red meat. *J. Intern. Med.* **2017**, *281*, 106–122. [CrossRef] [PubMed]
153. Escobedo-Monge, M.F.; Ayala-Macedo, G.; Sakihara, G.; Peralta, S.; Almaraz-Gomez, A.; Barrado, E.; Marugan-Miguelsanz, J.M. Effects of Zinc Supplementation on Nutritional Status in Children with Chronic Kidney Disease: A Randomized Trial. *Nutrients* **2019**, *11*, 2671. [CrossRef] [PubMed]
154. Tonelli, M.; Wiebe, N.; Thompson, S.; Kinniburgh, D.; Klarenbach, S.W.; Walsh, M.; Bello, A.K.; Faruque, L.; Field, C.; Manns, B.J.; et al. Trace element supplementation in hemodialysis patients: A randomized controlled trial. *BMC Nephrol.* **2015**, *16*, 52. [CrossRef]
155. Wang, L.J.; Wang, M.Q.; Hu, R.; Yang, Y.; Huang, Y.S.; Xian, S.X.; Lu, L. Effect of Zinc Supplementation on Maintenance Hemodialysis Patients: A Systematic Review and Meta-Analysis of 15 Randomized Controlled Trials. *Biomed. Res. Int.* **2017**, *2017*, 1024769. [CrossRef] [PubMed]
156. Kobayashi, H.; Abe, M.; Okada, K.; Tei, R.; Maruyama, N.; Kikuchi, F.; Higuchi, T.; Soma, M. Oral zinc supplementation reduces the erythropoietin responsiveness index in patients on hemodialysis. *Nutrients* **2015**, *7*, 3783–3795. [CrossRef] [PubMed]
157. El-Shazly, A.N.; Ibrahim, S.A.; El-Mashad, G.M.; Sabry, J.H.; Sherbini, N.S. Effect of zinc supplementation on body mass index and serum levels of zinc and leptin in pediatric hemodialysis patients. *Int. J. Nephrol. Renovasc. Dis.* **2015**, *8*, 159–163. [CrossRef] [PubMed]
158. Pakfetrat, M.; Shahroodi, J.R.; Zolgadr, A.A.; Larie, H.A.; Nikoo, M.H.; Malekmakan, L. Effects of zinc supplement on plasma homocysteine level in end-stage renal disease patients: A double-blind randomized clinical trial. *Biol. Trace Elem. Res.* **2013**, *153*, 11–15. [CrossRef]
159. Mazani, M.; Argani, H.; Rashtchizadeh, N.; Ghorbanihaghjo, A.; Hamdi, A.; Estiar, M.A.; Nezami, N. Effects of zinc supplementation on antioxidant status and lipid peroxidation in hemodialysis patients. *J. Ren. Nutr.* **2013**, *23*, 180–184. [CrossRef]
160. Guo, C.H.; Wang, C.L. Effects of zinc supplementation on plasma copper/zinc ratios, oxidative stress, and immunological status in hemodialysis patients. *Int. J. Med. Sci.* **2013**, *10*, 79–89. [CrossRef]
161. Rahimi-Ardabili, B.; Argani, H.; Ghorbanihaghjo, A.; Rashtchizadeh, N.; Naghavi-Behzad, M.; Ghorashi, S.; Nezami, N. Paraoxonase enzyme activity is enhanced by zinc supplementation in hemodialysis patients. *Ren. Fail.* **2012**, *34*, 1123–1128. [CrossRef] [PubMed]
162. Rashidi, A.A.; Salehi, M.; Piroozmand, A.; Sagheb, M.M. Effects of zinc supplementation on serum zinc and C-reactive protein concentrations in hemodialysis patients. *J. Ren. Nutr.* **2009**, *19*, 475–478. [CrossRef] [PubMed]
163. Nava, H.J.; Amato, D. Effect of zinc supplements on the levels of pre-albumin and transferrin in patients with dialysis. *Rev. Investig. Clín.* **2005**, *57*, 123–125.
164. Matson, A.; Wright, M.; Oliver, A.; Woodrow, G.; King, N.; Dye, L.; Blundell, J.; Brownjohn, A.; Turney, J. Zinc supplementation at conventional doses does not improve the disturbance of taste perception in hemodialysis patients. *J. Ren. Nutr.* **2003**, *13*, 224–228. [CrossRef]
165. Chevalier, C.A.; Liepa, G.; Murphy, M.D.; Suneson, J.; Vanbeber, A.D.; Gorman, M.A.; Cochran, C. The effects of zinc supplementation on serum zinc and cholesterol concentrations in hemodialysis patients. *J. Ren. Nutr.* **2002**, *12*, 183–189. [CrossRef]
166. Candan, F.; Gultekin, F.; Candan, F. Effect of vitamin C and zinc on osmotic fragility and lipid peroxidation in zinc-deficient haemodialysis patients. *Cell. Biochem. Funct.* **2002**, *20*, 95–98. [CrossRef] [PubMed]
167. Jern, N.A.; VanBeber, A.D.; Gorman, M.A.; Weber, C.G.; Liepa, G.U.; Cochran, C.C. The effects of zinc supplementation on serum zinc concentration and protein catabolic rate in hemodialysis patients. *J. Ren. Nutr.* **2000**, *10*, 148–153. [CrossRef]
168. Brodersen, H.P.; Holtkamp, W.; Larbig, D.; Beckers, B.; Thiery, J.; Lautenschlager, J.; Probst, H.J.; Ropertz, S.; Yavari, A. Zinc supplementation and hepatitis B vaccination in chronic haemodialysis patients: A multicentre study. *Nephrol. Dial. Transpl.* **1995**, *10*, 1780.
169. Group, K.W. KDOQI Clinical Practice Guideline for Nutrition in Children with CKD: 2008 update. Executive summary. *Am. J. Kidney Dis.* **2009**, *53*, S11–S104. [CrossRef]

170. Abraham, A.G.; Mak, R.H.; Mitsnefes, M.; White, C.; Moxey-Mims, M.; Warady, B.; Furth, S.L. Protein energy wasting in children with chronic kidney disease. *Pediatr. Nephrol.* **2014**, *29*, 1231–1238. [CrossRef] [PubMed]
171. McClave, S.A.; Taylor, B.E.; Martindale, R.G.; Warren, M.M.; Johnson, D.R.; Braunschweig, C.; McCarthy, M.S.; Davanos, E.; Rice, T.W.; Cresci, G.A.; et al. Guidelines for the Provision and Assessment of Nutrition Support Therapy in the Adult Critically Ill Patient: Society of Critical Care Medicine (SCCM) and American Society for Parenteral and Enteral Nutrition (A.S.P.E.N.). *JPEN J. Parenter. Enteral Nutr.* **2016**, *40*, 159–211. [CrossRef] [PubMed]
172. Kondrup, J.; Allison, S.P.; Elia, M.; Vellas, B.; Plauth, M.; Educational and Clinical Practice Committee; European Society of Parenteral and Enteral Nutrition (ESPEN). ESPEN guidelines for nutrition screening 2002. *Clin. Nutr.* **2003**, *22*, 415–421. [CrossRef]
173. Qu, X.; Yang, H.; Yu, Z.; Jia, B.; Qiao, H.; Zheng, Y.; Dai, K. Serum zinc levels and multiple health outcomes: Implications for zinc-based biomaterials. *Bioact. Mater.* **2020**, *5*, 410–422. [CrossRef] [PubMed]
174. Nishime, K.; Kondo, M.; Saito, K.; Miyawaki, H.; Nakagawa, T. Zinc Burden Evokes Copper Deficiency in the Hypoalbuminemic Hemodialysis Patients. *Nutrients* **2020**, *12*, 577. [CrossRef]

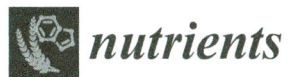

Review

Positive and Negative Aspects of Sodium Intake in Dialysis and Non-Dialysis CKD Patients

Yasuyuki Nagasawa

Department of Internal Medicine, Division of Kidney and Dialysis, Hyogo College of Medicine, 1-1 Mukogawa-Cho, Nishinomiya, Hyogo 663-8501, Japan; nagasawa@hyo-med.ac.jp; Tel.: +81-798-45-6521; Fax: +81-798-45-6880

Abstract: Sodium intake theoretically has dual effects on both non-dialysis chronic kidney disease (CKD) patients and dialysis patients. One negatively affects mortality by increasing proteinuria and blood pressure. The other positively affects mortality by ameliorating nutritional status through appetite induced by salt intake and the amount of food itself, which is proportional to the amount of salt under the same salty taste. Sodium restriction with enough water intake easily causes hyponatremia in CKD and dialysis patients. Moreover, the balance of these dual effects in dialysis patients is likely different from their balance in non-dialysis CKD patients because dialysis patients lose kidney function. Sodium intake is strongly related to water intake via the thirst center. Therefore, sodium intake is strongly related to extracellular fluid volume, blood pressure, appetite, nutritional status, and mortality. To decrease mortality in both non-dialysis and dialysis CKD patients, sodium restriction is an essential and important factor that can be changed by the patients themselves. However, under sodium restriction, it is important to maintain the balance of negative and positive effects from sodium intake not only in dialysis and non-dialysis CKD patients but also in the general population.

Keywords: hypertension; body weight; mortality; sodium; dialysis

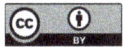

Citation: Nagasawa, Y. Positive and Negative Aspects of Sodium Intake in Dialysis and Non-Dialysis CKD Patients. *Nutrients* **2021**, *13*, 951. https://doi.org/10.3390/nu13030951

Academic Editor: Murielle Bochud

Received: 12 February 2021
Accepted: 12 March 2021
Published: 16 March 2021

Publisher's Note: MDPI stays neutral with regard to jurisdictional claims in published maps and institutional affiliations.

Copyright: © 2021 by the author. Licensee MDPI, Basel, Switzerland. This article is an open access article distributed under the terms and conditions of the Creative Commons Attribution (CC BY) license (https://creativecommons.org/licenses/by/4.0/).

1. Introduction

Sodium intake is related to extracellular fluid volume. Increased fluid volume increases blood pressure, resulting in hypertension. Moreover, excretion of sodium is also related to blood pressure. Increased sodium excretion in the kidneys requires elevated blood pressure in the glomeruli, also resulting in hypertension. Guyton described this phenomenon as a pressure–natriuresis relationship [1]. Therefore, sodium intake is strongly related to fluid volume (body weight) and hypertension. Hypertension is an important key factor in determining mortality. On the other hand, sodium intake is also related to nutrition. If someone eats more food, that person is usually ingesting more sodium. Moreover, sodium intake is correlated with appetite. Therefore, sodium intake is strongly related to nutrition, which is another important key factor determining mortality. There are two contradictory aspects of the effect of sodium intake: hypertension and nutrition (see Figure 1). This review describes the interaction between sodium intake, body weight, hypertension, nutrition, and mortality in chronic kidney disease patients, including dialysis patients.

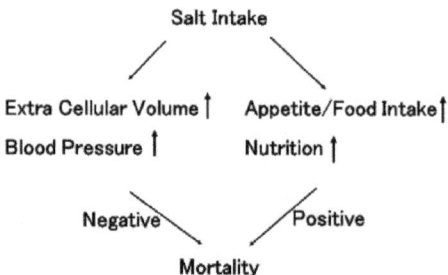

Figure 1. The influence of salt intake on mortality. Salt intake increases extracellular volume, resulting in increased blood pressure in both the general population and chronic kidney disease (CKD) patients, including dialysis patients. Hypertension is considered to worsen prognosis. This salt sensation higher in CKD patients than in the general population. In contrast, salt intake increase appetite. Under the same salt taste, salt intake is basically proportional to the amount of food intake. Good nutritional conditions improve prognosis. Therefore, salt intake has dual effects on prognosis, both negative and positive effects.

2. Interaction between Sodium Intake and Body Weight (Extracellular Volume) in Non-Dialysis CKD Patients

In extracellular fluid volume, osmotic presser is derived from sodium, glucose, and blood urea nitrogen concentrations. Among these osmolytes, sodium is the strongest determinate of osmotic pressure because sodium occupies a major portion of osmolytes in extracellular volume. After sodium intake, osmotic pressure should increase, resulting in strong thirst via the thirst center in the brain (see Figure 2). Water intake continues until osmotic pressure became normal, similar to physiological saline. After drinking water, extracellular volume increases to the same osmotic pressure as normal osmotic pressure in the extracellular fluid. After ingesting 9 g of salt, a person needs to drink 1000 mL of water to reach 0.9% physiological saline in the extracellular fluid (This person is ideal and fictional for this review). Edema is often observed after intake of excess sodium. In the general population, excretion of sodium in the kidneys increases just after consuming sodium [1]. Sodium excretion rapidly equalizes to sodium intake. However, in non-dialysis chronic kidney disease (CKD) patients, decreased kidney function prolongs the effect of sodium intake because the ability to excrete excess sodium is decreased, resulting in elevated blood pressure.

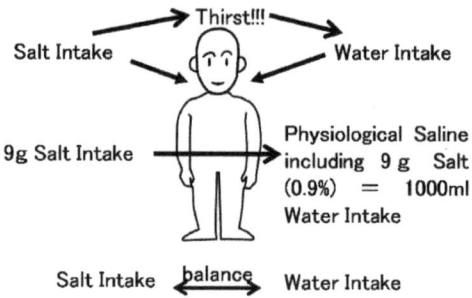

Figure 2. The balance between salt intake and water intake. Salt intake is balanced with water intake via the thirst center. After 9 g of salt intake, a person wants to drink 1000 mL water, resulting in 0.9% physiological saline in extracellular fluid. If the person does not drink enough water, the concentration of sodium will increase, resulting in strong thirst.

3. Interaction between Sodium Intake and Hypertension in Non-Dialysis CKD Patients

After sodium intake, the kidney increases sodium excretion via inducing elevated blood pressure. Known as Guyton's pressure–natriuresis curve [1], salt excretion is basically proportional to blood pressure. From renal aspects, blood pressure depends upon arterial resistance to glomeruli, such as renal artery stenosis, the coefficient of glomerular excess filtration and sodium reabsorption in distal tubules, regulated primarily by aldosterone (see Figure 3). The coefficient of glomerular excess filtration depends on the effective glomerular filtration surface and coefficient of penetration. In CKD patients, the effective glomerular filtration surface decreases, resulting in enhanced salt sensation. Indeed, CKD patients are reported to have strong salt sensation in response to food [2–5]. In the setting of increased salt sensitivity, excess sodium intake easily elevates blood pressure. Excess salt intake increases proteinuria via elevated internal glomerular pressure. Hypertension and proteinuria are important factors in determining the rate of worsening renal function. Decreasing blood pressure and proteinuria are important therapeutic targets. Excess sodium intake worsens both blood pressure and proteinuria, and inhibition of sodium intake decreases blood pressure and proteinuria at the same time (see Figure 4). Restriction of sodium intake is an important therapy in CKD patients.

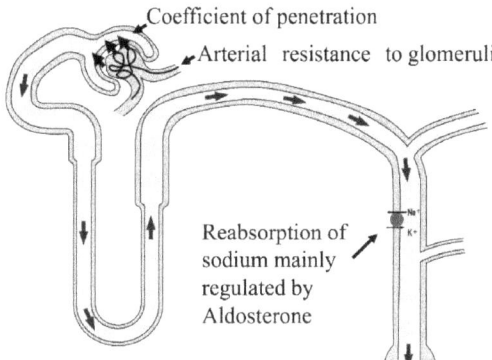

Figure 3. Determinates of blood pressure in the glomeruli. There are three elements that can determine blood pressure. One is arterial resistance to glomeruli, such as renovascular hypertension. The second is the coefficient of penetration, such as hypertension, in CKD patients. The third element is reabsorption of sodium in distal tubules, regulated primarily by aldosterone, such as primary aldosteronism. In CKD patients, the coefficient of penetration is not normal because this coefficient depends on the effective surface of the glomeruli.

4. Interaction among Sodium Intake, Appetite, and Nutrition in Non-Dialysis CKD Patients

The sensation of taste components consists of five factors: salt, sweet, sour, bitter, and umami. Salt is an important taste component and influences other components. Salt restriction also causes taste restriction. Moreover, salt and bitter taste acuity declines with age, while sweet and sour perception does not [6]. The prevalence of CKD in elderly patients is much higher than in the young population [7,8]. Therefore, most CKD patients suffer from low salt sensation. Moreover, CKD itself worsens the accuracy of salt and sour taste sensations [9,10], while the mechanism this abnormality of tastes induced by CKD remained unclear. Weakening salt sensation theoretically leads to more salt intake during free food intake. Typically, salt restriction worsens taste, and therefore causes loss of appetite. In CKD patients, this effect becomes larger due to decreased salt sensation. Under the same salt concentrations, salt restriction also means diet restriction. Salt intake in CKD patients is strongly correlated with phosphate intake, which is equal to protein intake [11]. Sodium restriction easily causes appetite loss and worsens nutrition status. However, salt restriction improves salt sensation [10,12]. Kusaba-K et al. reported that one week of sodium restriction dramatically improved salt sensation. Several reports have also supported that education on sodium intake improves salt sensation itself [9,10]. It was reported that educational hospitalization with enhanced salt reduction guidance reduced the risk of end-stage renal disease [13]. Sodium restriction seems to be effective under the control of nutritional status.

5. Interaction between Sodium Intake and Mortality in Non-Dialysis CKD Patients

Generally, excess sodium intake is considered an important life-threatening risk factor that can be improved by personal efforts. Excess salt intake necessitates induction of high blood pressure to increase salt excretion in the kidney according to the pressure-diuresis curve [1]. Excess sodium is believed to increase blood pressure, resulting in worsening mortality. According to this theory, the World Health Organization recommended restrictions on salt intake for the general population [14,15]. However, Martin O'Donnell et al. reported a U-curve effect of sodium intake on morality in the general population [16] (see Figure 5). This article reported that among 103,570 international subjects in eighteen countries, the relationship between sodium and potassium intake was evaluated by morning fasting urine with respect to mortality during a median follow-up of 8.2 years. Among the joint sodium and potassium excretion categories, the lowest risk of death and cardiovascular events occurred in the group with moderate sodium excretion and higher potassium excretion (3–5 g sodium/day = 7.6–12.7 g salt/day; 21.9% of cohort). Compared to this reference group, the combinations of low potassium with low sodium excretion (<3 g sodium/day $\leq$ 7.6 g salt/day) (hazard ratio 1.23 (1.11–1.37); 7.4% of cohort) and low potassium with high sodium excretion (>5 g sodium/day $\geq$ 12.7 g salt/day) (1.21 (1.11–1.32); 13.8% of cohort) were associated with the highest risk, followed by low sodium excretion and higher potassium excretion (<3 g sodium/day $\leq$ 7.6 g salt/day) (1.19 (1.02–1.38); 3.3% of cohort), and high sodium excretion and higher potassium excretion (1.10 (1.02–1.180); 29.6% of cohort). Higher potassium excretion attenuated the increased cardiovascular risk associated with high sodium excretion (P for interaction = 0.007). This report concluded that moderate sodium intake combined with high potassium intake is associated with the lowest risk of mortality and cardiovascular events. This J-shaped effect of sodium intake on mortality has also been reported in patients with cardiovascular events [17]. Martin O'Donnell et al. reported this phenomenon in the general population in several studies [18–20]. The finding that potassium intake attenuated the effect of sodium intake suggested that the low food intake induced by sodium restriction worsened mortality. However, after adjustment for nutritional factors, the effect of low sodium intake was still observed. The effect of sodium restriction, except for nutritional factors, ultimately remains unknown. However, one considerable mechanism is that imbalance of sodium intake and water intake may cause hyponatremia. Water intake is usually encouraged to avoid dehydration [21], especially in elderly subjects. Excess water intake, along with restricted sodium intake requires water diuresis with salt reabsorption in the kidney. In patients with several diseases, such as heart failure, chronic kidney disease, and liver failure, the kidney cannot provide sufficient water diuresis because high vasopressin levels induced by these disease conditions perturb proper water diuresis, resulting in hyponatremia. Hyponatremia is well known as a risk factor for worse mortality [22–26]. Of course, overload of sodium intake worsens mortality not only in heart failure patients but also in the general populations. Moreover, the effect of an overload of excess sodium intake in heart failure patients was markedly higher than in the general population [17]. Sodium restriction is essential in patients with many kinds of diseases, but in the case of sodium restriction, regular monitoring of serum sodium concentrations is also essential. Based on this evidence, sodium restriction in the general population has become controversial [27].

In non-dialysis CKD patients, the effect of excess sodium intake is more important than in the general population. Excess sodium intake increases blood pressure, especially glomerular blood pressure. Elevated permeable pressure in the glomeruli induced by excess sodium intake increases proteinuria [28], which is an important and classical risk factor for kidney disease progression. Moreover, excess sodium intake suppresses the renin–angiotensin system, resulting in cancelling the reno-protective effect of renin–angiotensin system blockers. Renin–angiotensin system blockers in conjunction with sodium restriction can decrease proteinuria more effectively than renin–angiotensin system blockers alone [28,29] (see Figure 4). Even in the case of diuretic use, which may decrease the amount of sodium in the body, sodium restriction could decrease proteinuria [28]. Theoretically, sodium restriction in chronic kidney disease patients should decrease proteinuria and blood pressure and therefore improve renal progression, resulting in improved mortality. The CRIC study, comprising an important chronic kidney disease cohort, reported the relationship between sodium intake evaluated by urinary sodium excretion and kidney disease progression or mortality [30]. Non-dialysis CKD patients with high sodium intake (more than 194.6 mmol sodium/day = 11.4 g salt/day) exhibited significantly worse renal prognosis. However, CKD patients with several categories of sodium intakes less than 194.6 mmol sodium/day (11.4 g salt/day) had almost the same kidney prognosis. Moreover, those CKD patients had the same mortality (see Figure 5). Apparently, non-dialysis CKD patients were more vulnerable to high salt intake than the general population (see Figure 5), but there were no significant differences between CKD patients with low salt intake and those with moderate salt intake, most likely because CKD patients are a high-risk group of hyponatremia who were encouraged to drink water to avoid dehydration, and sodium restriction may easily cause hyponatremia, resulting in a worsening prognosis. In CKD patients, mild sodium restriction (less than 194.6 mmol = 11.4 salt/day) is essential with regular sodium concentration monitoring.

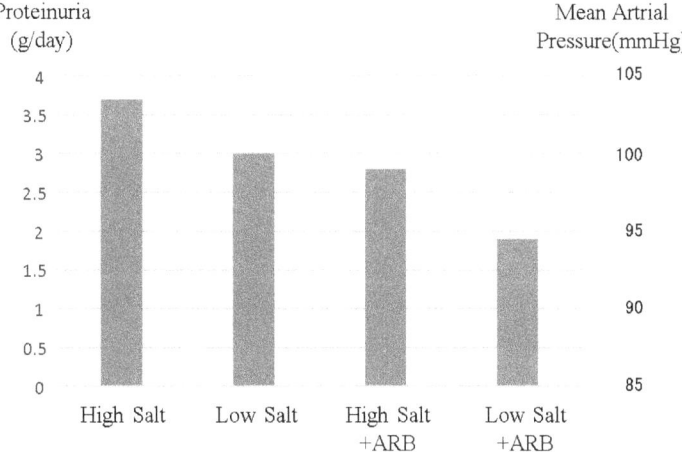

Figure 4. Changes in proteinuria and blood pressure induced by salt intake and angiotensin-receptor blocker administration. High salt intake increases both blood pressure and proteinuria. Although angiotensin-receptor blockers are well known to reduce blood pressure and proteinuria, resulting in reno-protective effects, high salt intake reduces these renoprotective effects. This image was made from data reported by Vogt et al. [28], but this phenomenon is common in CKD patients.

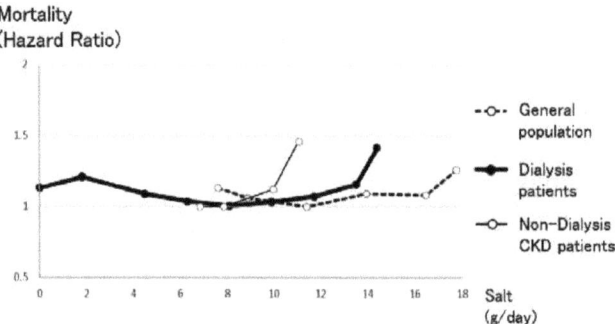

Figure 5. The relationship between salt intake and mortality in the general population, non-dialysis CKD patients and dialysis patients. The right line shows the relationship between salt intake and mortality in the general population, which was made from data reported by O'Donnell et al. [16]. Intake of more than 17.8 g salt/day made the prognosis significantly worse after diet adjustments, while intake of less than 7.6 g salt/day also made the prognosis worse. The center bold line shows the relationship between salt intake and mortality in dialysis patients, which was made from the relationship between intradialysis body weight gain and mortality reported by the Japan Society of Dialysis Therapy. Intake of more than 12.6 g salt/day made the prognosis significantly worse after diet adjustments, while intake of less than 5.4 g salt/day also made the prognosis worse. The left line shows the relationship between salt intake and mortality in non-dialysis CKD patients, which was made from data reported by the CRIC cohort study [30]. Non-dialysis CKD patients were more vulnerable to salt intake than the other groups, likely because excess sodium intake increases blood pressure and proteinuria, resulting in worsening prognosis. Simple comparisons should be considered because these three lines refer to different cohorts that originate in different countries, with different observation periods and numbers.

6. Summary of Interaction between Sodium Intake, Body Weight, Hypertension, Nutrition, and Mortality in Non-Dialysis CKD Patients

Sodium intake theoretically has dual effects on prognosis, including both harmful effects and beneficial effects (see Figure 1). Sodium intake is believed to induce hypertension, resulting in poor prognosis. In contrast, sodium intake increases appetite, resulting in improved nutrition and good prognosis. In fact, a U-shaped relationship between sodium intake and mortality support these dual effects in the general population (see Figure 5).

In CKD patients, sodium intake exerts more important effects on prognosis. Sodium intake increases not only blood pressure but also proteinuria, resulting in both poor renal prognosis and life expectancy. In contrast, sodium intake increases appetite, resulting in good nutritional status. In dialysis patients, the obesity paradox is well known [31,32]. This paradox involves a higher body mass index (BMI) causing a better prognosis in dialysis patients, while in the general population, a higher BMI causes a poor prognosis by increasing cardiovascular events [33]. This obesity paradox is also observed in non-dialysis CKD patients [34] (see Figure 6). Another Japanese non-dialysis CKD cohort also reported that low BMI (18.4–20.3) was associated with significant risk of all-cause mortality and infection-related death [35]. Therefore, nutritional factors are very important for CKD patients. Obesity is considered to have negative effects on the progression of kidney disease through elevation of eGFR, hypertension, and proteinuria. Exercise has reno-protective effects [36,37]. However, obesity seemed to cancel out these renoprotective effects [38]. It is important to maintain a balance between nutritionally good conditions and bad conditions induced by obesity. Sodium restriction is necessary for CKD patients to decrease proteinuria and preserve kidney function, but in cases of sodium restriction, nutritional factors, and hyponatremia should be considered.

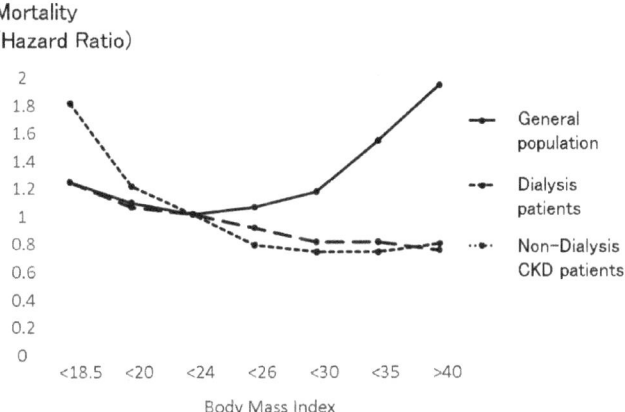

Figure 6. The relationship between body mass index and mortality in the general population, non-dialysis CKD patients and dialysis patients. The upper U-shaped line shows the relationship between body mass index (BMI) and mortality in the general population, which was made from data reported based on 900,000 subjects [33]. The line indicates the average mortality in men and in women. The effect of BMI on mortality in women was smaller than in men in all BMI categories. High BMI was associated with high mortality in the general population, while low BMI was also associated with high mortality. The middle line shows the relationship between BMI and mortality in dialysis patients reported by Kalantar-Zadeh et al. [31]. Higher BMI in dialysis patients consistently improves prognosis in dialysis patients. This divergence from the relationship in the general population was named the "obesity paradox". The bottom line shows the relationship between BMI and mortality in non-dialysis CKD patients reported by Navaneethan-SD et al. [34]. The obesity paradox was observed in non-dialysis patients. Simple comparisons should be considered because these three lines refer to different cohorts that have different countries of origin, observation periods, and numbers.

7. Interaction between Sodium Intake and Body Weight (Intradialysis Increase in Body Weight) in Dialysis CKD Patients

In dialysis patients, salt and water intake should be balanced (see Figure 2). When dialysis patients ingest salt for additional taste during meals, the sodium concentration increases. In such cases, sodium concentrations tend to increase and cause strong thirst via the thirst center in the brain. This thirst continues until the sodium concentration becomes normal, similar to physiological saline solution (isotonic sodium chloride solution). Sodium intake should be completely balanced with water intake via the thirst center. Nine grams of sodium chloride intake requires subsequent intake of 1000 mL water, resulting in physiological saline (0.9% sodium chloride solution). In non-dialysis CKD patients, urine attenuates this volume increase induced by sodium, but in dialysis patients, sodium intake induces exactly this volume retention because the kidneys are not functioning properly.

In dialysis patients, salt removal should also be balanced with water removal (see In dialysis patients, salt removal should also be balanced with water removal (see Figure 7). The sodium concentration in dialysate is usually the same as the serum sodium concentration (140 mEq/L), meaning that during dialysis, sodium cannot move to the dialysate. During dialysis, water is usually removed. This water includes sodium, whose concentration should be equal to the serum sodium concentration. Water and salt are removed at the same time during the dialysis process as physiological saline is removed. Therefore, in dialysis patients the intake of sodium and water is basically equal to the removal of sodium and water during the dialysis session because these patients have lost kidney function (see Figures 2 and 7).

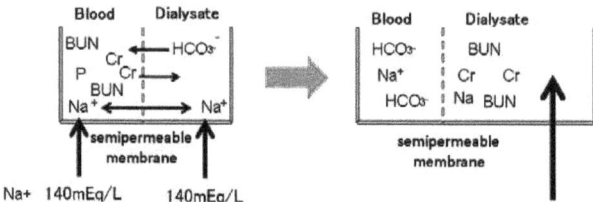

Figure 7. Removal of sodium during dialysis sessions. Small molecular substances, such as blood urea nitrogen and phosphate creatinine, are moved to the dialysate according to the concentration gradient. Bicarbonate also moves to the blood from the dialysate according to the concentration gradient. The sodium concentration in the dialysate is 140 mEq/L. The serum sodium concentration is also approximately 140 mEq/L. Therefore, sodium cannot move from the blood to the dialysate through the semipermeable membrane in the dialyzer. However, water removal during dialysis sessions includes 140 mEq/L sodium. Water removal during dialysis sessions means sodium removal at the same time.

Generally, estimation of sodium intake is very difficult because the precise intake and sodium concentration of each meal are usually unknown. However, estimation of water intake, including water in food, is far easier because intradialysis body weight gain is equal to the water intake. The amount of salt intake can be estimated using water intake because salt intake is basically balanced with water intake. Reports of the Japanese dialysis patient registry, which are provided by the Japanese Society of Dialysis Therapy, published the relationship between the increase in body weight during the dialysis interval and mortality one year later. A 3% body weight increase to a 7% body weight increase reportedly resulted in a good prognosis, according to the relationship between body weight increase and mortality after adjustment for fundamental factors, the amount of dialysis therapy and nutritional factors (see Figure 8). If the body weight of the dialysis patient was 60 kg, a 3% body weight increase meant 1800 g. Therefore, 1800 g divided by 3 days equals to 600 g, and 600 g divided by 1000 mL physiological saline, including 9 g salt, yields 5.4 g salt. This calculation means that approximately 6 g salt (=2.36 g sodium) per day is essential for a 60 kg dialysis patient. In contrast, in 60 kg dialysis patients, a 7% body weight increase was 4200 g. 4200 g divided by 3 days equals 1400 g, and 1400 g divided by 1000 mL physiological saline, including 9 g sodium chloride, yields 12.6 g salt. This calculation means that 60 kg dialysis patients can ingest 12.6 g salt (=4.96 g sodium) per day safely. (These 60 kg dialysis patients are ideal and fictional for this review).

There is a pitfall in the method to determine the recommended salt intake. The reason the standard salt intake can be calculated by intradialysis body weight gain depends on thirst. If people drink water when they are not thirsty, the estimation of sodium intake based on intradialysis body weight gain would not make sense. Drinking without thirst typically involves alcohol drinks. If a patient drinks a 350 g can of beer every day, these patients drank a total of 1050 g of water during the interval of dialysis (3 days), resulting in a total salt intake of 9.4 g during those periods. If a patient drank two bottles of beer every day, these patients ingested 3798 g of water during hemodialysis intervals, resulting in a salt intake of 11.3 g a day, which means that this patient could not eat anything with salt, except for the beer. (These drunken dialysis patients are ideal and fictional for this review). If the patient truly wants to drink alcohol, the patient should choose an alcohol drink including a high concentration of alcohol, such as whisky without water. If dialysis patients drink a small amount of alcohol, their thirst after eating food with salt should be suppressed, and their serum sodium concentration with stay within normal ranges. In the case of sick individuals, patients tend to ingest food, including much water, such as soup, rice porridge (Okayu), and oatmeal. These kinds of food also reduce the capacity of salt intake.

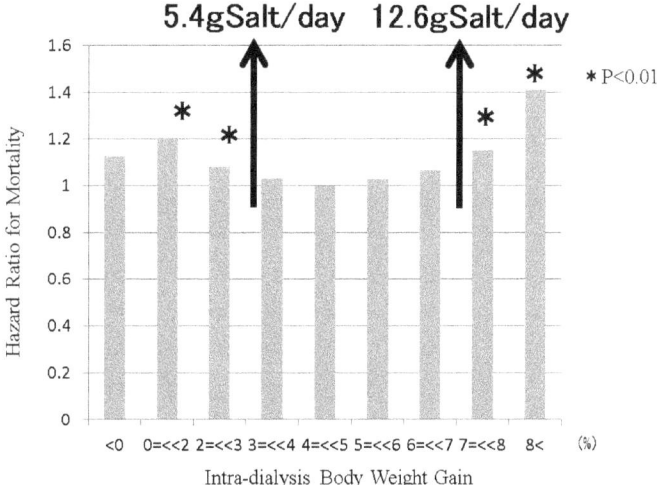

Figure 8. The relationship between intradialysis body weight gain and mortality in dialysis patients. Sodium intake is balanced with water intake via the thirst center. Sodium removal is balanced with water removal during dialysis session. Therefore, intradialysis salt intake can be estimated from intradialysis body weight gain. The Japanese Society of Dialysis Therapy reported the relationship between intradialysis body weight gain and mortality at 1 year as surveillance of dialysis patients by the Japan Society of Dialysis Therapy 2009.12.31. From 3% to 7% of intradialysis body weight gain, the mortality of dialysis patients remained good. From estimations from this intradialysis body weight gain, dialysis patients can maintain good conditions from 5.4 g salt/day (=2.1 g sodium/day) intake to 12.6 g salt/day (=5.0 g sodium/day) intake, if the body weight of the dialysis patient is 60 kg.

In the case of hypernatremia, strong thirst induces water consumption, resulting in normalization of hypernatremia. This system can work in both normal subjects and hemodialysis patients. In contrast, in the case of hyponatremia, activation of the renin–angiotensin–aldosterone system along with inhibition of vasopressin induces upregulation of salt retention in the kidney without water retention, resulting in normalization of hyponatremia. This system works in subjects without kidney disease, but in dialysis patients, this system does not work because patients have lost kidney function. Moreover, salt removal in dialysis patients is performed by salt with the removal of water during dialysis therapy. The balance between the removal of salt and water is basically constant to ensure serum sodium concentrations similar to physiological saline. Under hyponatremic conditions, thirst cannot correct the balance between water intake and salt intake. Therefore, dialysis patients are prone to developing hyponatremia. The Japan Society of Dialysis Therapy reported that predialysis hyponatremia was associated with worse mortality after one year (see Figure 9). Moreover, hyponatremia in dialysis patients can be corrected by dialysis therapy because sodium moves from the dialysate to serum according to the sodium concentration gradient. This means that dialysis patients with hyponatremia receive salt through dialysis therapy, while those patients restrict salt in food. Rapid correction of serum sodium by dialysis therapy increases serum osmolality, possibly resulting in several ill reactions, such as general fatigue, headache, osmotic demyelination syndrome, and so on. Hyponatremia itself has been reported to have a strong relationship with worse prognosis in several disease conditions [22–26]. If hyponatremia is observed in dialysis patients, the balance between water intake and salt intake should be checked. Overdose of water intake or overrestriction of salt intake along with relative overdose of water results in hyponatremia.

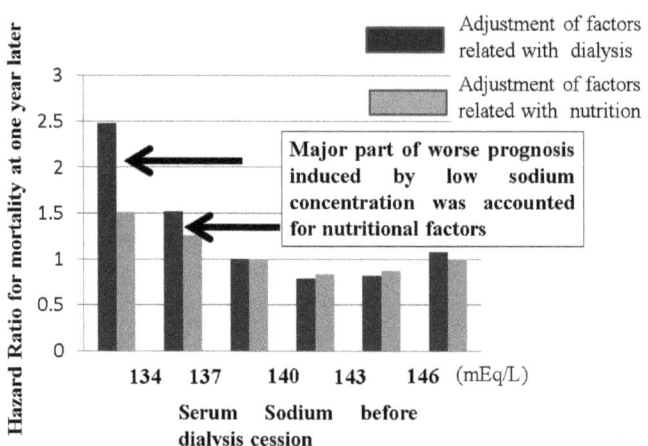

Figure 9. The relationship between serum sodium concentration before dialysis sessions and mortality in dialysis patients. The Japanese Society of Dialysis Therapy reported the relationship between serum sodium concentration before dialysis sessions and mortality at 1 year as surveillance of dialysis patients by the Japan Society of Dialysis Therapy 2009.12.31. Dialysis patients with less than 137 mEq/L sodium concentrations exhibited poor prognosis, but this negative effect induced by low sodium concentration could be adjusted by nutritional factors, meaning that the low sodium concentration in dialysis patients usually indicates poor nutritional intake. Water intake without proper salt easily induces hyponatremia in dialysis patients. In the case of hyponatremia in dialysis patients, the balance between sodium and water intake should be monitored to improve nutritional status.

8. Interaction between Sodium Intake and Hypertension in Dialysis CKD Patients

Sodium intake is directly related to extracellular fluid volume in dialysis patients via the thirst center, as shown in Figure 2. Increased fluid volume caused the elevation of blood pressure. Indeed, blood pressure just before dialysis session tended to be higher than after dialysis session. Elasticity of blood vessels can buffer this volume effect, but atherosclerosis, which is very common in dialysis patents, prevents this buffering effect. Therefore, hypertension before dialysis session is very common, but in terms of this hypertension in dialysis patients, there is another paradox regarding hypertension in the general population [39,40]. A reverse effect of blood pressure on mortality in dialysis patients was reported in 56,388 incident dialysis patients [41]. In this report, dialysis patients whose blood pressure was less than 120 mmHg had the worst prognosis, those with 120–140 mmHg blood pressure had the second worst prognosis, and there were no differences in prognosis in those with 140–160, 160–180, 180–200, and more than 200 mmHg blood pressure. Another study also reported that in 37,069 dialysis patients, those with less than 115 mmHg systolic blood pressure had the worst mortality, while those with more than 135 mmHg systolic pressure had a good prognosis [42]. Another study in 5433 dialysis patients reported that systolic pressure greater than 180 mmHg improved prognosis [43]. While hypertension itself has been classically considered a risk factor for cardiovascular events [44–48], the role of hypertension as a risk factor for mortality has been controversial [43,49–53] The reverse effect of blood pressure on mortality in dialysis patients is similar to the reverse effect of BMI on mortality, which is well known as the obesity paradox and is discussed above. One of the possible mechanisms is that after initiation of dialysis, nutritional factors, which can be related to BMI and hypertension induced by intradialysis food and sodium intake, are more important than classical cardiovascular event risk factors [54]. Another possible mechanism is that hypertension before dialysis session makes dialysis therapy safe and comfortable until end of scheduled dialysis session time because hypotension during dialysis session sometimes required the termination of dialysis session. KDOQI comments on the 2017 ACC/AHA hypertension guidelines described that the treatment of targets of hypertension in dialysis patients cannot be proposed due to the lack of clinical trial evidence [55]. The Japanese Society of Hypertension described that the Japanese guidelines for hypertension cannot be applied to dialysis patients due to the specific and distinct conditions of dialysis patients.

9. Interaction among Sodium Intake, Appetite and Nutrition in Dialysis CKD Patients

Salt sensation in dialysis patients is reported to be worse than that in non-dialysis CKD patients [56]. Theoretically, dialysis patients with salt taste dysfunction ingest more salt than is appropriate to gain sufficient salty taste, possibly resulting in an increase in intradialytic body weight gain. However, there were no changes in intradialytic body weight gain between dialysis patients with or without salt sensation dysfunction [57]. This report indicates that food intake, including salt intake, depends not only on salt sensation dysfunction but also on other factors. One possible factor related to appetite is zinc. Zinc deficiency is common in dialysis patients, and zinc deficiency causes a decrease in the sensation of taste, including salt taste. Moreover, zinc is related to many enzymatic activities related to protein synthesis; therefore, zinc deficiency is reportedly related to nutritional status. In fact, zinc supplementation ameliorated nutritional status [58] in a randomized control study. If dialysis patients suffer from appetite loss and a small increase in intradialysis body weight gain, there is the possibility that too much salt restriction retards food intake through appetite loss, which may also be caused by zinc deficiency.

10. Interaction between Sodium Intake and Body Weight (Nutritional Status) and Mortality in Dialysis CKD Patients

Estimation of the amount of sodium intake is difficult; therefore, reports on the relationship between sodium intake in the diet and mortality are limited. Post hoc analysis of the HEMO study reported that increased dietary sodium intake, which was estimated using a history of food intake by dietitians, was independently associated with greater mortality among hemodialysis subjects [59]. Although there were no descriptions of sodium intake in quartiles, only the fourth category of dialysis patients who might ingest more than 4 g sodium a day (=10 g salt intake a day) exhibited significantly higher risk. Moreover, this article reported that sodium intake was strongly associated with caloric intake, but the adjustment of nutritional status was not sufficient. In this study, only weight was reported rather than BMI, while albumin was selected.

Sodium intake is strongly correlated with food intake. Under the same salt sensation, sodium intake is proportional to food intake. Sufficient food intake ameliorates nutritional status. The question is whether a better nutritional status can overcome the negative effects caused by excess sodium intake, such as an increase in intradialytic body weight and hypertension. As well-known as the obesity paradox, high BMI in dialysis patients attenuates mortality (see Figure 6). This obesity paradox was first reported in heart failure patients [60]. Recently, the obesity paradox was observed in many energy wasting diseases, such as COPD and cancers, especially esophageal cancer [33]. The reason the obesity paradox is observed in many energy-wasting diseases is that a stock of energy can sustain energy-wasting conditions and make it possible to overcome several illness conditions, such as infectious diseases and cardiovascular diseases [54]. In dialysis patients, body weight gain ameliorated mortality. Surprisingly, in obesity dialysis patients whose BMI was greater than 30, body weight gain indicated better prognosis [61], and body weight loss indicated poor prognosis. The improvement of prognosis induced by body weight was attenuated by BMI, but good nutritional status could overcome the negative effects induced by obesity, even in obese dialysis patients with a BMI greater than 30. Unless excess sodium intake ameliorates the nutritional condition, sodium intake itself should be acceptable.

11. Summary of Interactions between Sodium Intake, Body Weight, Hypertension, Nutrition, and Mortality in Dialysis CKD Patients

In dialysis CKD patients, sodium intake is directly related to intradialytic body weight gain via the thirst center, resulting in hypertension before hemodialysis sessions. However, this hypertension does not worsen the prognosis of dialysis patients. Sodium intake is also directly related to nutrition status via the appetite center. Moreover, the amount of sodium intake is basically proportional to food intake under the same salt taste conditions. Therefore, sodium intake may improve nutritional status. In dialysis patients, both obesity and body weight gain improve prognosis through good nutritional conditions. Sodium intake has both good and bad effects in dialysis CKD patients, as well as in non-CKD patients. However, in dialysis patients, the good effect of sodium basically overcomes the bad effect from the perspective of mortality.

A comfortable dialysis session and safe control of life-limiting biochemical parameters may exert opposite effects from the good nutritional status induced by food intake. Salt intake causes an increase in intradialytic body weight gain, requiring prolonged dialysis time because the time-averaged removal of water is limited. Protein intake, including phosphate intake, may cause hyperphosphoremia, increasing the risk of cardiovascular events. Fruit and vegetable intake may cause hyperkalemia [62], which is famously a risk factor for sudden death (see Figure 10). The standard nutritional intake has not been changed for a long time (see Table 1). This standard is similar to the nutritional guidelines in many countries [63–65]. The reason for the unchanged nutritional guidelines was that these guidelines were based on comfortable and safe control of dialysis session and the lives of dialysis patients, which were physiologically unchanged. However, recent advances in drug- and technology-related dialysis therapy may change the physiological limitation of nutritional intake. New phosphate binders and calcium-sensing receptor agonists have become available, which increase protein intake [66,67]. Indeed, protein intake with phosphate binders could improve nutritional factors in the short term [68]. New potassium binders have also become available, making safe fruit and vegetable intake possible [69]. Moreover, it was recently reported that a high frequency of fruit and vegetable intake in dialysis patients improved prognosis [70]. Fruits and vegetables are considered to have good effects on mortality [71]. Potassium intake was not related to hyperkalemia in either non-dialysis CKD patients or dialysis patients [72]. The upper limit of sodium is much higher than the target of sodium intake in the nutritional standard, as discussed in the above section. Food intake, including sodium intake, should be encouraged in dialysis CKD patients to improve nutritional status, resulting in a better prognosis.

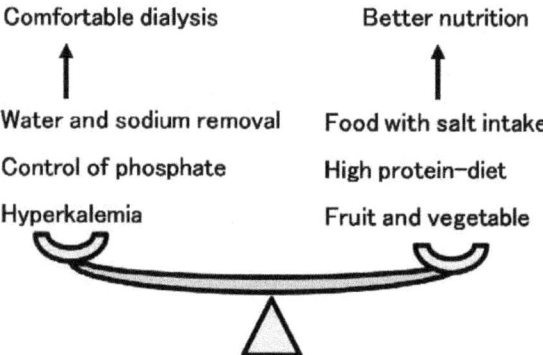

Figure 10. The balance of food and salt intake between comfortable dialysis and better nutrition. Comfortable dialysis therapy is sometimes contrary to better nutritional intake. Sufficient food intake with proper salt taste increases intradialytic body weight gain, resulting in prolonged dialysis session time. A high-protein diet easily induces hyperphosphatemia, resulting in vascular calcification and cardiovascular events. Healthy fruit and vegetable intake induces hyperkalemia.

Table 1. Standard nutritional intake in hemodialysis patients in Japan.

Energy	30–35 kcal/kg (*)(**)
Protein	0.9–1.2 g/kg (*)
Salt	less than 6 g (***)
Water	Minimum requirement
Potassium	less than 2000 mg
Phosphate	less than Protein (g) × 15 mg

* Standard Body Weight (BMI = 22) ** Depending on sex, age, physical activity *** Depending on urine volume, physical activity, body weight, nutritional status, increase of body weight between HD sessions. This recommendation was published by a committee for nutritional factors in the Japanese Society of Dialysis Therapy, including the authors. The original recommendation was written by Nakao, T., Kanno, Y., Nagasawa, Y., Kanazawa, Y., Akib, T., Sanaka, K., Standard nutritional intake in maintained dialysis patients. *J. Jpn. Soc. Dial. Ther.* **2014**, *47*, 287–291. (In Japanese) [65].

12. Conclusions: Important Gaps in Awareness of Sodium Intake between Non-Dialysis and Dialysis CKD Patients

Sodium intake has both a good effect on improving nutritional effects and a bad effect on increasing fluid volume, which causes hypertension and increases proteinuria. In non-dialysis CKD patients, doctors should pay attention to the balance between the positive and negative effects of sodium restriction, while in dialysis patients, the good effect of sodium intake basically overcomes the bad effect of sodium intake because nutritional status is an important issue in dialysis patients.

Recently, frailty and protein-energy wasting have been recognized as serious problems in dialysis patients [73,74]. Frailty worsens prognosis in dialysis and non-dialysis CKD patients [75]. Nutritional intervention in frail dialysis patients is an important and practical therapy [76,77]. However, restriction of sodium intake sometimes prevents sufficient food intake. In dialysis CKD patients, a good effect of sodium intake basically overcomes the bad effect because nutritional status limits the prognosis of dialysis patients, while in non-CKD patients, the balance between the positive and negative effects of sodium intake is important because restriction of sodium decreases blood pressure and proteinuria, resulting in preserving kidney function. There was no evidence of the beginning of the change in sodium intake between non-dialysis CKD patients and dialysis patients. However, the report that weight loss in non-dialysis patients worsened prognosis after initiation of dialysis therapy [78] indicated that sodium restriction in non-dialysis CKD patients should sometimes be re-evaluated and relaxed at the time of weight loss as well as during hyponatremia. There are important gaps in awareness of sodium intake between non-dialysis and dialysis CKD patients. Sodium restriction may be allowed in cases of maintaining good nutritional status and normal serum sodium levels in CKD patients, including dialysis patients.

Funding: This research received no external funding.

Institutional Review Board Statement: Not applicable.

Informed Consent Statement: Not applicable.

Acknowledgments: I deeply thank Masaaki Inaba, a chairman of 65th Annual Meeting of Japan Society of Dialysis Therapy. I thank Noriko Echigoya, Division of Kidney and Dialysis, Department of Internal Medicine, Hyogo College of Medicine, for assistance of illustrations. The main message in this review was presented in the symposium in the meeting. This work was supported by JSPS KAKENHI Grant Number JP17K09721, JP19K10098, JP20K10225, JP20ek0109479, and AMED Grant Number JP20ek0109479.

Conflicts of Interest: The author declares no conflict of interest.

References

1. Hall, J.E.; Hall, M.E. Chapter 19—Role of the Kidney in Long-Term control of arterial pressure in hypertension: The integrated system for arterial pressure regulation. In *Guyton and Hall Textbook of Medical Physiology*, 14th ed.; Elsevier: Amsterdam, The Netherlands, 2020; pp. 229–244.
2. Bovee, D.M.; Cuevas, C.A.; Zietse, R.; Danser, A.H.J.; Mirabito Colafella, K.M.; Hoorn, E.J. Salt-sensitive hypertension in chronic kidney disease: Distal tubular mechanisms. *Am. J. Physiol. Ren. Physiol.* **2020**, *319*, F729–F745. [CrossRef]
3. Komnenov, D.; Levanovich, P.E.; Rossi, N.F. Hypertension Associated with Fructose and High Salt: Renal and Sympathetic Mechanisms. *Nutrients* **2019**, *11*, 569. [CrossRef] [PubMed]
4. Furusho, T.; Uchida, S.; Sohara, E. The WNK signaling pathway and salt-sensitive hypertension. *Hypertens. Res.* **2020**, *43*, 733–743. [CrossRef] [PubMed]
5. Kimura, G.; Dohi, Y.; Fukuda, M. Salt sensitivity and circadian rhythm of blood pressure: The keys to connect CKD with cardiovascular events. *Hypertens. Res.* **2010**, *33*, 515–520. [CrossRef]
6. Winkler, S.; Garg, A.K.; Mekayarajjananonth, T.; Bakaeen, L.G.; Khan, E. Depressed taste and smell in geriatric patients. *J. Am. Dent. Assoc.* **1999**, *130*, 1759–1765. [CrossRef]
7. Hill, N.R.; Fatoba, S.T.; Oke, J.L.; Hirst, J.A.; O'Callaghan, C.A.; Lasserson, D.S.; Hobbs, F.D.R. Global Prevalence of Chronic Kidney Disease—A Systematic Review and Meta-Analysis. *PLoS ONE* **2016**, *11*, e0158765. [CrossRef]
8. Imai, E.; Horio, M.; Iseki, K.; Yamagata, K.; Watanabe, T.; Hara, S.; Ura, N.; Kiyohara, Y.; Hirakata, H.; Moriyama, T.; et al. Prevalence of chronic kidney disease (CKD) in the Japanese general population predicted by the MDRD equation modified by a Japanese coefficient. *Clin. Exp. Nephrol.* **2007**, *11*, 156–163. [CrossRef] [PubMed]
9. McMahon, E.J.; Campbell, K.L.; Bauer, J.D. Taste perception in kidney disease and relationship to dietary sodium intake. *Appetite* **2014**, *83*, 236–241. [CrossRef] [PubMed]
10. Kim, T.H.; Kim, Y.H.; Bae, N.Y.; Kang, S.S.; Lee, J.B.; Kim, S.B. Salty taste thresholds and preference in patients with chronic kidney disease according to disease stage: A cross-sectional study. *Nutr. Diet.* **2018**, *75*, 59–64. [CrossRef]
11. Humalda, J.K.; Keyzer, C.A.; Binnenmars, S.H.; Kwakernaak, A.J.; Slagman, M.C.; Laverman, G.D.; Bakker, S.J.; de Borst, M.H.; Navis, G.J. Concordance of dietary sodium intake and concomitant phosphate load: Implications for sodium interventions. *Nutr. Metab. Cardiovasc. Dis.* **2016**, *26*, 689–696. [CrossRef] [PubMed]
12. Kusaba, T.; Mori, Y.; Masami, O.; Hiroko, N.; Adachi, T.; Sugishita, C.; Sonomura, K.; Kimura, T.; Kishimoto, N.; Nakagawa, H.; et al. Sodium restriction improves the gustatory threshold for salty taste in patients with chronic kidney disease. *Kidney Int.* **2009**, *76*, 638–643. [CrossRef] [PubMed]
13. Ota, Y.; Kitamura, M.; Tsuji, K.; Torigoe, K.; Yamashita, A.; Abe, S.; Muta, K.; Uramatsu, T.; Obata, Y.; Furutani, J.; et al. Risk Reduction for End-Stage Renal Disease by Dietary Guidance Using the Gustatory Threshold Test for Salty Taste. *Nutrients* **2020**, *12*, 2703. [CrossRef] [PubMed]
14. WHO. *Guideline: Sodium Intake for Adults and Children*; WHO: Geneva, Switzerland, 2012.
15. Powles, J.; Fahimi, S.; Micha, R.; Khatibzadeh, S.; Shi, P.; Ezzati, M.; Engell, R.E.; Lim, S.S.; Danaei, G.; Mozaffarian, D.; et al. Global, regional and national sodium intakes in 1990 and 2010: A systematic analysis of 24 h urinary sodium excretion and dietary surveys worldwide. *BMJ Open* **2013**, *3*, e003733. [CrossRef]
16. O'Donnell, M.; Mente, A.; Rangarajan, S.; McQueen, M.J.; O'Leary, N.; Yin, L.; Liu, X.; Swaminathan, S.; Khatib, R.; Rosengren, A.; et al. Joint association of urinary sodium and potassium excretion with cardiovascular events and mortality: Prospective cohort study. *BMJ* **2019**, *364*, l772. [CrossRef]
17. O'Donnell, M.J.; Yusuf, S.; Mente, A.; Gao, P.; Mann, J.F.; Teo, K.; McQueen, M.; Sleight, P.; Sharma, A.M.; Dans, A.; et al. Urinary sodium and potassium excretion and risk of cardiovascular events. *JAMA* **2011**, *306*, 2229–2238. [CrossRef] [PubMed]
18. O'Donnell, M.; Mente, A.; Rangarajan, S.; McQueen, M.J.; Wang, X.; Liu, L.; Yan, H.; Lee, S.F.; Mony, P.; Devanath, A.; et al. Urinary sodium and potassium excretion, mortality, and cardiovascular events. *N. Engl. J. Med.* **2014**, *371*, 612–623. [CrossRef] [PubMed]
19. Mente, A.; O'Donnell, M.; Rangarajan, S.; Dagenais, G.; Lear, S.; McQueen, M.; Diaz, R.; Avezum, A.; Lopez-Jaramillo, P.; Lanas, F.; et al. Associations of urinary sodium excretion with cardiovascular events in individuals with and without hypertension: A pooled analysis of data from four studies. *Lancet* **2016**, *388*, 465–475. [CrossRef]
20. Mente, A.; O'Donnell, M.; Rangarajan, S.; McQueen, M.; Dagenais, G.; Wielgosz, A.; Lear, S.; Ah, S.T.L.; Wei, L.; Diaz, R.; et al. Urinary sodium excretion, blood pressure, cardiovascular disease, and mortality: A community-level prospective epidemiological cohort study. *Lancet* **2018**, *392*, 496–506. [CrossRef]
21. Armstrong, L.E.; Johnson, E.C. Water intake, water balance, and the elusive daily water requirement. *Nutrients* **2018**, *10*, 1928. [CrossRef]
22. Hoorn, E.J.; Zietse, R. Hyponatremia and mortality: Moving beyond associations. *Am. J. Kidney Dis.* **2013**, *62*, 139–149. [CrossRef]
23. Wald, R.; Jaber, B.L.; Price, L.L.; Upadhyay, A.; Madias, N.E. Impact of hospital-associated hyponatremia on selected outcomes. *Arch. Intern. Med.* **2010**, *170*, 294–302. [CrossRef]
24. Gheorghiade, M.; Rossi, J.S.; Cotts, W.; Shin, D.D.; Hellkamp, A.S.; Pina, I.L.; Fonarow, G.C.; DeMarco, T.; Pauly, D.F.; Rogers, J.; et al. Characterization and prognostic value of persistent hyponatremia in patients with severe heart failure in the ESCAPE Trial. *Arch. Intern. Med.* **2007**, *167*, 1998–2005. [CrossRef]

25. Londoño, M.-C.; Cárdenas, A.; Guevara, M.; Quinto, L.; de Las Heras, D.; Navasa, M.; Rimola, A.; Garcia-Valdecasas, J.-C.; Arroyo, V.; Gines, P. MELD score and serum sodium in the prediction of survival of patients with cirrhosis awaiting liver transplantation. *Gut* **2007**, *56*, 1283–1290. [CrossRef] [PubMed]
26. Konishi, M.; Haraguchi, G.; Ohigashi, H.; Sasaoka, T.; Yoshikawa, S.; Inagaki, H.; Ashikaga, T.; Isobe, M. Progression of hyponatremia is associated with increased cardiac mortality in patients hospitalized for acute decompensated heart failure. *J. Card. Fail.* **2012**, *18*, 620–625. [CrossRef] [PubMed]
27. O'Donnell, M.; Mente, A.; Alderman, M.H.; Brady, A.J.B.; Diaz, R.; Gupta, R.; Lopez-Jaramillo, P.; Luft, F.C.; Luscher, T.F.; Mancia, G.; et al. Salt and cardiovascular disease: Insufficient evidence to recommend low sodium intake. *Eur. Heart J.* **2020**, *41*, 3363–3373. [CrossRef] [PubMed]
28. Vogt, L.; Waanders, F.; Boomsma, F.; de Zeeuw, D.; Navis, G. Effects of dietary sodium and hydrochlorothiazide on the antiproteinuric efficacy of losartan. *J. Am. Soc. Nephrol.* **2008**, *19*, 999–1007. [CrossRef]
29. Nishiyama, A.; Kobori, H. Independent regulation of renin-angiotensin-aldosterone system in the kidney. *Clin. Exp. Nephrol.* **2018**, *22*, 1231–1239. [CrossRef]
30. He, J.; Mills, K.T.; Appel, L.J.; Yang, W.; Chen, J.; Lee, B.T.; Rosas, S.E.; Porter, A.; Makos, G.; Weir, M.R.; et al. Urinary Sodium and Potassium Excretion and CKD Progression. *J. Am. Soc. Nephrol.* **2016**, *27*, 1202–1212. [CrossRef]
31. Kalantar-Zadeh, K.; Kopple, J.D.; Kilpatrick, R.D.; McAllister, C.J.; Shinaberger, C.S.; Gjertson, D.W.; Greenland, S. Association of morbid obesity and weight change over time with cardiovascular survival in hemodialysis population. *Am. J. Kidney Dis.* **2005**, *46*, 489–500. [CrossRef]
32. Kakiya, R.; Shoji, T.; Tsujimoto, Y.; Tatsumi, N.; Hatsuda, S.; Shinohara, K.; Kimoto, E.; Tahara, H.; Koyama, H.; Emoto, M.; et al. Body fat mass and lean mass as predictors of survival in hemodialysis patients. *Kidney Int.* **2006**, *70*, 549–556. [CrossRef]
33. Prospective Studies Collaboration. Whitlock, G.; Lewington, S.; Sherliker, P.; Clarke, R.; Emberson, J.; Halsey, J.; Qizilbash, N.; Collins, R.; Peto, R. Body-mass index and cause-specific mortality in 900 000 adults: Collaborative analyses of 57 prospective studies. *Lancet* **2009**, *373*, 1083–1096. [CrossRef]
34. Navaneethan, S.D.; Schold, J.D.; Arrigain, S.; Kirwan, J.P.; Nally, J.V., Jr. Body mass index and causes of death in chronic kidney disease. *Kidney Int.* **2016**, *89*, 675–682. [CrossRef] [PubMed]
35. Yamamoto, T.; Nakayama, M.; Miyazaki, M.; Sato, H.; Matsushima, M.; Sato, T.; Ito, S. Impact of lower body mass index on risk of all-cause mortality and infection-related death in Japanese chronic kidney disease patients. *BMC Nephrol.* **2020**, *21*, 244. [CrossRef] [PubMed]
36. Yamamoto, R.; Ito, T.; Nagasawa, Y.; Matsui, K.; Egawa, M.; Nanami, M.; Isaka, Y.; Okada, H. Efficacy of aerobic exercise on the cardiometabolic and renal outcomes in patients with chronic kidney disease: A systematic review of randomized controlled trials. *J. Nephrol.* **2021**, *34*, 155–164. [CrossRef] [PubMed]
37. Oguchi, H.; Tsujita, M.; Yazawa, M.; Kawaguchi, T.; Hoshino, J.; Kohzuki, M.; Ito, O.; Yamagata, K.; Shibagaki, Y.; Sofue, T. The efficacy of exercise training in kidney transplant recipients: A meta-analysis and systematic review. *Clin. Exp. Nephrol.* **2019**, *23*, 275–284. [CrossRef]
38. Nagasawa, Y.; Yamamoto, R.; Shinzawa, M.; Hasuike, Y.; Kuragano, T.; Isaka, Y.; Nakanishi, T.; Iseki, K.; Yamagata, K.; Tsuruya, K.; et al. Body Mass Index Modifies an Association between Self-Reported Regular Exercise and Proteinuria. *J. Atheroscler. Thromb.* **2016**, *23*, 402–412. [CrossRef]
39. Kalantar-Zadeh, K.; Kilpatrick, R.D.; McAllister, C.J.; Greenland, S.; Kopple, J.D. Reverse epidemiology of hypertension and cardiovascular death in the hemodialysis population: The 58th annual fall conference and scientific sessions. *Hypertension* **2005**, *45*, 811–817. [CrossRef] [PubMed]
40. Kalantar-Zadeh, K.; Kilpatrick, R.D.; Kopple, J.D. Reverse epidemiology of blood pressure in dialysis patients. *Kidney Int.* **2005**, *67*, 2067. [CrossRef]
41. Li, Z.; Lacson, E., Jr.; Lowrie, E.G.; Ofsthun, N.J.; Kuhlmann, M.K.; Lazarus, J.M.; Levin, N.W. The epidemiology of systolic blood pressure and death risk in hemodialysis patients. *Am. J. Kidney Dis.* **2006**, *48*, 606–615. [CrossRef]
42. Klassen, P.S.; Lowrie, E.G.; Reddan, D.N.; DeLong, E.R.; Coladonato, J.A.; Szczech, L.A.; Lazarus, J.M.; Owen, W.F., Jr. Association between pulse pressure and mortality in patients undergoing maintenance hemodialysis. *JAMA* **2002**, *287*, 1548–1555. [CrossRef]
43. Port, F.K.; Hulbert-Shearon, T.E.; Wolfe, R.A.; Bloembergen, W.E.; Golper, T.A.; Agodoa, L.Y.; Young, E.W. Predialysis blood pressure and mortality risk in a national sample of maintenance hemodialysis patients. *Am. J. Kidney Dis.* **1999**, *33*, 507–517. [CrossRef]
44. Rostand, S.G.; Kirk, K.A.; Rutsky, E.A. Relationship of coronary risk factors to hemodialysis-associated ischemic heart disease. *Kidney Int.* **1982**, *22*, 304–308. [CrossRef] [PubMed]
45. Tomita, J.; Kimura, G.; Inoue, T.; Inenaga, T.; Sanai, T.; Kawano, Y.; Nakamura, S.; Baba, S.; Matsuoka, H.; Omae, T. Role of systolic blood pressure in determining prognosis of hemodialyzed patients. *Am. J. Kidney Dis.* **1995**, *25*, 405–412. [CrossRef]
46. Kimura, G.; Tomita, J.; Nakamura, S.; Uzu, T.; Inenaga, T. Interaction between hypertension and other cardiovascular risk factors in survival of hemodialyzed patients. *Am. J. Hypertens.* **1996**, *9*, 1006–1012. [CrossRef]
47. Foley, R.N.; Parfrey, P.S.; Harnett, J.D.; Kent, G.M.; Murray, D.C.; Barre, P.E. Impact of hypertension on cardiomyopathy, morbidity and mortality in end-stage renal disease. *Kidney Int.* **1996**, *49*, 1379–1385. [CrossRef]
48. Mazzuchi, N.; Carbonell, E.; Fernandez-Cean, J. Importance of blood pressure control in hemodialysis patient survival. *Kidney Int.* **2000**, *58*, 2147–2154. [CrossRef]

49. Schomig, M.; Eisenhardt, A.; Ritz, E. Controversy on optimal blood pressure on haemodialysis: Normotensive blood pressure values are essential for survival. *Nephrol. Dial. Transplant.* **2001**, *16*, 469–474. [CrossRef]
50. London, G.M. Controversy on optimal blood pressure on haemodialysis: Lower is not always better. *Nephrol. Dial. Transplant.* **2001**, *16*, 475–478. [CrossRef]
51. Lucas, M.F.; Quereda, C.; Teruel, J.L.; Orte, L.; Marcen, R.; Ortuno, J. Effect of hypertension before beginning dialysis on survival of hemodialysis patients. *Am. J. Kidney Dis.* **2003**, *41*, 814–821. [CrossRef]
52. Turner, J.M.; Peixoto, A.J. Blood pressure targets for hemodialysis patients. *Kidney Int.* **2017**, *92*, 816–823. [CrossRef]
53. Agarwal, R.; Flynn, J.; Pogue, V.; Rahman, M.; Reisin, E.; Weir, M.R. Assessment and management of hypertension in patients on dialysis. *J. Am. Soc. Nephrol.* **2014**, *25*, 1630–1646. [CrossRef] [PubMed]
54. Wanner, C.; Amann, K.; Shoji, T. The heart and vascular system in dialysis. *Lancet* **2016**, *388*, 276–284. [CrossRef]
55. Kramer, H.J.; Townsend, R.R.; Griffin, K.; Flynn, J.T.; Weiner, D.E.; Rocco, M.V.; Choi, M.J.; Weir, M.R.; Chang, T.I.; Agarwal, R.; et al. KDOQI US Commentary on the 2017 ACC/AHA Hypertension Guideline. *Am. J. Kidney Dis.* **2019**, *73*, 437–458. [CrossRef] [PubMed]
56. Marquez-Herrera, R.M.; Nunez-Murillo, G.K.; Ruiz-Gurrola, C.G.; Gomez-Garcia, E.F.; Orozco-Gonzalez, C.N.; Cortes-Sanabria, L.; Cueto-Manzano, A.M.; Rojas-Campos, E. Clinical Taste Perception Test for Patients With End-Stage Kidney Disease on Dialysis. *J. Ren. Nutr.* **2020**, *30*, 79–84. [CrossRef]
57. Tanaka, M.; Nishiwaki, H.; Kado, H.; Doi, Y.; Ihoriya, C.; Omae, K.; Tamagaki, K. Impact of salt taste dysfunction on interdialytic weight gain for hemodialysis patients; a cross-sectional study. *BMC Nephrol.* **2019**, *20*, 121. [CrossRef]
58. Escobedo-Monge, M.F.; Ayala-Macedo, G.; Sakihara, G.; Peralta, S.; Almaraz-Gomez, A.; Barrado, E.; Marugan-Miguelsanz, J.M. Effects of Zinc Supplementation on Nutritional Status in Children with Chronic Kidney Disease: A Randomized Trial. *Nutrients* **2019**, *11*, 2671. [CrossRef]
59. Mc Causland, F.R.; Waikar, S.S.; Brunelli, S.M. Increased dietary sodium is independently associated with greater mortality among prevalent hemodialysis patients. *Kidney Int.* **2012**, *82*, 204–211. [CrossRef]
60. Curtis, J.P.; Selter, J.G.; Wang, Y.; Rathore, S.S.; Jovin, I.S.; Jadbabaie, F.; Kosiborod, M.; Portnay, E.L.; Sokol, S.I.; Bader, F.; et al. The obesity paradox: Body mass index and outcomes in patients with heart failure. *Arch. Intern. Med.* **2005**, *165*, 55–61. [CrossRef]
61. Cabezas-Rodriguez, I.; Carrero, J.J.; Zoccali, C.; Qureshi, A.R.; Ketteler, M.; Floege, J.; London, G.; Locatelli, F.; Gorriz, J.L.; Rutkowski, B.; et al. Influence of body mass index on the association of weight changes with mortality in hemodialysis patients. *Clin. J. Am. Soc. Nephrol.* **2013**, *8*, 1725–1733. [CrossRef] [PubMed]
62. Nomura, N.; Shoda, W.; Uchida, S. Clinical importance of potassium intake and molecular mechanism of potassium regulation. *Clin. Exp. Nephrol.* **2019**, *23*, 1175–1180. [CrossRef] [PubMed]
63. Ikizler, T.A.; Burrowes, J.D.; Byham-Gray, L.D.; Campbell, K.L.; Carrero, J.J.; Chan, W.; Fouque, D.; Friedman, A.N.; Ghaddar, S.; Goldstein-Fuchs, D.J.; et al. KDOQI Clinical Practice Guideline for Nutrition in CKD: 2020 Update. *Am. J. Kidney Dis.* **2020**, *76*, S1–S107. [CrossRef] [PubMed]
64. Combe, C.; McCullough, K.P.; Asano, Y.; Ginsberg, N.; Maroni, B.J.; Pifer, T.B. Kidney Disease Outcomes Quality Initiative (K/DOQI) and the Dialysis Outcomes and Practice Patterns Study (DOPPS): Nutrition guidelines, indicators, and practices. *Am. J. Kidney Dis.* **2004**, *44*, 39–46. [CrossRef]
65. Nakao, T.; Kanno, Y.; Nagasawa, Y.; Kanazawa, Y.; Akib, T.; Sanaka, K.; Watanabe, Y.; Masakane, I.; Tmoro, M.; Hirakata, H.; et al. Standard nutritional intake in maintained dialysis patients. *J. Jpn. Soc. Dial. Ther.* **2014**, *47*, 287–291.
66. Barreto, F.C.; Barreto, D.V.; Massy, Z.A.; Drueke, T.B. Strategies for Phosphate Control in Patients With CKD. *Kidney Int. Rep.* **2019**, *4*, 1043–1056. [CrossRef] [PubMed]
67. Rastogi, A.; Bhatt, N.; Rossetti, S.; Beto, J. Management of Hyperphosphatemia in End-Stage Renal Disease: A New Paradigm. *J. Ren. Nutr.* **2021**, *31*, 21–34. [CrossRef] [PubMed]
68. Rhee, C.M.; You, A.S.; Koontz Parsons, T.; Tortorici, A.R.; Bross, R.; St-Jules, D.E.; Jing, J.; Lee, M.L.; Benner, D.; Kovesdy, C.P.; et al. Effect of high-protein meals during hemodialysis combined with lanthanum carbonate in hypoalbuminemic dialysis patients: Findings from the FrEDI randomized controlled trial. *Nephrol. Dial. Transplant.* **2017**, *32*, 1233–1243. [CrossRef]
69. Sussman, E.J.; Singh, S.; Clegg, D.; Palmer, B.F.; Kalantar-Zadeh, K. Let Them Eat Healthy: Can Emerging Potassium Binders Help Overcome Dietary Potassium Restrictions in Chronic Kidney Disease? *J. Ren. Nutr.* **2020**, *30*, 475–483. [CrossRef]
70. Saglimbene, V.M.; Wong, G.; Ruospo, M.; Palmer, S.C.; Garcia-Larsen, V.; Natale, P.; Teixeira-Pinto, A.; Campbell, K.L.; Carrero, J.J.; Stenvinkel, P.; et al. Fruit and Vegetable Intake and Mortality in Adults undergoing Maintenance Hemodialysis. *Clin. J. Am. Soc. Nephrol.* **2019**, *14*, 250–260. [CrossRef]
71. Lapuente, M.; Estruch, R.; Shahbaz, M.; Casas, R. Relation of Fruits and Vegetables with Major Cardiometabolic Risk Factors, Markers of Oxidation, and Inflammation. *Nutrients* **2019**, *11*, 2381. [CrossRef]
72. Ramos, C.I.; Gonzalez-Ortiz, A.; Espinosa-Cuevas, A.; Avesani, C.M.; Carrero, J.J.; Cuppari, L. Does dietary potassium intake associate with hyperkalemia in patients with chronic kidney disease? *Nephrol. Dial. Transplant.* **2020**. [CrossRef]
73. Koppe, L.; Fouque, D.; Kalantar-Zadeh, K. Kidney cachexia or protein-energy wasting in chronic kidney disease: Facts and numbers. *J. Cachexia Sarcopenia Muscle* **2019**, *10*, 479–484. [CrossRef] [PubMed]

74. Carrero, J.J.; Thomas, F.; Nagy, K.; Arogundade, F.; Avesani, C.M.; Chan, M.; Chmielewski, M.; Cordeiro, A.C.; Espinosa-Cuevas, A.; Fiaccadori, E.; et al. Global Prevalence of Protein-Energy Wasting in Kidney Disease: A Meta-analysis of Contemporary Observational Studies From the International Society of Renal Nutrition and Metabolism. *J. Ren. Nutr.* **2018**, *28*, 380–392. [CrossRef] [PubMed]
75. Johansen, K.L.; Chertow, G.M.; Jin, C.; Kutner, N.G. Significance of frailty among dialysis patients. *J. Am. Soc. Nephrol.* **2007**, *18*, 2960–2967. [CrossRef]
76. Nagasawa, Y.; Kanno, Y. Nutritional Interventions in Dialysis Patients. In *Recent Advances of Sarcopenia and Frailty in CKD*; Springer: Singapore, 2020; pp. 147–163.
77. Robinson, S.; Granic, A.; Sayer, A.A. Nutrition and Muscle Strength, As the Key Component of Sarcopenia: An Overview of Current Evidence. *Nutrients* **2019**, *11*, 2942. [CrossRef]
78. Ku, E.; Kopple, J.D.; Johansen, K.L.; McCulloch, C.E.; Go, A.S.; Xie, D.; Lin, F.; Hamm, L.L.; He, J.; Kusek, J.W.; et al. Longitudinal Weight Change During CKD Progression and Its Association with Subsequent Mortality. *Am. J. Kidney Dis.* **2018**, *71*, 657–665. [CrossRef] [PubMed]

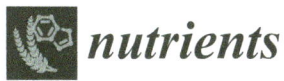

Review

Application of Magnetic Resonance Imaging in the Evaluation of Nutritional Status: A Literature Review with Focus on Dialysis Patients

Tsutomu Inoue [1], Eito Kozawa [2], Masahiro Ishikawa [3] and Hirokazu Okada [1,*]

1. Department of Nephrology, Faculty of Medicine, Saitama Medical University, Saitama 350-0495, Japan; t_inoue@saitama-med.ac.jp
2. Department of Radiology, Faculty of Medicine, Saitama Medical University, Saitama 350-0495, Japan; 8kozawa@saitama-med.ac.jp
3. School of Biomedical Engineering, Faculty of Health and Medical Care, Saitama Medical University, Saitama 350-1241, Japan; ishikawa@saitama-med.ac.jp
* Correspondence: hirookda@saitama-med.ac.jp; Tel.: +81-49-276-1611

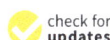

Citation: Inoue, T.; Kozawa, E.; Ishikawa, M.; Okada, H. Application of Magnetic Resonance Imaging in the Evaluation of Nutritional Status: A Literature Review with Focus on Dialysis Patients. *Nutrients* **2021**, *13*, 2037. https://doi.org/10.3390/nu13062037

Academic Editor: Riccardo Caccialanza

Received: 19 May 2021
Accepted: 11 June 2021
Published: 14 June 2021

Publisher's Note: MDPI stays neutral with regard to jurisdictional claims in published maps and institutional affiliations.

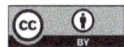

Copyright: © 2021 by the authors. Licensee MDPI, Basel, Switzerland. This article is an open access article distributed under the terms and conditions of the Creative Commons Attribution (CC BY) license (https:// creativecommons.org/licenses/by/ 4.0/).

Abstract: Magnetic resonance imaging (MRI) is indispensable in clinical medicine for the morphological and tomographic evaluation of many parenchymal organs. With varied imaging methods, diverse biological information, such as the perfusion volume and measurements of metabolic products, can be obtained. In addition to conventional MRI for morphological assessment, diffusion-weighted MRI/diffusion tensor imaging is used to evaluate white matter structures in the brain; arterial spin labeling is used for cerebral blood flow evaluation; magnetic resonance elastography for fatty liver and cirrhosis evaluation; magnetic resonance spectroscopy for evaluation of metabolites in specific regions of the brain; and blood oxygenation level-dependent imaging for neurological exploration of eating behavior, obesity, and food perception. This range of applications will continue to expand in the future. Nutritional science is a multidisciplinary and all-inclusive field of research; therefore, there are many different applications of MRI. We present a literature review of MRI techniques that can be used to evaluate the nutritional status, particularly in patients on dialysis. We used MEDLINE as the information source, conducted a keyword search in PubMed, and found that, as a nutritional evaluation method, MRI has been used frequently to comprehensively and quantitatively evaluate muscle mass for the determination of body composition.

Keywords: magnetic resonance imaging; diffusion tensor imaging; arterial spin labeling; blood oxygenation level-dependent; nutritional status; dialysis patients

1. Introduction

1.1. The Origins of Medical Magnetic Resonance Imaging (MRI)

Medical magnetic resonance imaging (MRI) was established in the 1970s as a tomographic imaging method for the human body, and its full-scale clinical implementation began in the 1980s. Since then, the technology of medical imaging hardware has progressed by leaps and bounds; the development of versatile imaging methods has likewise been actively pursued. Currently, MRI has become an indispensable diagnostic imaging method in the medical field.

1.2. Principles and History of MRI

MRI is based on the physical phenomenon of nuclear magnetic resonance (NMR). In some types of nuclei, such as the hydrogen nucleus (referred to as "proton" or "1H" as it is a nucleus that consists solely of a proton; the number "1" indicates the mass number and the atomic number is often omitted), which rotates along the axis of rotation, the + charge of the nucleus generates a magnetic field. When a strong magnetic field in a certain direction is applied to the nucleus, it starts to rotate with an angular momentum called "Larmor precession", that is, a cone about the direction of the magnetic field, and each nucleus has its own frequency. When radio waves of the same frequency as the precession are applied to the nucleus, a resonance phenomenon called NMR causes radio waves to absorb energy. Once the radio waves are turned off after the resonance phenomenon, the nucleus returns to its original state while releasing energy. By capturing this energy released as an electrical signal, an NMR signal is obtained. NMR is a technique used to investigate molecular structures, various intermolecular interactions, and molecular motion states and is used in a wide range of fields, such as polymer chemistry, biochemistry, and medicine.

In comparison to NMR, which has zero-dimensional information with no positional identification, MRI can be defined as a positionally-identified NMR measurement method. There is a law that states that the resonant frequency of an atom is proportional to the strength of the magnetic field. By combining a strong magnetic field with magnetic fields of different strengths, depending on the position (a gradient magnetic field), it was discovered that any position in space could be accurately determined using the strength of the magnetic field, and this NMR phenomenon became the principle of tomography. This discovery occurred 30 years after that of NMR. Although it uses the resonance phenomenon of atomic nuclei, it has nothing to do with radioactivity; thus, the term MRI came to be used idiomatically without the N in NMR.

The MRI technology has progressed dramatically since its introduction into clinical practice, and the number of clinical applications has increased accordingly, driving the development of the technology further. The principles and imaging methods of medical MRI have been documented previously [1]. The advantages of MRI include the absence of ionizing radiation, good soft-tissue contrast with multiple imaging methods, and the ability to reconstruct any cross-section with similar image quality, based on the imaging principle. This is limited to not only two-dimensional but also three-dimensional reconstruction. In addition, because the basic principle, the magnetic resonance (MR) signal, depends on various physical parameters, MRI can display morphological and structural information, as well as provide a wide range of functional information using diffusion, perfusion, and frequency decomposition techniques. Currently, clinical MRI observes water molecules (mainly consisting of hydrogen atoms), which is the most abundant constituent of living organisms, although it is also possible to collect signals from carbon and sodium atoms. Due to this diversity of imaging methods, the clinical applications of MRI are not just limited to use in neurology or psychiatry, but rather extend to the examination of the abdominal organs, heart, musculoskeletal system, and body fat.

1.3. MRI and Nutrition Research

The role of MRI in nutrition includes the measurement of organ volumes, analysis of constituent components (hard tissues, such as bones; soft tissues, such as fat and muscles), and acquisition of location information, such as the distribution of these components, through its function as a tomographic imaging method. Because of the objective, quantitative, and predominantly non-invasive nature of MRI, repeated evaluations are possible, and changes after interventions can be assessed. In the past, nutritional assessments using MRI were focused mainly on the fat and muscle mass; thus, there was no significant difference in the subject of assessment between an MRI and an X-ray computed tomography (CT) scan, except for the fact that no ionizing radiation was used in MRI.

However, with the introduction of high magnetic fields in clinical MR machines and advances in analytical technology, imaging methods exclusive to MRI technology are now being used in the field of nutrition, such as functional MRI (fMRI), e.g., blood oxygenation level-dependent (BOLD) MRI, diffusion-weighted imaging (DWI) methods, including diffusion tensor imaging (DTI), and MR spectroscopy (MRS). In view of this technical and historical background about the advances in MRI technology, this article presents a literature review of the clinical applications of fMRI in nutrition research.

2. Materials and Methods

A literature search was conducted using PubMed for the medical database MEDLINE, produced by the National Library of Medicine (NLM). The search was conducted on 28 December 2020. Articles published before the year 2000 were not included in the study.

First, we searched for studies in which MRI was used to assess the nutritional status of patients on dialysis. To prevent missing out on relevant articles, we used a free word search using the following search terms in all the fields: "magnetic resonance imaging," "nutrition," and "dialysis". Thirty-two published papers were identified from the search. Of these, only nine reported the use of MRI for nutritional assessment (the others reported its use for the diagnosis of comorbidities or complications) and were suitable for our review; thus, there were limitations of the evidence, and we opined that if we were to conduct a systematic review, the scarce number of studies limited only to patients on dialysis would severely underestimate the relevance of MRI as a tool for the evaluation of nutritional status. Contrastingly, there were many research papers on the use of MRI in the assessment of nutritional indices if we did not limit the search only to patients on dialysis, and we opted for a literature review study design.

Therefore, we conducted a search for articles, in which MRI was the main topic of the study, as "magnetic resonance imaging [MeSH Major Topic]". We then searched for articles that included "nutrition" as a free word in the abstract or title to narrow down the target articles. Furthermore, we searched only for research papers targeting humans ("nutrition" [Title/Abstract] AND "magnetic resonance imaging" [MeSH Major Topic] AND "humans" [Filter]). Case reports were excluded from the study. Consequently, 68 articles were found, and their titles and abstracts were reviewed. We excluded papers where MRI was used to detect diseases, that is, where MRI was performed for a purpose different from nutritional evaluation. However, research reports with MRIs of the brain or organs were incorporated if they were intended for nutritional evaluation. For the review, we also searched for relevant articles in the reference lists of the included articles. Only articles in English were included in the study.

3. Results and Discussion

3.1. Summary of Search Results

MRI is mainly used in clinical medicine for tomographic imaging of living organisms; however, in nutritional research, its most common use was found to be the analysis of body composition, such as muscle and adipose tissue. In a nutritional assessment, the excellent soft-tissue contrast of an MRI was used to evaluate the body composition of the human body. In addition to soft-tissue imaging, MRI was performed to evaluate the volume of abdominal organs and the brain. This method takes advantage of the MRI as an imaging test; however, a MRI, in addition to tomography, is capable of extracting a variety of biological information by devising an imaging sequence. BOLD MRI, diffusion-weighted MRI, DTI, arterial spin labeling (ASL), magnetic resonance elastography (MRE), and MRS were considered to be either non-morphological MRI or fMRI based on the content of the articles and reviews included in this literature review (Table 1). The following are some observations drawn from specific examples from the search results.

Table 1. A summary of the various MRI methods used in nutrition-related clinical studies reviewed in this article.

Imaging Procedure	Primary Evaluation Objective	Example of Use	Nutrition-Related Clinical Study Included
Conventional MRI	Structural Evaluation based on proton distribution.	• Measurement of the location and volume of adipose tissue and muscle tissue. • Assessment of the volume of the brain and other parenchymal organs.	Addeman, B.T. et al. [2] Molfino, A. et al. [3] Fischer, K. et al. [4] Maskarinec, G. et al. [5] Ishihara, S. et al. [6] Abe, T. et al. [7] Spinnato, P. et al. [8] Carrero, J.J. et al. [9] Johansen, K.L. et al. [10] Morrell, G.R. et al. [11] Gamboa, J.L. et al. [12] Martinson, M. et al. [13] Delgado, C. et al. [14] Wells, C.I. et al. [15] Salinari, S. et al. [16] Carter, M. et al. [17] Yang, Y.X. et al. [18] de van der Schueren, M.A. et al. [19] Bourdel-Marchasson, I. et al. [20]
Diffusion Tensor Imaging	Evaluation of microstructure in the tissue based on the anisotropy of thermal diffusion of protons.	• Assessment of the degree of degeneration and development of cerebral white matter based on nerve fiber structure.	Drew, D.A. et al. [21] Witte, A.V. et al. [22] Ottolini, K.M. et al. [23] Blesa, M. et al. [24] Coviello, C. et al. [25] Shen, Q. et al. [26]
Arterial Spin Labeling	Evaluation of tissue perfusion using magnetically labeled protons as an endogenous tracer	• Assessment of the changes in regional blood flow in the brain	de Rooij, S.R. et al. [27] Lamport, D.J. et al. [28] Presley, T.D. et al. [29] Vidyasagar, R. et al. [30] Rickenbacher, E. et al. [31] Khalili-Mahani, N. et al. [32] Strang, N.M. et al. [33] Marxen, M. et al. [34]
Magnetic Resonance Elastography	Evaluation of organ elasticity based on strain when the organ is vibrated.	• Evaluation of progression of liver diseases, such as cirrhosis, fatty liver, etc. It mainly evaluates changes due to fibrosis of organs.	Furlan, A. et al. [35]
Magnetic Resonance Spectroscopy	Evaluation of the amount and spatial distribution of various molecular compounds, based on the principles of NMR.	• Evaluation of various metabolites in the brain, including N-acetyl aspartate, γ-aminobutyric acid, glutamine, and lactate, by 1H-MRS.	Artzi, M. et al. [36] Park, Y. et al. [37] Choi, I.Y. et al. [38] Cheng, Y. et al. [39]
Blood Oxygenation Level Dependent-MRI	Assessment of brain activation sites via increased regional cerebral blood flow from changes in deoxyhemoglobin concentration.	• Identification of changes in activity and functional areas of the brain associated with appetite, nutritional intake, and eating behavior.	Belaich, R. et al. [40] van Opstal, A.M. et al. [41] Hawton, K. et al. [42] Dong, D. et al. [43]

3.2. MRI for Structural Evaluation: MRI-Based Assessment of Body Fat Distribution

Assessment of body fat composition could be performed using imaging techniques, including radiography, CT, and MRI (Figure 1) [44,45]. MRI was reported to accurately and reliably assess body fat distribution and characteristics [46,47]. T1-weighted imaging was reported to differentiate between the proton signals from water and fat owing to their different T1 relaxation times. Adipose tissue appeared bright on T1-weighted images, and this feature was used for the quantification of subcutaneous adipose tissue, visceral adipose tissue, bone marrow fat, and intermuscular adipose tissue. In addition, T1-weighted imaging was used to assess muscular fat infiltration in neuromuscular disorders [2,48]. The use of MRI for the evaluation of adipose tissue was reviewed and reported [49].

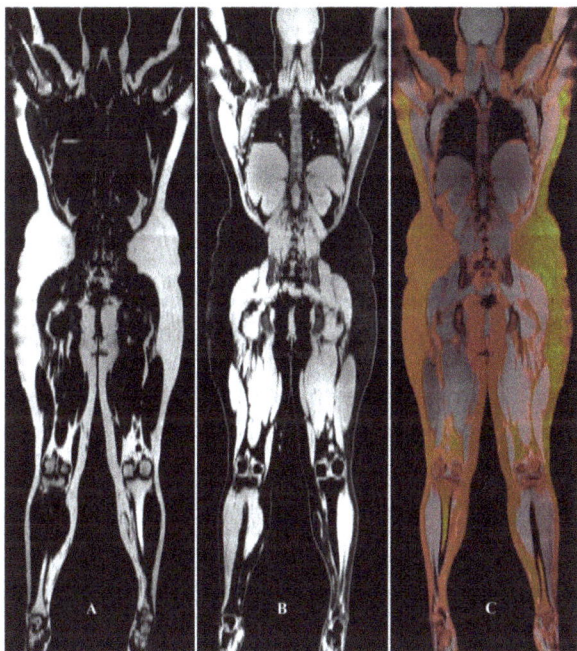

Figure 1. Separated fat (**A**) and water (**B**) MRI of an obese individual. Panel (**C**) depicts the fat overlayed in color on the water grayscale image. From Seabolt et al. (2015), with permission.

In patients on dialysis, albumin and prealbumin were reported to be associated with nutritional and inflammatory statuses. Molfino et al. [3] evaluated the contribution of adiposity to prealbumin levels in patients receiving dialysis. Of 48 patients receiving hemodialysis, the total skeletal muscle mass and visceral and subcutaneous adipose tissues were measured using MRI. Prealbumin was positively associated with visceral adipose tissue and negatively associated with interleukin-6 (IL-6). In contrast, albumin was positively associated with the normalized protein catabolic rate (nPCR) and negatively associated with IL-6, but not with any measure of adiposity. Prealbumin, similar to albumin, was associated with markers of nutrition (nPCR) and inflammation, although, unlike albumin, prealbumin levels were positively associated with visceral adiposity [3].

Regarding other reports not limited to patients on dialysis, two studies were reviewed that investigated the relationship between diet and the volume of adipose tissue in various locations (for example: visceral, subcutaneous abdominal, and trunk adipose tissues), and MRI was used to quantify the adipose tissue [4,5]. There has also been a report of fatty deposits in the liver that were assessed by MRI on the basis of the liver signal intensity [50]. These reports aimed to compare the associations of dietary patterns with liver fat contents. Moreover, there is an interesting report about fat tissue in the epidural space (epidural fat (EF), Figure 2) [6]. Overt accumulation of EF, referred to as spinal epidural lipomatosis (SEL), can compress the spinal cord, leading to the development of neurological symptoms, such as lower back pain. MRI is useful for the evaluation of EF; studies in which MRI was used have shown that it is statistically significantly associated with metabolic syndrome (Table 2) [6] and visceral and liver fat deposition [6–8].

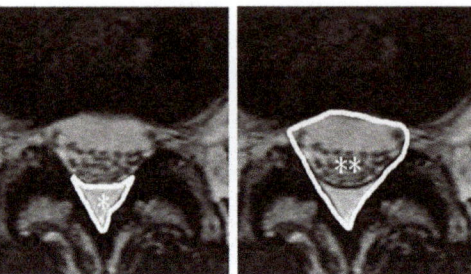

Figure 2. Cross-sectional area of epidural fat (EF) * and the spinal canal **. From Ishihara et al. (2019), with permission.

Table 2. Association of metabolic syndrome with SEL.

		Prevalence of SEL	p Value with Chi-Square Test	Odds Ratio *	95% CI	p Value *
Metabolic syndrome	No (N = 267)	7.1% (N = 19)	<0.01	Ref.		0.01
	Yes (N = 57)	19.3% (N = 11)		3.9	1.5–9.8	

CI, confidence interval; SEL, spinal epidural lipomatosis; Ref., reference value. * Adjusted for age, gender, smoking habit, and drinking history. From Ishihara et al. (2019), with permission.

3.3. MRI for Structural Evaluation: Evaluation of Muscle Mass by MRI

Because the resonance frequency of protons in water and in fat is different, MRI can distinguish between the two; therefore, MRIs can provide high contrast between fat and water, which allows for an accurate assessment of muscle mass. Skeletal muscle mass and function were reported to be negatively affected by a variety of conditions inherent to chronic kidney disease (CKD) and dialysis treatment in a study. Skeletal muscle mass and function served as indicators of the nutritional and clinical state of patients with CKD, and low values or derangements over time were strong predictors of poor patient outcomes [9]. However, muscle size and function can be affected by different factors, may decline at different rates, and may have different patient implications. Therefore, operational definitions of frailty and sarcopenia have emerged to encompass these two dimensions of muscle health, that is, size and functionality.

Johansen et al. [10] investigated 38 patients on dialysis and 19 healthy sedentary controls and used an MRI of the lower leg to determine the total cross-sectional area and the area of contractile and non-contractile tissues of the ankle dorsiflexor muscles. Patients on dialysis were less active and walked more slowly than the control subjects. The total muscle compartment cross-sectional area was not significantly different between patients on dialysis and the healthy controls; however, the contractile cross-sectional area was smaller in the dialysis patients even after adjustment for age, sex, and physical activity. Significant atrophy and increased non-contractile tissue were present in the muscles of patients undergoing dialysis [10].

Another research group used MRI to accurately assess muscle mass [11]. They recruited 105 adult participants on maintenance hemodialysis. The psoas, paraspinous, and mid-thigh muscle areas were measured using an MRI, and the lean body mass was measured using a dual-energy absorptiometry scan. The results showed that the psoas, paraspinous, and mid-thigh muscle areas were associated with an increase in lean body mass. The psoas muscle area provided a better measure of whole-body muscle mass than the paraspinous muscle area but was a slightly inferior measurement to the mid-thigh measurement. This study showed that, in body composition studies, a single axial MRI at the L4–L5 level can be used to provide information on both fat and muscle.

Gamboa et al. [12] used MRI to investigate whether the combination of nutritional supplementation and resistance exercise would have additive effects on muscle mass. They found that six months of nutritional supplementation during hemodialysis increased the muscle protein net balance and mid-thigh fat area. Three months of nutritional supplementation also increased the markers of mitochondrial content in the muscle. They concluded that the study was underpowered for the detection of differences; the combination of nutritional supplementation and exercise failed to show further benefit in protein accretion or muscle cross-sectional area [12]. Other studies have used MRI as a method to measure muscle mass in patients on dialysis [13,14].

Wells et al. [15] studied the relationship between total body protein and the cross-sectional skeletal muscle area in liver cirrhosis using MRI and found that overhydration influenced the skeletal muscle area. Although this report was not a study on dialysis patients, it provided interesting suggestions that need to be taken into consideration when measuring muscle mass in dialysis patients with excess fluid volume.

3.4. MRI for Structural Evaluation: Simultaneous Evaluation of Multiple Tissues by MRI

As mentioned above, because MRI depicts water and fat separately with good contrast, it is also possible to assess muscle mass and fat components simultaneously. Similar body compositions were obtained in a comparative evaluation using MRI and the bioimpedance method [16].

A similar study was reported in patients on dialysis [17]. This study used multi-frequency bioimpedance spectroscopy (BIS) of the arm and whole body to estimate muscle mass and subcutaneous adipose tissue in patients receiving hemodialysis by comparing these results with those of MRI. Total body and arm muscle mass and subcutaneous adipose tissue were measured using MRI. Correlations between MRI and the BIS model were high for the arm and whole body subcutaneous adipose tissues and arm and whole-body muscle mass. The results of this study indicated that total body muscle mass and subcutaneous adipose tissue can be predicted accurately, using arm BIS models with the advantages of convenience and portability, and it could be useful in assessing the nutritional status of hemodialysis patients.

MRI can also quantify the fatty components in the bone marrow [51], liver, and muscle. A study used quantitative MRI to assess yearly disease progression in patients with facioscapulohumeral muscular dystrophy type 1 [52]. The MRI Dixon technique (a T1-weighted imaging method for fat suppression with capabilities of enhancing the contrast between water and fat) was used to evaluate muscle fat replacement. The result showed that MRI detected the progression of the disease, often before changes could be appreciated in strength and functional tests. Considering the ability of MRI to measure fat and muscle simultaneously, the authors expected that MRI will also be useful in accurately classifying sarcopenia. It is noteworthy that the results of the MRI evaluation significantly correlated with a clinical diagnosis of normal obesity, sarcopenia, and sarcopenic obesity [18].

3.5. MRI for Structural Evaluation: Measurement of the Size of Organs by MRI

There have been reports of MRI being used to measure the volume of various organs accurately, including the brain. Conventional brain MRI can also be a useful method to study the relationship between the nutritional status and the degree of brain degeneration and atrophy.

A study, not conducted on patients with CKD, reported that malnutrition and lower vitamin B1 and B12 levels were independently associated with a risk of white matter hyperintensities in brain MRI [19]. There are studies that have performed simultaneous assessment of the brain and skeletal muscle or brain and fat. Bourdel-Marchasson et al. [20] evaluated both the brain and muscles of participants using a T1-weighted MRI. Sarcopenia features were more frequent in frail subjects than in prefrail subjects and were associated with a decrease in gray matter volumes involved in motor control [20].

3.6. Diffusion-Weighted MRI and Diffusion Tensor Imaging

DWI is an MRI technique that utilizes the diffusion phenomenon caused by the Brownian motion of water molecules in tissues. It was first reported by Le Bihan in 1986 [53]. It is now an indispensable imaging method for the diagnosis of acute cerebral infarction. Cellular edema is induced in acute cerebral infarction, and the extracellular fluid space becomes narrow. Therefore, the movement of water molecules in the extracellular fluid space is restricted, and the signal is higher than that of the surrounding brain parenchyma. Similarly, in cancerous tissues, the cell density is high, and the intercellular space is narrowed, resulting in a strong high-intensity signal. The apparent diffusion coefficient can be calculated from the results of imaging with two or more different b-values; although this coefficient is a quantitative value of DWI, it is relative to the image and not standardized.

While the apparent diffusion coefficient map of DWI is useful for assessing acute strokes and malignancies, its use in the field of nutritional science is less common. DTI, an extension of DWI technology, is a means of assessing nerve fiber structure in the white matter and spinal cord [54] and is often used to investigate the relationship between nutrition and the cranial nerves.

The DWI is an imaging method that documents the degree of diffusion of water molecules due to thermal motion. Diffusion usually occurs in a disordered manner, that is, if there is no structure that hinders diffusion, the diffusion direction of a certain proton is three-dimensionally equivalent in all directions and is spherical. This is called isotropic diffusion. However, when there is a structure that restricts the movement of protons, the direction of diffusion is biased, which is called anisotropic diffusion. Taking the central nervous system as an example, nerve fibers are regularly arranged in the same direction in the white matter. In such a structure, it can be considered that protons diffuse easily along the axons but not in the direction across the thick lipid-covered nerve fibers. The anisotropic diffusion index is called the fractional anisotropy (FA) value. Using this principle, a method called DTI was devised for imaging the course of nerve fibers in the brain and spinal cord.

In a study that compared brain structures using DTI in patients on hemodialysis to individuals without known kidney disease, using FA and mean diffusivity, patients on hemodialysis had a significantly lower FA across multiple white matter fiber tracts. Similarly, patients on hemodialysis had significantly higher mean diffusivity in multiple anterior brain regions. In patients on hemodialysis, white matter disease in the anterior parts of the brain is more common than in the posterior parts compared to that in controls without kidney disease. This pattern of injury is similar to that observed in aging, suggesting that developing CKD, and finally, kidney failure, may result in a phenotype consistent with accelerated aging [21].

A research report, not limited to only patients on dialysis, evaluated the beneficial effects of long-chain omega-3 polyunsaturated fatty acids (LC-n3-FA) on white matter microstructural integrity based on the FA value [22]. Other similar studies reported that breast milk feeding in low-birth-weight infants was associated with increased FA values in the white matter, which implied an improved structural connectivity of developing networks in the white matter [23,24]. This means that feeding of breast milk is linked to improved neurodevelopmental outcomes. In addition to breast milk, MRI studies have shown that adequate caloric intake, including fat, during infancy is important for the volume of cortical gray matter and the degree of white matter development, which was evaluated by DTI [25]. Using DTI, the influence of alcohol use during adolescence on white matter microstructure was investigated [26]. Decreased FA was found in moderate-to-heavy drinking men, which suggested the association between alcohol use and neural development.

As described above, DTI can be used to assess nutrition, brain development, and atrophy through the evaluation of brain microstructure and is considered to be a particularly useful tool for obtaining information on white matter.

3.7. Arterial Spin Labeling

Perfusion is the tissue blood flow at the capillary level and plays an important role in transporting gases, such as oxygen and carbon dioxide, and supplying local energy. It can be evaluated by the contrast effect of the organs and tissues by the contrast medium. MRI is performed using a gadolinium contrast medium. Instead of these extrinsic tracers, the ASL method magnetically labels the blood flowing into the organs and uses it as an intrinsic tracer [55]. The "contrast effect" is low; hence, the signal-to-noise ratio is low. Based on this principle, it uses the difference between the magnetically-labeled state and un-magnetically-labeled state; thus, ASL is a subtraction image in principle. With the spread of MR equipment and a static magnetic field of 3.0 Tesla, this imaging method has become clinically feasible. It is a completely non-invasive method because perfusion images can be obtained without using a contrast medium, and it can be said that it is an excellent diagnostic imaging method that takes advantage of MRI.

Although the following studies were not conducted on patients with CKD, their findings suggested an association between nutrition and cerebral blood flow. A study found that prenatal undernutrition was associated with differences in brain perfusion during older age evaluated using ASL [27]. Early nutritional deprivation may cause irreversible damage to the brain and may affect cognitive function in older adults. The effects of flavonoids, dietary nitrate, and caffeine on brain perfusion have also been evaluated using ASL [28–30]. ASL also demonstrated clearly that alcohol increased cerebral perfusion [31,32]. It has also been confirmed that the degree of increase in cerebral blood flow varies from region to region [45,46]. In interventional studies, the same subject can be evaluated repeatedly because ASL does not require the use of contrast media.

3.8. Magnetic Resonance Elastography

MRE is an imaging method used to evaluate the elasticity and viscosity of living organisms using MRI. The basic principle was reported in the journal Science in 1995 [56], as follows: protons, which are the basis of MR signals, are rotating, and the signals obtained from protons by MR equipment are vector quantities. Usually, the "magnitude" is imaged. This is why they are called "T1-weighted images" or "proton-weighted images." However, MRE can be said to use the phase information, that is, the "phase contrast-based" MRI technique. In practice, MRE requires ordinary MR equipment, a vibration generator (a speaker that generates air vibrations, a tube that transmits the vibrations, and a pad that attached to the thorax), and software for image analysis. It is mostly used to evaluate the liver. It is used to evaluate fibrosis in liver cirrhosis because vibrations are transmitted faster in hard materials. In nutritional research, MRE is mostly used to evaluate fatty liver and assess the degree of progression of cirrhosis [35].

3.9. Magnetic Resonance Spectroscopy

MRS is a non-invasive method for measuring the composition and quantity of compounds in tissues and detecting the amount and spatial distribution of various molecular compounds, which are involved in metabolism [57]. It has already been mentioned that atoms, such as 1H (protons), have a Larmor precession at a specific frequency when placed in a static magnetic field. This frequency depends on the magnitude of the static magnetic field. Even for the same proton, the magnitude of the static magnetic field acting on the proton will differ owing to differences in electron distribution caused by the influence of surrounding atoms and substituents (this is called the "shielding effect"). As a result, protons in water and those in lactic acid, for example, have different resonance frequencies, even if the static magnetic field added by the apparatus is the same. This difference in frequency is called a chemical shift. When MR signals are collected for protons, the signals from protons in water molecules overwhelmingly dominate the entire signal. However, by precisely resolving the frequency, signals from protons in other compounds can be captured. This is the basic principle of MRS. Unlike NMR systems that analyze compounds, medical MR equipment has a small static magnetic field; thus, 1H-MRS is mainly used for protons. In proton MRS (1H-MRS), the targets of measurement are creatine, choline, N-acetyl-acetate, citrate, lactate, and lipids [58]. In addition, when using a high-magnetic field device, it is expected that it will be possible to measure substances related to energy metabolism, such as ATP, based on signals from 31P (phosphorus).

Several studies, not limited to patients with chronic kidney disease, utilizing the MRS, have reported about the relationship between brain metabolism and nutrition. Normal brain cells depend on glucose metabolism, yet they have the flexibility to switch to the usage of ketone bodies during caloric restriction. In contrast, tumor cells lack genomic and metabolic flexibility and are largely dependent on glucose levels. Hence, a ketogenic diet (KD) has been suggested as a therapeutic option for malignant brain cancer. A 1H-MRS was, in fact, able to visualize the effects of treatment in patients with brain tumors who adhered to a KD [36]. Moreover, a 1H-MRS detected metabolic effects in different brain regions caused by food consumption [37]. It was also reported that dairy food consumption was associated with cerebral glutathione concentrations in older adults [38]. These data showed that the 1H-MRS is a non-invasive tool suitable for nutritional assessment. Cheng et al. used a 1H-MRS and a dual-echo in-phase and out-phase MRI (dual-echo MRI) to assess the effects of dietary nutrient intake on hepatic lipid content [39]. In their conclusion, hepatic fat content was associated with high-energy, high-fat, and high-saturated fatty acid intake, quantified by 1H-MRS and dual-echo MRI. The method of simultaneously evaluating the same organ under multiple conditions is also called "multiparametric MRI" and is currently attracting attention as a multifaceted evaluation method unique to MRI that is not possible with X-ray CT.

3.10. Blood Oxygenation Level-Dependent–MRI

BOLD MRI is an MRI technique originally used to study the active areas of the brain [59]. Many studies have been reported on areas of brain activity related to taste, smell, and food perception, and many of the papers are closer to neuroscience research than nutrition research. As for reports related to nutritional science, there are many studies examining the relationship between dietary content, overeating, obesity, and central nervous system, especially brain function.

In a study, functional BOLD-MRI maps of the motor area were obtained from a patient receiving hemodialysis before and after a hemodialysis session. This report demonstrated a decrease in the maximum intensity of BOLD response, while the BOLD area increased in the primary motor cortex after hemodialysis. These changes were involved with oxidative stress levels. It is known that oxidative stress is systematically increased in patients on hemodialysis after the hemodialysis process. The BOLD-fMRI shows a remarkable sensitivity to brain plasticity and reorganization of the functional control of the studied cortical area. The results also confirmed the superiority of the BOLD-MRI compared with the biological method used for assessing oxidative stress generated by hemodialysis [40].

A report, not about patients receiving dialysis, was based on the fact that the human brain is essential for regulating the intake of food and beverages by balancing energy homeostasis with reward perception. Using BOLD MRI, the effects of ingestion of glucose, fructose, sucrose, and sucralose (a non-caloric artificial sweetener) on the magnitude of brain responses was investigated. The results demonstrated that, while the brain responded directly and readily to glucose as a preferred source of energy in the brain, it may not have responded as efficiently to other sugars [41]. Other research results on the relationship between eating behavior and brain activity using BOLD MRI have also been reported [42,43] and are considered to be important basic research results for effective diet planning from the aspects of brain science and behavior.

4. Conclusions

Relevant observations from multiple published reports on the plethora of uses of MRI in nutritional science research have been summarized in this article, along with an overview of the principles of each imaging method. For morphological assessment, MRI has been widely reported to be useful for body composition analysis and can provide comprehensive and quantitative assessment values. Since it is a completely non-invasive method that does not use ionizing radiation, it is expected to have an increasingly wider application than X-ray CT. DTI was frequently used in conjunction with conventional MRI to evaluate the structure of cerebral white matter. ASL was reported to be an important evaluation method for cerebral blood flow because it does not use contrast media and has a relatively wide evaluation range. Although the constituents that can be evaluated with MRS are limited, the evaluation of metabolic products has been demonstrated to provide important information that cannot be obtained using urine or blood tests, because MRS involves location information. BOLD MRI, referred to as an fMRI of the brain, has been found to provide information on the neuroscience of eating behavior and cognition related to eating, olfaction, vision, and appetite. Nutritional science is a multidisciplinary and comprehensive field of research; therefore, there are many different applications of MRI. The use of MRI as a candidate evaluation tool is recommended for future research.

Author Contributions: Conceptualization, T.I., E.K., and M.I.; original draft preparation, T.I.; review and editing, H.O. All authors have read and agreed to the published version of the manuscript.

Funding: This research was supported by AMED, Grant Number 20ek0210122h0002, 19ek0210122h0001.

Institutional Review Board Statement: Not applicable.

Informed Consent Statement: Not applicable.

Data Availability Statement: Not applicable.

Acknowledgments: The authors would like to thank T. Iso, M. Fukuoka, and W. Kosakai for their technical assistance with the experiments.

Conflicts of Interest: The authors declare no conflict of interest. The sponsors had no role in the design, execution, interpretation, or writing of the study.

References

1. Moser, E.; Stadlbauer, A.; Windischberger, C.; Quick, H.H.; Ladd, M.E. Magnetic resonance imaging methodology. *Eur. J. Nucl. Med. Mol. Imaging* **2009**, *36* (Suppl. S1), S30–S41. [CrossRef]
2. Addeman, B.T.; Kutty, S.; Perkins, T.G.; Soliman, A.S.; Wiens, C.N.; McCurdy, C.M.; Beaton, M.D.; Hegele, R.A.; McKenzie, C.A. Validation of volumetric and single-slice MRI adipose analysis using a novel fully automated segmentation method. *J. Magn. Reson. Imaging* **2015**, *41*, 233–241. [CrossRef]
3. Molfino, A.; Heymsfield, S.B.; Zhu, F.; Kotanko, P.; Levin, N.W.; Dwyer, T.; Kaysen, G.A. Prealbumin is associated with visceral fat mass in patients receiving hemodialysis. *J. Ren. Nutr.* **2013**, *23*, 406–410. [CrossRef]
4. Fischer, K.; Moewes, D.; Koch, M.; Muller, H.P.; Jacobs, G.; Kassubek, J.; Lieb, W.; Nothlings, U. MRI-determined total volumes of visceral and subcutaneous abdominal and trunk adipose tissue are differentially and sex-dependently associated with patterns of estimated usual nutrient intake in a northern German population. *Am. J. Clin. Nutr.* **2015**, *101*, 794–807. [CrossRef]
5. Maskarinec, G.; Lim, U.; Jacobs, S.; Monroe, K.R.; Ernst, T.; Buchthal, S.D.; Shepherd, J.A.; Wilkens, L.R.; Le Marchand, L.; Boushey, C.J. Diet quality in midadulthood predicts visceral adiposity and liver fatness in older ages: The Multiethnic Cohort Study. *Obesity* **2017**, *25*, 1442–1450. [CrossRef] [PubMed]
6. Ishihara, S.; Fujita, N.; Azuma, K.; Michikawa, T.; Yagi, M.; Tsuji, T.; Takayama, M.; Matsumoto, H.; Nakamura, M.; Matsumoto, M.; et al. Spinal epidural lipomatosis is a previously unrecognized manifestation of metabolic syndrome. *Spine J.* **2019**, *19*, 493–500. [CrossRef] [PubMed]
7. Abe, T.; Miyazaki, M.; Ishihara, T.; Kanezaki, S.; Notani, N.; Kataoka, M.; Tsumura, H. Spinal epidural lipomatosis is associated with liver fat deposition and dysfunction. *Clin. Neurol. Neurosurg.* **2019**, *185*, 105480. [CrossRef]
8. Spinnato, P.; Ponti, F.; de Pasqua, S. MRI diagnosis of obesity-related spinal epidural lipomatosis. *Can. J. Neurol. Sci.* **2020**, *47*, 124–125. [CrossRef] [PubMed]
9. Carrero, J.J.; Johansen, K.L.; Lindholm, B.; Stenvinkel, P.; Cuppari, L.; Avesani, C.M. Screening for muscle wasting and dysfunction in patients with chronic kidney disease. *Kidney Int.* **2016**, *90*, 53–66. [CrossRef] [PubMed]
10. Johansen, K.L.; Shubert, T.; Doyle, J.; Soher, B.; Sakkas, G.K.; Kent-Braun, J.A. Muscle atrophy in patients receiving hemodialysis: Effects on muscle strength, muscle quality, and physical function. *Kidney Int.* **2003**, *63*, 291–297. [CrossRef]
11. Morrell, G.R.; Ikizler, T.A.; Chen, X.; Heilbrun, M.E.; Wei, G.; Boucher, R.; Beddhu, S. Psoas muscle cross-sectional area as a measure of whole-body lean muscle mass in maintenance hemodialysis patients. *J. Ren. Nutr.* **2016**, *26*, 258–264. [CrossRef]

12. Gamboa, J.L.; Deger, S.M.; Perkins, B.W.; Mambungu, C.; Sha, F.; Mason, O.J.; Stewart, T.G.; Ikizler, T.A. Effects of long-term intradialytic oral nutrition and exercise on muscle protein homeostasis and markers of mitochondrial content in patients on hemodialysis. *Am. J. Physiol. Ren. Physiol.* **2020**, *319*, F885–F894. [CrossRef]
13. Martinson, M.; Ikizler, T.A.; Morrell, G.; Wei, G.; Almeida, N.; Marcus, R.L.; Filipowicz, R.; Greene, T.H.; Beddhu, S. Associations of body size and body composition with functional ability and quality of life in hemodialysis patients. *Clin. J. Am. Soc. Nephrol.* **2014**, *9*, 1082–1090. [CrossRef] [PubMed]
14. Delgado, C.; Doyle, J.W.; Johansen, K.L. Association of frailty with body composition among patients on hemodialysis. *J. Ren. Nutr.* **2013**, *23*, 356–362. [CrossRef]
15. Wells, C.I.; McCall, J.L.; Plank, L.D. Relationship between total body protein and cross-sectional skeletal muscle area in liver cirrhosis is influenced by overhydration. *Liver Transpl.* **2019**, *25*, 45–55. [CrossRef]
16. Salinari, S.; Bertuzzi, A.; Mingrone, G.; Capristo, E.; Pietrobelli, A.; Campioni, P.; Greco, A.V.; Heymsfield, S.B. New bioimpedance model accurately predicts lower limb muscle volume: Validation by magnetic resonance imaging. *Am. J. Physiol. Endocrinol. Metab.* **2002**, *282*, E960–E966. [CrossRef]
17. Carter, M.; Zhu, F.; Kotanko, P.; Kuhlmann, M.; Ramirez, L.; Heymsfield, S.B.; Handelman, G.; Levin, N.W. Assessment of body composition in dialysis patients by arm bioimpedance compared to MRI and 40K measurements. *Blood Purif.* **2009**, *27*, 330–337. [CrossRef] [PubMed]
18. Yang, Y.X.; Chong, M.S.; Lim, W.S.; Tay, L.; Yew, S.; Yeo, A.; Tan, C.H. Validity of estimating muscle and fat volume from a single MRI section in older adults with sarcopenia and sarcopenic obesity. *Clin. Radiol.* **2017**, *72*, 427.e9–427.e14. [CrossRef]
19. De van der Schueren, M.A.; Lonterman-Monasch, S.; Van der Flier, W.M.; Kramer, M.H.; Maier, A.B.; Muller, M. Malnutrition and Risk of Structural Brain Changes Seen on Magnetic Resonance Imaging in Older Adults. *J. Am. Geriatr. Soc.* **2016**, *64*, 2457–2463. [CrossRef] [PubMed]
20. Bourdel-Marchasson, I.; Catheline, G.; Regueme, S.; Danet-Lamasou, M.; Barse, E.; Ratsimbazafy, F.; Rodriguez-Manas, L.; Hood, K.; Sinclair, A.J. Frailty and brain-muscle correlates in older people with type 2 diabetes: A structural-MRI explorative study. *J. Nutr. Health Aging* **2019**, *23*, 637–640. [CrossRef]
21. Drew, D.A.; Koo, B.B.; Bhadelia, R.; Weiner, D.E.; Duncan, S.; la Garza, M.M.; Gupta, A.; Tighiouart, H.; Scott, T.; Sarnak, M.J. White matter damage in maintenance hemodialysis patients: A diffusion tensor imaging study. *BMC Nephrol.* **2017**, *18*, 213. [CrossRef]
22. Witte, A.V.; Kerti, L.; Hermannstadter, H.M.; Fiebach, J.B.; Schreiber, S.J.; Schuchardt, J.P.; Hahn, A.; Floel, A. Long-chain omega-3 fatty acids improve brain function and structure in older adults. *Cereb. Cortex* **2014**, *24*, 3059–3068. [CrossRef] [PubMed]
23. Ottolini, K.M.; Andescavage, N.; Kapse, K.; Jacobs, M.; Limperopoulos, C. Improved brain growth and microstructural development in breast milk-fed very low birth weight premature infants. *Acta Paediatr.* **2020**, *109*, 1580–1587. [CrossRef] [PubMed]
24. Blesa, M.; Sullivan, G.; Anblagan, D.; Telford, E.J.; Quigley, A.J.; Sparrow, S.A.; Serag, A.; Semple, S.I.; Bastin, M.E.; Boardman, J.P. Early breast milk exposure modifies brain connectivity in preterm infants. *Neuroimage* **2019**, *184*, 431–439. [CrossRef]
25. Coviello, C.; Keunen, K.; Kersbergen, K.J.; Groenendaal, F.; Leemans, A.; Peels, B.; Isgum, I.; Viergever, M.A.; de Vries, L.S.; Buonocore, G.; et al. Effects of early nutrition and growth on brain volumes, white matter microstructure, and neurodevelopmental outcome in preterm newborns. *Pediatr. Res.* **2018**, *83*, 102–110. [CrossRef]
26. Shen, Q.; Heikkinen, N.; Karkkainen, O.; Grohn, H.; Kononen, M.; Liu, Y.; Kaarre, O.; Zhang, Z.; Tan, C.; Tolmunen, T.; et al. Effects of long-term adolescent alcohol consumption on white matter integrity and their correlations with metabolic alterations. *Psychiatry Res. Neuroimaging* **2019**, *294*, 111003. [CrossRef]
27. De Rooij, S.R.; Mutsaerts, H.; Petr, J.; Asllani, I.; Caan, M.W.A.; Groot, P.; Nederveen, A.J.; Schwab, M.; Roseboom, T.J. Late-life brain perfusion after prenatal famine exposure. *Neurobiol. Aging* **2019**, *82*, 1–9. [CrossRef]
28. Lamport, D.J.; Pal, D.; Macready, A.L.; Barbosa-Boucas, S.; Fletcher, J.M.; Williams, C.M.; Spencer, J.P.; Butler, L.T. The effects of flavanone-rich citrus juice on cognitive function and cerebral blood flow: An acute, randomised, placebo-controlled cross-over trial in healthy, young adults. *Br. J. Nutr.* **2016**, *116*, 2160–2168. [CrossRef] [PubMed]
29. Presley, T.D.; Morgan, A.R.; Bechtold, E.; Clodfelter, W.; Dove, R.W.; Jennings, J.M.; Kraft, R.A.; King, S.B.; Laurienti, P.J.; Rejeski, W.J.; et al. Acute effect of a high nitrate diet on brain perfusion in older adults. *Nitric Oxide* **2011**, *24*, 34–42. [CrossRef] [PubMed]
30. Vidyasagar, R.; Greyling, A.; Draijer, R.; Corfield, D.R.; Parkes, L.M. The effect of black tea and caffeine on regional cerebral blood flow measured with arterial spin labeling. *J. Cereb. Blood Flow Metab.* **2013**, *33*, 963–968. [CrossRef]
31. Rickenbacher, E.; Greve, D.N.; Azma, S.; Pfeuffer, J.; Marinkovic, K. Effects of alcohol intoxication and gender on cerebral perfusion: An arterial spin labeling study. *Alcohol* **2011**, *45*, 725–737. [CrossRef] [PubMed]
32. Khalili-Mahani, N.; van Osch, M.J.; Baerends, E.; Soeter, R.P.; de Kam, M.; Zoethout, R.W.; Dahan, A.; van Buchem, M.A.; van Gerven, J.M.; Rombouts, S.A. Pseudocontinuous arterial spin labeling reveals dissociable effects of morphine and alcohol on regional cerebral blood flow. *J. Cereb. Blood Flow Metab.* **2011**, *31*, 1321–1333. [CrossRef]
33. Strang, N.M.; Claus, E.D.; Ramchandani, V.A.; Graff-Guerrero, A.; Boileau, I.; Hendershot, C.S. Dose-dependent effects of intravenous alcohol administration on cerebral blood flow in young adults. *Psychopharmacology* **2015**, *232*, 733–744. [CrossRef]
34. Marxen, M.; Gan, G.; Schwarz, D.; Mennigen, E.; Pilhatsch, M.; Zimmermann, U.S.; Guenther, M.; Smolka, M.N. Acute effects of alcohol on brain perfusion monitored with arterial spin labeling magnetic resonance imaging in young adults. *J. Cereb. Blood Flow Metab.* **2014**, *34*, 472–479. [CrossRef]

35. Furlan, A.; Tublin, M.E.; Yu, L.; Chopra, K.B.; Lippello, A.; Behari, J. Comparison of 2D shear wave elastography, transient elastography, and MR elastography for the diagnosis of fibrosis in patients with nonalcoholic fatty liver disease. *Am. J. Roentgenol.* **2020**, *214*, W20–W26. [CrossRef] [PubMed]
36. Artzi, M.; Liberman, G.; Vaisman, N.; Bokstein, F.; Vitinshtein, F.; Aizenstein, O.; Ben Bashat, D. Changes in cerebral metabolism during ketogenic diet in patients with primary brain tumors: (1)H-MRS study. *J. Neurooncol.* **2017**, *132*, 267–275. [CrossRef] [PubMed]
37. Park, Y.; Zhao, T.; Miller, N.G.; Kim, S.B.; Accardi, C.J.; Ziegler, T.R.; Hu, X.; Jones, D.P. Sulfur amino acid-free diet results in increased glutamate in human midbrain: A pilot magnetic resonance spectroscopic study. *Nutrition* **2012**, *28*, 235–241. [CrossRef] [PubMed]
38. Choi, I.Y.; Lee, P.; Denney, D.R.; Spaeth, K.; Nast, O.; Ptomey, L.; Roth, A.K.; Lierman, J.A.; Sullivan, D.K. Dairy intake is associated with brain glutathione concentration in older adults. *Am. J. Clin. Nutr.* **2015**, *101*, 287–293. [CrossRef] [PubMed]
39. Cheng, Y.; Zhang, K.; Chen, Y.; Li, Y.; Li, Y.; Fu, K.; Feng, R. Associations between dietary nutrient intakes and hepatic lipid contents in NAFLD patients quantified by (1)H-MRS and dual-echo MRI. *Nutrients* **2016**, *8*, 527. [CrossRef] [PubMed]
40. Belaich, R.; Boujraf, S.; Housni, A.; Maaroufi, M.; Batta, F.; Magoul, R.; Sqalli, T.; Errasfa, M.; Tizniti, S. Assessment of hemodialysis impact by polysulfone membrane on brain plasticity using BOLD-fMRI. *Neuroscience* **2015**, *288*, 94–104. [CrossRef]
41. Van Opstal, A.M.; Kaal, I.; Van den Berg-Huysmans, A.A.; Hoeksma, M.; Blonk, C.; Pijl, H.; Rombouts, S.; Van der Grond, J. Dietary sugars and non-caloric sweeteners elicit different homeostatic and hedonic responses in the brain. *Nutrition* **2019**, *60*, 80–86. [CrossRef]
42. Hawton, K.; Ferriday, D.; Rogers, P.; Toner, P.; Brooks, J.; Holly, J.; Biernacka, K.; Hamilton-Shield, J.; Hinton, E. Slow down: Behavioral and physiological effects of reducing eating rate. *Nutrients* **2018**, *11*, 50. [CrossRef] [PubMed]
43. Dong, D.; Wang, Y.; Jackson, T.; Chen, S.; Wang, Y.; Zhou, F.; Chen, H. Impulse control and restrained eating among young women: Evidence for compensatory cortical activation during a chocolate-specific delayed discounting task. *Appetite* **2016**, *105*, 477–486. [CrossRef]
44. Seabolt, L.A.; Welch, E.B.; Silver, H.J. Imaging methods for analyzing body composition in human obesity and cardiometabolic disease. *Ann. NY Acad. Sci.* **2015**, *1353*, 41–59. [CrossRef] [PubMed]
45. Wang, H.; Chen, Y.E.; Eitzman, D.T. Imaging body fat: Techniques and cardiometabolic implications. *Arterioscler. Thromb. Vasc. Biol.* **2014**, *34*, 2217–2223. [CrossRef]
46. Hu, H.H.; Kan, H.E. Quantitative proton MR techniques for measuring fat. *NMR Biomed.* **2013**, *26*, 1609–1629. [CrossRef]
47. Machann, J.; Horstmann, A.; Born, M.; Hesse, S.; Hirsch, F.W. Diagnostic imaging in obesity. *Best Pract. Res. Clin. Endocrinol. Metab.* **2013**, *27*, 261–277. [CrossRef] [PubMed]
48. Mercuri, E.; Pichiecchio, A.; Allsop, J.; Messina, S.; Pane, M.; Muntoni, F. Muscle MRI in inherited neuromuscular disorders: Past, present, and future. *J. Magn. Reson. Imaging* **2007**, *25*, 433–440. [CrossRef]
49. Baum, T.; Cordes, C.; Dieckmeyer, M.; Ruschke, S.; Franz, D.; Hauner, H.; Kirschke, J.S.; Karampinos, D.C. MR-based assessment of body fat distribution and characteristics. *Eur. J. Radiol.* **2016**, *85*, 1512–1518. [CrossRef]
50. Koch, M.; Borggrefe, J.; Barbaresko, J.; Groth, G.; Jacobs, G.; Siegert, S.; Lieb, W.; Muller, M.J.; Bosy-Westphal, A.; Heller, M.; et al. Dietary patterns associated with magnetic resonance imaging-determined liver fat content in a general population study. *Am. J. Clin. Nutr.* **2014**, *99*, 369–377. [CrossRef]
51. Gao, Y.; Zong, K.; Gao, Z.; Rubin, M.R.; Chen, J.; Heymsfield, S.B.; Gallagher, D.; Shen, W. Magnetic resonance imaging-measured bone marrow adipose tissue area is inversely related to cortical bone area in children and adolescents aged 5–18 years. *J. Clin. Densitom.* **2015**, *18*, 203–208. [CrossRef] [PubMed]
52. Andersen, G.; Dahlqvist, J.R.; Vissing, C.R.; Heje, K.; Thomsen, C.; Vissing, J. MRI as outcome measure in facioscapulohumeral muscular dystrophy: 1-year follow-up of 45 patients. *J. Neurol.* **2017**, *264*, 438–447. [CrossRef]
53. Le Bihan, D.; Breton, E.; Lallemand, D.; Grenier, P.; Cabanis, E.; Laval-Jeantet, M. MR imaging of intravoxel incoherent motions: Application to diffusion and perfusion in neurologic disorders. *Radiology* **1986**, *161*, 401–407. [CrossRef] [PubMed]
54. Jeon, T.; Fung, M.M.; Koch, K.M.; Tan, E.T.; Sneag, D.B. Peripheral nerve diffusion tensor imaging: Overview, pitfalls, and future directions. *J. Magn. Reson. Imaging* **2018**, *47*, 1171–1189. [CrossRef] [PubMed]
55. Telischak, N.A.; Detre, J.A.; Zaharchuk, G. Arterial spin labeling MRI: Clinical applications in the brain. *J. Magn. Reson. Imaging* **2015**, *41*, 1165–1180. [CrossRef] [PubMed]
56. Muthupillai, R.; Lomas, D.J.; Rossman, P.J.; Greenleaf, J.F.; Manduca, A.; Ehman, R.L. Magnetic resonance elastography by direct visualization of propagating acoustic strain waves. *Science* **1995**, *269*, 1854–1857. [CrossRef]
57. Buonocore, M.H.; Maddock, R.J. Magnetic resonance spectroscopy of the brain: A review of physical principles and technical methods. *Rev. Neurosci.* **2015**, *26*, 609–632. [CrossRef]
58. Mountford, C.; Lean, C.; Malycha, P.; Russell, P. Proton spectroscopy provides accurate pathology on biopsy and in vivo. *J. Magn. Reson. Imaging* **2006**, *24*, 459–477. [CrossRef]
59. Bandettini, P.A. Twenty years of functional MRI: The science and the stories. *Neuroimage* **2012**, *62*, 575–588. [CrossRef]

MDPI
St. Alban-Anlage 66
4052 Basel
Switzerland
Tel. +41 61 683 77 34
Fax +41 61 302 89 18
www.mdpi.com

Nutrients Editorial Office
E-mail: nutrients@mdpi.com
www.mdpi.com/journal/nutrients

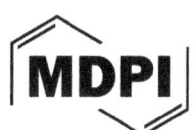

www.ingramcontent.com/pod-product-compliance
Lightning Source LLC
LaVergne TN
LVHW070157120526
838202LV00013BA/1331